For Tom,

with marvelous memories of the time with me in the offices when he was still a resident and with the hope that it will not be long before he returns to New York University and New York City

Bernie Ackerman

who has great admiration for him

April 14, 1984 —
Palm Springs

Differential Diagnosis in Dermatopathology

A. Bernard Ackerman, M.D.

Professor of Dermatology and Pathology, Director of Dermatopathology,
New York University School of Medicine, Adjunct Professor of Pathology,
New York University College of Dentistry, Consultant Dermatopathologist,
Department of Pathology, Memorial Sloan-Kettering Cancer Center,
New York City

JOHN NIVEN, M.D.

Staff Physician, Department of Dermatology
Mount Sinai Medical Center of Greater Miami

JANE M. GRANT-KELS, M.D.

Chief, Division of Dermatology, Department of Medicine;
Director of Dermatopathology
Assistant Professor of Medicine, Pathology and Pediatrics
The University of Connecticut School of Medicine
Farmington, Connecticut

LEA & FEBIGER   PHILADELPHIA

1982

Lea & Febiger
600 Washington Square
Philadelphia, Pa. 19106
U.S.A.

Library of Congress Cataloging in Publication Data

Ackerman, A. Bernard, 1936–
    Differential diagnosis in dermatopathology.

    Includes bibliographical references and index.
    1. Skin—Diseases—Diagnosis.   2. Dermatology—Atlases.
3. Diagnosis, Differential.   I. Niven, John, 1945–   .   II. Grant-
Kels, Jane M. III. Title. [DNLM: 1. Skin diseases—Diagnosis. 2. Di-
agnosis, Differential. WR 140 A182d]
RL105.A25   616.5′075   81-5982
ISBN 0-8121-0800-0   AACR2

PRINTED IN THE UNITED STATES OF AMERICA
Print Number: 3 2 1

To
RUDOLF BAER
whose magnificent spirit helped make
this book possible
—and so much more

Preface

ALTHOUGH there are now several textbooks of dermatopathology in English,[1–8] none is especially designed to help pathologists and dermatologists to differentiate by microscopy between skin diseases that are similar histologically but are different clinically and in biologic course. Probably no other organ has as many diseases that histologically look alike as does the skin.[9] Among these are an ever-increasing number of benign inflammatory diseases that masquerade microscopically as malignant neoplasms (pseudo-malignancies) and, in reverse, malignant neoplasms that histologically simulate benign conditions (pseudo-benignancies). In addition, within the categories of hamartomatous malformations, abnormal autochthonous deposits, alopecias, vesicular and bullous disease, and neoplasias in general, there are many problems in differential diagnosis that may be resolved if only one attends to subtle histologic distinctions. Many of the major problems of histologic differential diagnosis in dermatopathology, as we perceive them, are listed in the Contents.

In this work, apparent histologic similarities are contrasted in a manner that establishes criteria for differentiating them. These distinctions are presented in capsule and table form by emphatic telegraphic statements. Photomicrographs of contrasted diseases that differentiate strikingly the histologic features are reproduced in low and high magnification. Clinical photographs permit the reader, particularly the pathologist, to visualize the pathologic condition in the gross.

The discussions that follow the tabulated points and counterpoints expatiate first on the histologic features that each pair of contrasted diseases have in common, and then on the correlations between their histologic and clinical appearances, their usual clinical courses and, lastly, their histologic differential diagnoses. For simplification and teaching purposes, we have tended to use the classical presentation of fully developed lesions as our models.

We derived criteria by laboriously examining tens, scores, and sometimes hundreds of histologic examples of the contrasted diseases. We were not swayed by traditional interpretations, although we did not deliberately and completely disregard them. No bibliography accompanies any of the 45 sections because the data presented here are our own.

During the years in which this book was evolving, I was fortunate to collaborate with two energetic Fellows in Dermatopathology, Drs. John Niven and Jane Grant-Kels. Dr. Niven collated the slides for histologic study and helped to prepare the first of many drafts of the manuscript. Dr. Grant-Kels collated the clinical pictures and was responsible for the photomicrography. As has been the case for virtually all of my writings during the past eight years, Dr. Morris Leider kindly, carefully, and critically edited this manuscript from Preface to Glossary. A special word of thanks is also due Drs. Helmut Kerl and Hans Kresbach of the Department of Dermatology at the University of Graz for kindly permitting us to use some of their clinical photographs, and to Dr. James Rasmussen of the Department of Dermatology at the University of Michigan for the clinical photograph of staphylococcal scalded skin syndrome, Dr. William Mahoney for the clinical photograph of hidradenoma papilliferum, Dr. George Popkin for the clinical photograph of trichoepitheliomas, and Dr. Phillip Frost for the clinical photograph of bullous congenital ichthyosiform erythroderma. I also appreciate the efforts of Tom Colaiezzi and Ken Bussy of Lea & Febiger, who shepherded the work from manuscript to bound book—a book designed by the incomparable Howard King, painstakingly and lovingly.

We hope that this book will be a useful adjunct to Sherlockian solving of histologic puzzles in dermatopathology and will enable differential diagnosis to become specific diagnosis.

A. BERNARD ACKERMAN

New York City

1. Ackerman, A.B.: *Histologic Diagnosis of Inflammatory Skin Diseases*, Lea & Febiger, Philadelphia, 1978.
2. Allen, C.: *The Skin. A Clinicopathologic Treatise*, The C.V. Mosby Company, St. Louis, 1974.
3. Graham, J.H., Johnson, W.C., Helwig, E.B.: *Dermal Pathology*, Harper and Row Publishers, Hagerstown, Maryland, 1972.
4. Lever, L., Shaumberg-Lever, G.: *Histopathology of the Skin*, J.B. Lippincott Co., Philadelphia-Toronto, Fifth Edition, 1975.
5. Milne, J.A.: *An Introduction to the Diagnostic Histopathology of the Skin*, Williams and Wilkins, Baltimore, 1972.
6. Montgomery, H.: *Dermatopathology Volumes I and II*, Harper and Row Publishers, New York, Evanston and London, 1967.
7. Okun, M., Edelstein, L.: *Gross and Microscopic Pathology of the Skin*, Dermatopathology Foundation Press, Boston, 1976.
8. Pinkus, H., Mehregan, A.H.: *A Guide to Dermatopathology*, Appleton-Century-Crofts, New York, 1975.
9. Connors, R.C., Ackerman, A.B.: Pseudomalignancies, in *Cancer Dermatology*, edited by F. Helm. Lea & Febiger, Philadelphia, 1979.

Contents

Contents

DIFFERENTIAL DIAGNOSIS IN DERMATOPATHOLOGY

1. Psoriasis

vs. Nummular Dermatitis

Psoriasis	*Nummular Dermatitis*
1. Confluent parakeratosis	1. Focal scale-crust
2. Granular layer mostly absent	2. Granular layer mostly intact
3. Regular psoriasiform hyperplasia (rete ridges of even lengths)	3. Irregular psoriasiform hyperplasia (rete ridges of unequal lengths)
4. Suprapapillary plates thinned	4. Suprapapillary plates not thinned
5. Pallor of keratinocytes in uppermost spinous zone	5. No pallor of epidermal keratinocytes
6. Slight spongiosis early; no microvesicles	6. Spongiosis evolves into microvesiculation
7. Neutrophils within the epidermis, especially in parakeratotic foci	7. No neutrophils within the epidermis (unless eroded or impetiginized)
8. Increased number of mitotic figures above the basal layer	8. Approximately normal number of mitotic figures above the basal layer
9. Blood vessels in the papillary dermis markedly tortuous (i.e., seemingly increased in number) and nearly touching the epidermis	9. Blood vessels in the papillary dermis dilated, but not tortuous and not nearly touching the epidermis
10. Sparse superficial perivascular lympho-histiocytic infiltrate with few neutrophils; no eosinophils usually	10. Moderately dense superficial lympho-histiocytic infiltrate, often with many eosinophils; no neutrophils usually

Psoriasis

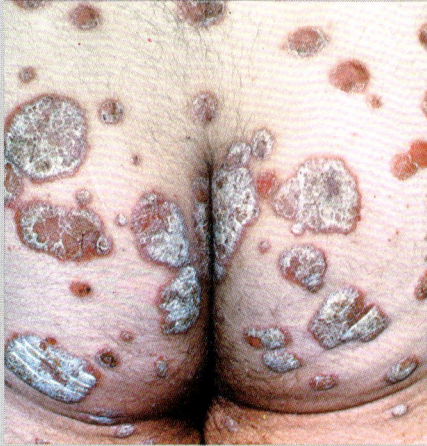

Nummular Dermatitis

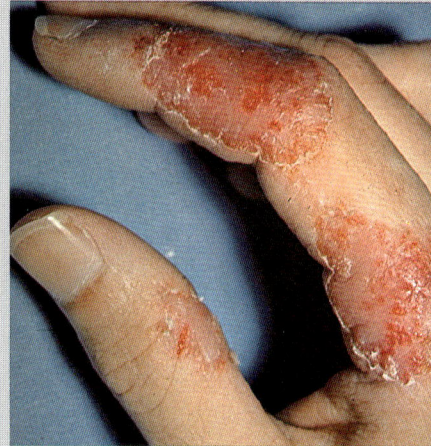

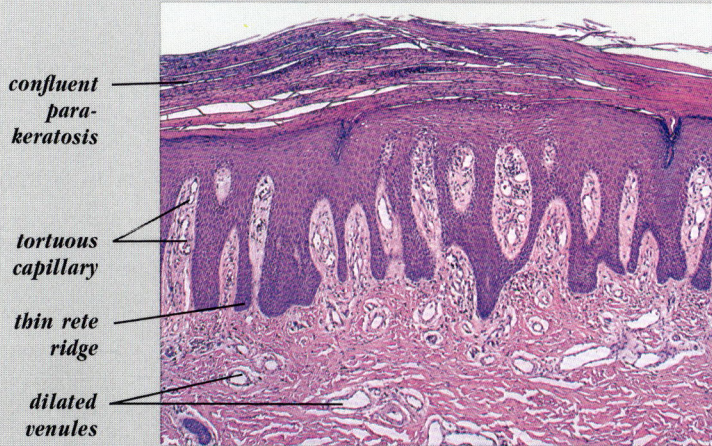

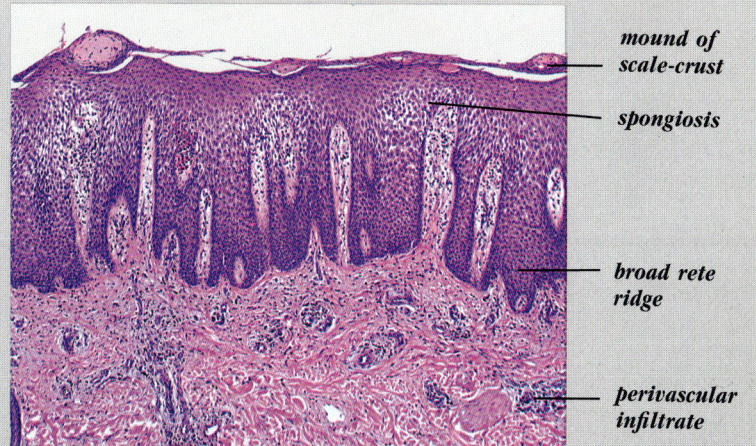

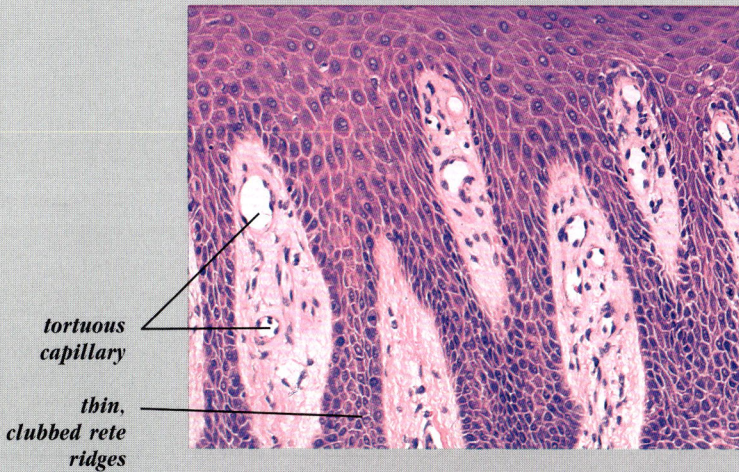

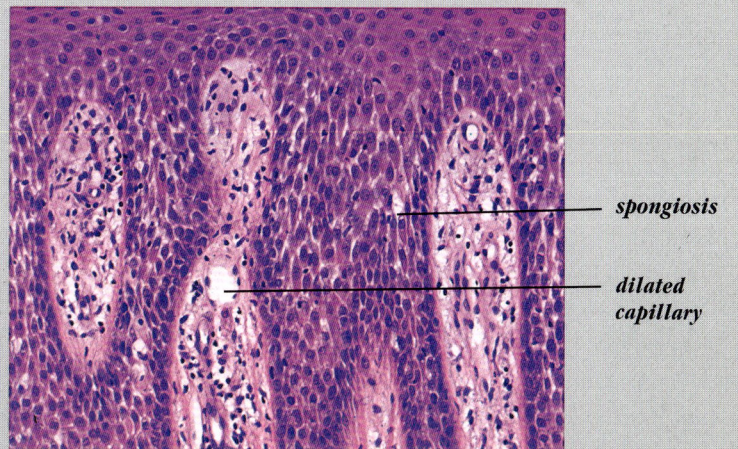

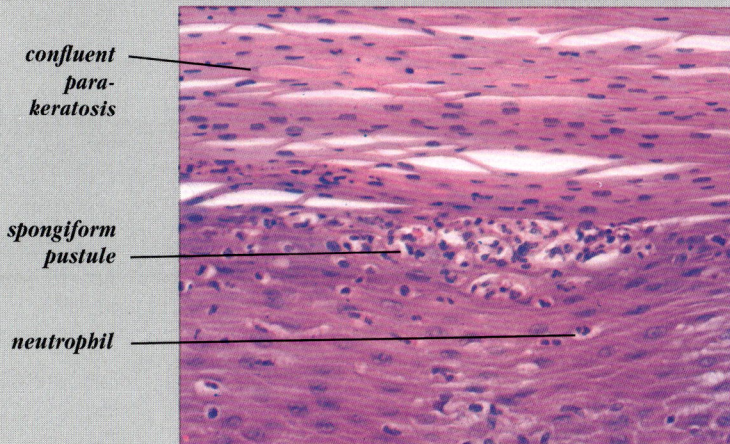

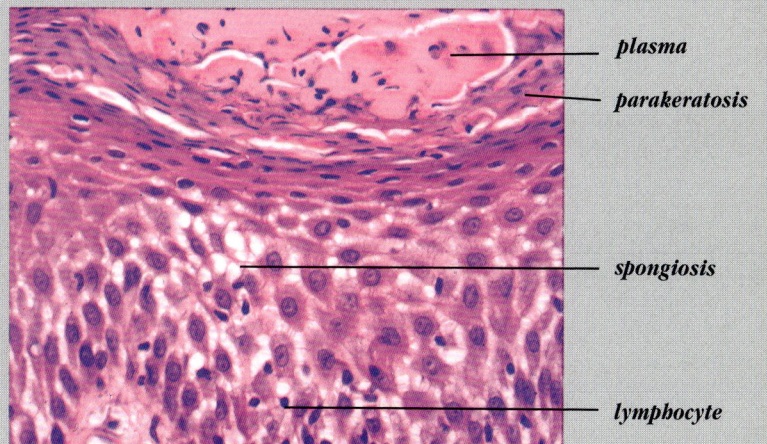

confluent para-keratosis

tortuous capillary

thin rete ridge

dilated venules

mound of scale-crust

spongiosis

broad rete ridge

perivascular infiltrate

tortuous capillary

thin, clubbed rete ridges

spongiosis

dilated capillary

confluent para-keratosis

spongiform pustule

neutrophil

plasma

parakeratosis

spongiosis

lymphocyte

THESE two diseases share histologic features in common, namely, some parakeratosis, psoriasiform hyperplasia, edema of the papillary dermis, and an inflammatory-cell infiltrate around dilated blood vessels of the superficial plexus. Eruptive lesions of psoriasis, like those of nummular dermatitis, are even marked by spongiosis.

The histological changes enumerated above apply only to fully developed active lesions of psoriasis and nummular dermatitis, i.e., scaly, reddish plaques in the case of psoriasis and tense vesicles surmounting reddish, crusted, coin-shaped plaques in the case of nummular dermatitis. Both diseases have a wide spectrum of pathological features clinically and histologically, as would be expected for conditions whose lesions last for weeks or months (and even years for psoriasis).

Clinically, psoriasis begins as tiny, reddish macules that soon enlarge and become slightly elevated and scaly. Early guttate (drop-sized) psoriatic lesions gradually enlarge centrifugally and may attain huge proportions. Nummular dermatitis starts as reddish macules that soon become scratched because of intense pruritus, leaving eroded, crusted, coin-shaped plaques. When persistently rubbed, the lesions of nummular dermatitis become lichenified (superimposition of lichen simplex chronicus). The lesions of both diseases in resolution may leave some hyperpigmentation.

Salient histologic features of early guttate lesions of psoriasis are:

1. Mounds of parakeratosis containing neutrophils at their summits
2. Neutrophils in intra- and subcorneal (Munro) or spongiform pustules (Kogoj)
3. Normal granular layer, except beneath parakeratotic foci
4. Normal suprapapillary plates
5. Slight epidermal hyperplasia
6. Slight spongiosis
7. Marked edema of the papillary dermis
8. Superficial infiltrate of lymphocytes, histiocytes, neutrophils, and extravasated erythrocytes around widely dilated capillaries and venules, and inflammatory cells scattered in the dermal papillae. A few erythrocytes may be present focally within the epidermis.

The early acute lesions of nummular dermatitis are characterized histologically by:

1. Normal or focally parakeratotic cornified layer
2. Focal spongiosis, sometimes diffuse

3. Slight epidermal hyperplasia
4. Edema of the papillary dermis
5. Superficial infiltrate of lymphocytes, histiocytes, and often numerous eosinophils around dilated blood vessels and interstitially in the papillary dermis.

Biopsy from the center of a long-standing or resolving plaque of psoriasis shows histologically:

1. Rather confluent compact orthokeratosis with only focal parakeratosis
2. Granular zone mostly of normal thickness
3. Supra-papillary plates of normal thickness
4. Psoriasiform epidermal hyperplasia with rete ridges of approximately equal length
5. Tortuous capillaries in the papillary dermis
6. Sparse to moderately dense superficial perivascular lympho-histiocytic infiltrate

Late chronic lesions of nummular dermatitis are marked histologically by:

1. Compact orthokeratosis with focal parakeratosis
2. Irregular psoriasiform epidermal hyperplasia with rete ridges of uneven lengths
3. Thickened papillary dermis with coarse collagen bundles arranged in vertical streaks parallel to the elongated rete ridges, i.e., signs of lichen simplex chronicus
4. Moderately dense superficial perivascular mixed inflammatory-cell infiltrate of lymphocytes, histiocytes (including melanophages), plasma cells, and eosinophils.

Lichen simplex chronicus is often superimposed upon longstanding lesions of nummular dermatitis and less commonly upon those of psoriasis. In these instances the histologic evidences of persistent rubbing, namely, a papillary dermis markedly thickened by coarse collagen fibers arranged in vertical streaks, may obscure the underlying nummular dermatitis or psoriasis. Helpful clues to discerning the underlying process as nummular dermatitis are slight spongiosis within the psoriasiform epidermis, crusts as well as scales, and some eosinophils within the infiltrate in the upper part of the dermis. Clues that the underlying process is psoriasis are neutrophils in the parakeratotic cornified layer and tortuous blood vessels in the papillary dermis.

2. Pityriasis Rosea
vs. Guttate Parapsoriasis

Pityriasis Rosea	*Guttate Parapsoriasis*
1. Parakeratosis in mounds	1. Scale-crusts in mounds
2. Spongiosis prominent usually	2. Slight or no spongiosis
3. Slight epidermal hyperplasia	3. Little or no epidermal hyperplasia
4. Marked edema of the papillary dermis often	4. Little or no edema of the papillary dermis
5. Few or many extravasated erythrocytes in the dermal papillae (and sometimes in the epidermis)	5. No extravasated erythrocytes
6. Moderately dense superficial perivascular lympho-histiocytic infiltrate with eosinophils occasionally	6. Sparse superficial perivascular lympho-histiocytic infiltrate without eosinophils
7. Melanophages occasionally	7. Melanophages rarely

Pityriasis Rosea

Guttate Parapsoriasis

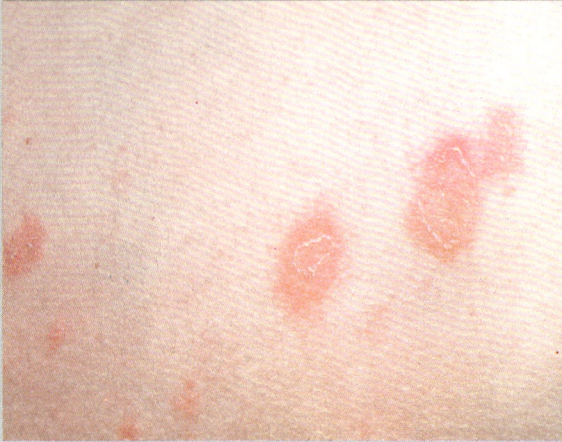

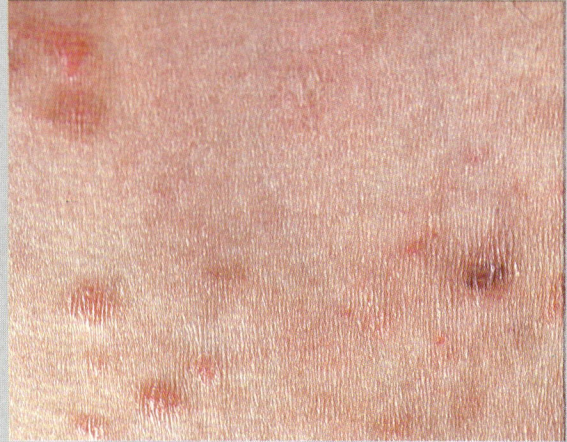

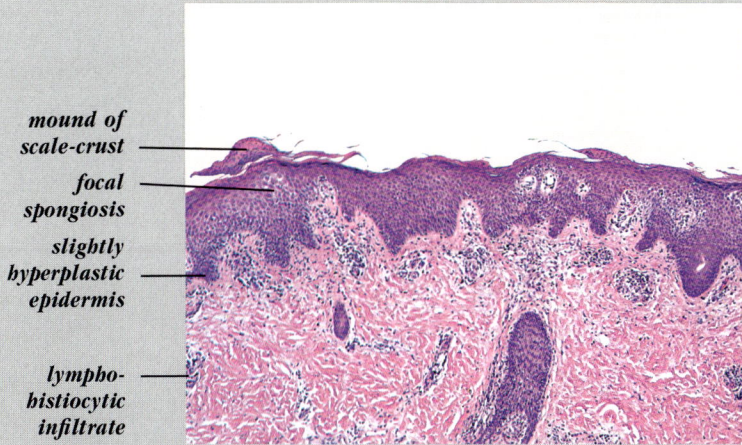

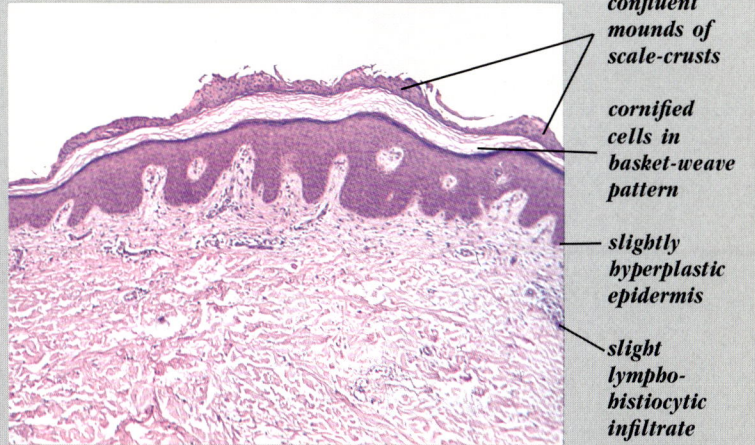

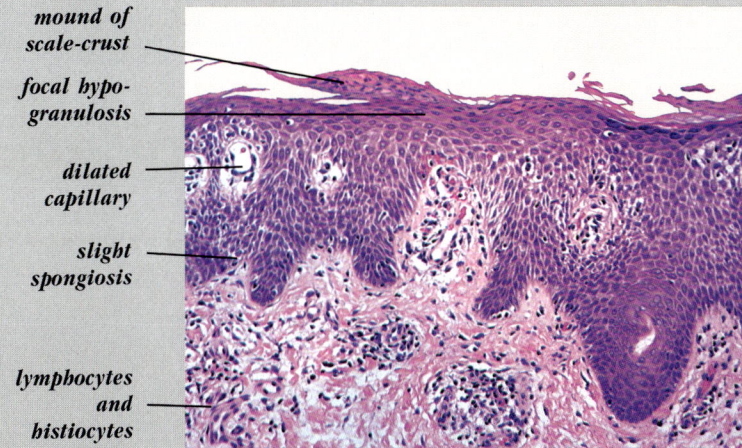

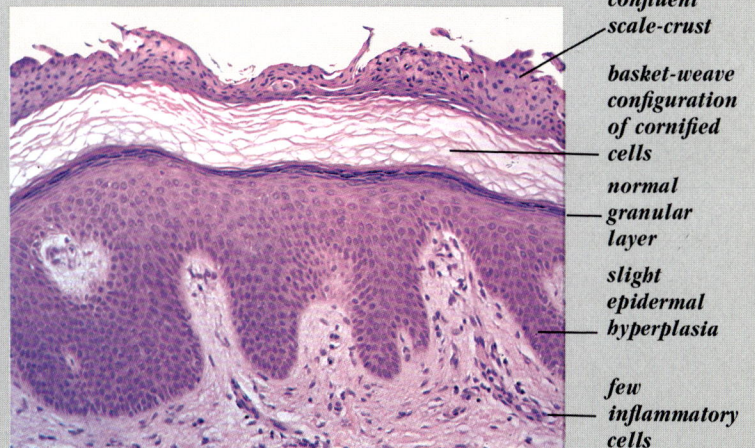

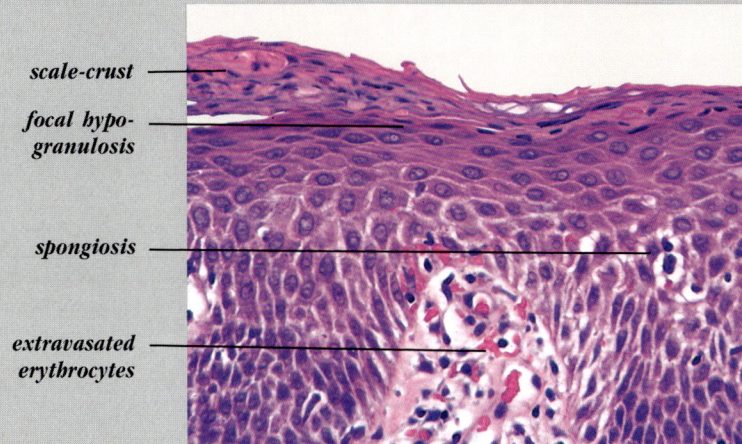

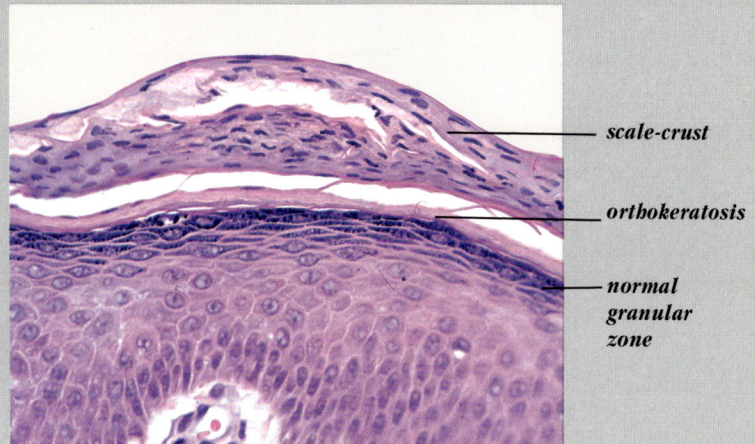

Pityriasis Rosea (left column labels):

- mound of scale-crust
- focal spongiosis
- slightly hyperplastic epidermis
- lympho-histiocytic infiltrate

- mound of scale-crust
- focal hypo-granulosis
- dilated capillary
- slight spongiosis
- lymphocytes and histiocytes

- scale-crust
- focal hypo-granulosis
- spongiosis
- extravasated erythrocytes

Guttate Parapsoriasis (right column labels):

- confluent mounds of scale-crusts
- cornified cells in basket-weave pattern
- slightly hyperplastic epidermis
- slight lympho-histiocytic infiltrate

- confluent scale-crust
- basket-weave configuration of cornified cells
- normal granular layer
- slight epidermal hyperplasia
- few inflammatory cells

- scale-crust
- orthokeratosis
- normal granular zone

P ITYRIASIS rosea and guttate parapsoriasis have more histiologic features in common than they have differences. Both have a superficial, perivascular, predominantly lympho-histiocytic infiltrate, spongiosis, and parakeratosis. They differ primarily in that pityriasis rosea has a denser infiltrate, extravasated erythrocytes, more noticeable spongiosis, and more epidermal hyperplasia. Another difference is a greater tendency to formation of scale-crusts in guttate parapsoriasis. In some instances, however, it may be difficult or impossible to differentiate between them histologically.

Pityriasis rosea tends to involve the torso from the neck to the knees and to consist of oval to round, salmon-pink papules and plaques with delicate scales that separate at their peripheries and remain adherent at their centers. On the trunk the lesions align themselves along the lines of cleavage of the skin (Langer's lines). Days or a week or two before the eruption, a larger, scaly lesion ("mother" or "herald" patch) generally appears. Biopsy of this larger lesion reveals histologic changes similar to the later smaller lesions of pityriasis rosea, but the perivascular inflammatory-cell infiltrate is often both superficial and deep, there is less spongiosis, and epidermal hyperplasia is more psoriasiform. Pityriasis rosea usually resolves spontaneously without treatment in about six to nine weeks.

Clinically, guttate parapsoriasis consists of widespread drop-sized, pink or tan papules covered by fine, wafer-like scales. The lesions are not pruritic, but they are indefinitely persistent and refractory to treatment. Histologically, guttate parapsoriasis, although fundamentally a spongiotic dermatitis, usually shows little or no spongiosis within the epidermis in a routine section. The finding of plasma in the scale-crusts, however, implies that spongiosis had been present in the underlying epidermis.

We consider digitate dermatosis to be a variant of guttate parapsoriasis. Clinically, it consists of large elongated scaly patches situated mostly on or near the trunk and that persist despite treatments of various kinds. Histologically, digitate dermatosis is indistinguishable from guttate parapsoriasis.

Superficial types of gyrate erythemas (e.g., erythema annulare centrifugum) also must be considered in the histological differential diagnosis of pityriasis rosea. Both diseases are characterized by a superficial perivascular lympho-histiocytic infiltrate, edema of the papillary dermis, spongiosis, and focal parakeratosis. Although histologically it is often impossible to distinguish between pityriasis rosea and superficial gyrate erythemas, clinically they are readily differentiated from guttate parapsoriasis. Lesions of pityriasis rosea and erythema annulare centrifugum are both characterized clinically by oral shapes and collarettes of scales at their peripheries. The rare vesicular variant of pityriasis rosea must be differentiated histologically from subacute allergic contact dermatitis, subacute nummular dermatitis, and subacute "id" reactions. Although this differentiation is not always possible, vesicular pityriasis rosea tends to have less epidermal hyperplasia and fewer eosinophils.

3. Lichen Planus
vs. Lichen Planus-like Keratosis

Lichen Planus	*Lichen Planus-like Keratosis*
1. Compact orthokeratosis	1. Compact orthokeratosis and focal parakeratosis
2. Granular zone thickened in wedge shapes	2. Granular zone thickened and thinned focally; not wedge-shaped usually
3. Irregular, jagged epidermal hyperplasia	3. Variably hyperplastic, sometimes thinned epidermis; not jagged
4. Keratinocytic nuclei not atypical	4. Keratinocytic nuclei in lower part of epidermis often atypical
5. Dense band-like lympho-histiocytic infiltrate with melanophages in upper dermis	5. Dense band-like lympho-histiocytic infiltrate with occasional plasma cells and/or eosinophils in upper dermis
6. Infiltrate obscures dermo-epidermal interface along entire length of lesion	6. Infiltrate obscures dermo-epidermal interface intermittently
7. Solar elastosis not usual	7. Solar elastosis usual
8. No solar lentigo contiguous to lesion	8. Solar lentigo usually contiguous to lesion

Lichen Planus

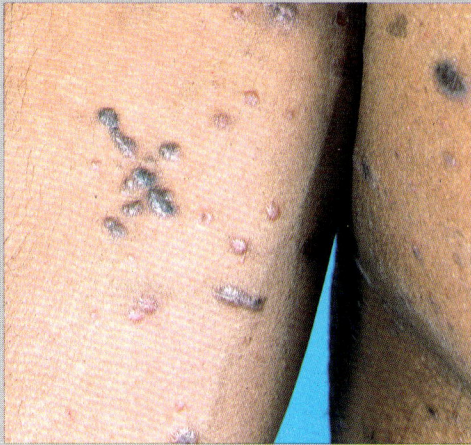

Lichen Planus-like Keratosis

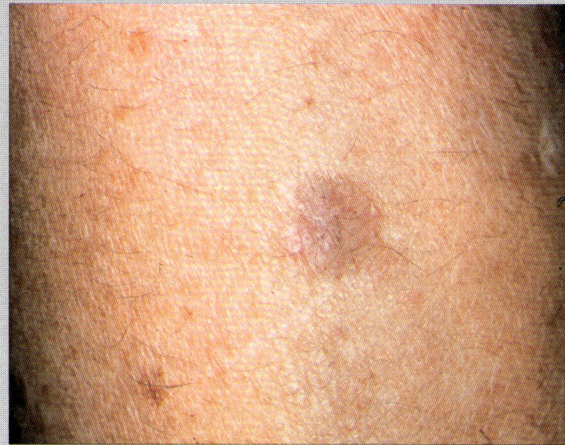

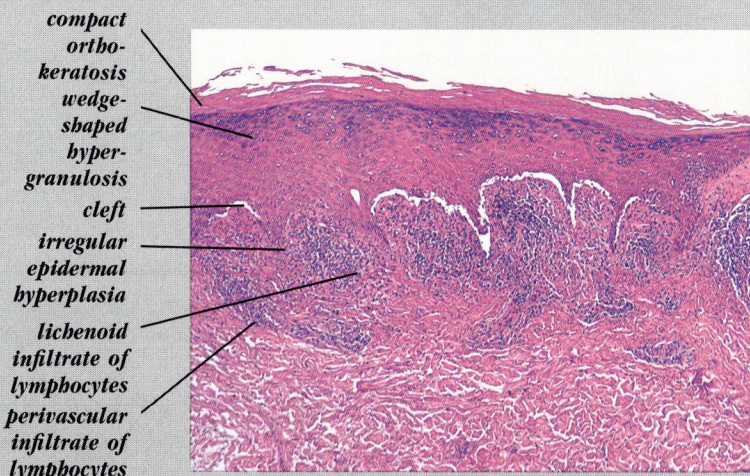

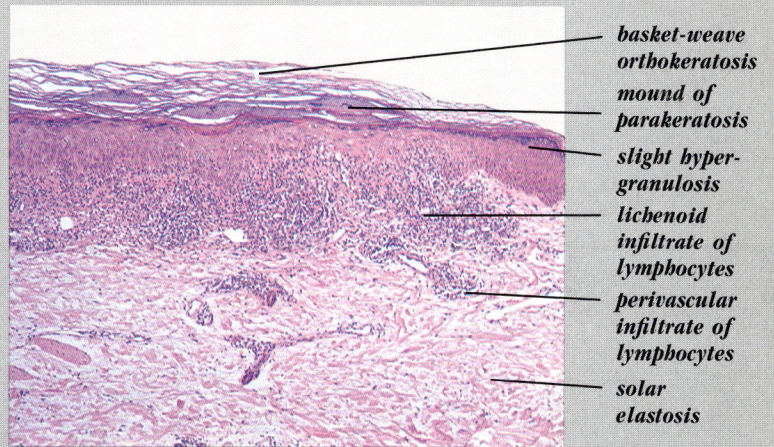

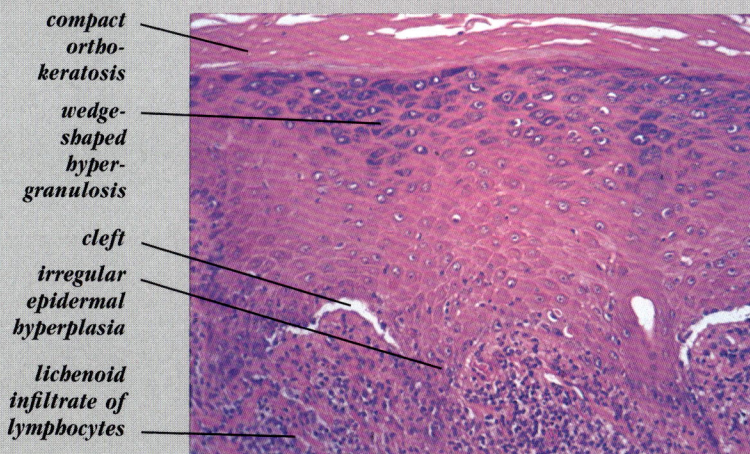

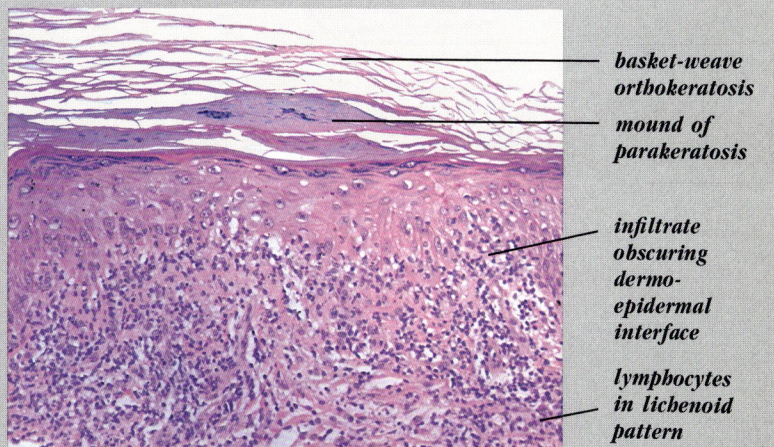

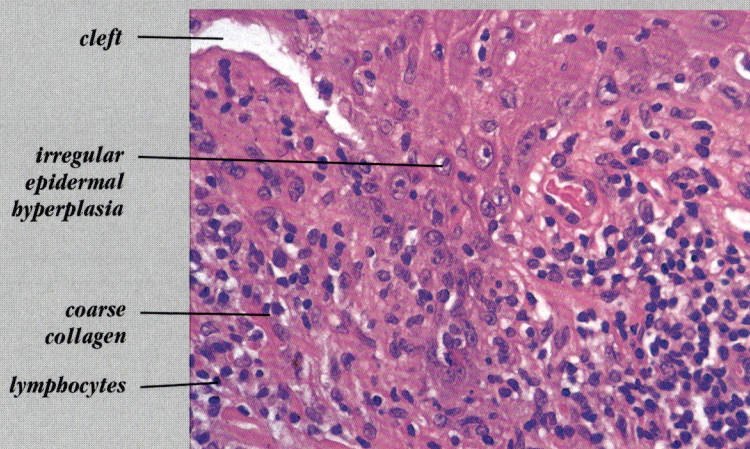

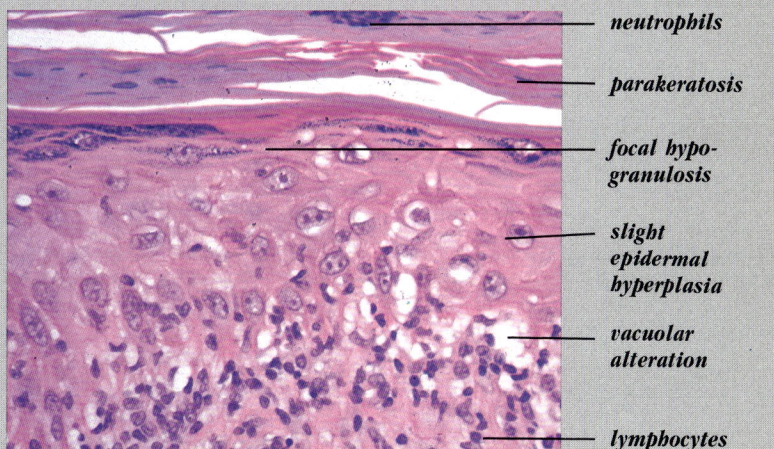

compact ortho-keratosis

wedge-shaped hyper-granulosis

cleft

irregular epidermal hyperplasia

lichenoid infiltrate of lymphocytes

perivascular infiltrate of lymphocytes

basket-weave orthokeratosis

mound of parakeratosis

slight hyper-granulosis

lichenoid infiltrate of lymphocytes

perivascular infiltrate of lymphocytes

solar elastosis

compact ortho-keratosis

wedge-shaped hyper-granulosis

cleft

irregular epidermal hyperplasia

lichenoid infiltrate of lymphocytes

basket-weave orthokeratosis

mound of parakeratosis

infiltrate obscuring dermo-epidermal interface

lymphocytes in lichenoid pattern

cleft

irregular epidermal hyperplasia

coarse collagen

lymphocytes

neutrophils

parakeratosis

focal hypo-granulosis

slight epidermal hyperplasia

vacuolar alteration

lymphocytes

THE lichen planus-like keratosis is often confused histologically with lichen planus. Ostensibly, both are superficial perivascular dermatitides with lichenoid infiltrates that obscure the dermo-epidermal junction where there are vacuolar alteration and necrotic keratinocytes (interface dermatitides, lichenoid types). Lichen planus-like keratosis begins as a solar lentigo and, in time, is associated with a dense lichenoid inflammatory-cell infiltrate. Lichen planus-like keratosis is usually removed by shave excision technique and the lesion generally extends broadly from one end of the specimen to the other. In contrast, a lesion of lichen planus is usually biopsied by punch excision technique and, more often than not, the lesion does not extend across the width of even a 4 mm specimen.

Clinically, a lichen planus-like keratosis usually develops as a solitary, reddish-brown, scaly lesion, predilectively on sun-exposed skin, especially the chest and arms of older persons. The lesion is often misdiagnosed clinically as basal-cell carcinoma. In time, lichen planus-like keratosis may regress spontaneously.

Lichen planus presents itself as a pruritic, widespread eruption of flat-topped, shiny, violaceous, polygonal papules. The disease may involve mucous membranes, nails, and hair follicles (lichen plano-pilaris). Although there are many variants of lichen planus (e.g., atrophic, hypertrophic, bullous) most have in common the following histologic features:

1. Compact orthokeratosis
2. Hypergranulosis in wedge shape
3. "Saw-tooth" irregular epidermal hyperplasia
4. Necrotic keratinocytes (Civatte bodies, hyaline bodies) at the dermo-epidermal junction
5. Vacuolar alteration at the dermo-epidermal junction
6. Dense, band-like lympho-histiocytic infiltrate with melanophages in the upper dermis obscuring the interface between epidermis and dermis
7. Coarse collagen bundles in the thickened papillary dermis

In atrophic (resolving or resolved) lichen planus, the epidermis is thinned and the cellular infiltrate in the dermis is relatively scant. In hypertrophic lichen planus, the epidermis and papillary dermis are both markedly thickened by superimposition of features of lichen simplex chronicus (from persistent rubbing). Bullous lichen planus may not show the band-like inflammatory-cell infiltrate characteristic of ordinary lichen planus, because the blister forms so quickly that the lesion has no chance to become fully developed. The effect is most common on the legs. In lichen planus-like drug eruptions there may be eosinophils and plasma cells in the dermal infiltrate, many necrotic keratinocytes in a thinned epidermis, focal hypogranulosis, and parakeratosis.

Other lichenoid inflammatory-cell infiltrates that must be differentiated from lichen planus and lichen planus-like keratosis are lichenoid photodermatitis (such as may be induced by thiazides), lichenoid drug eruptions (such as caused by gold), lichenoid discoid lupus erythematosus, and the lichenoid form of persistent pigmented purpuric dermatitis (Gougerot and Blum).

Why an apparently banal solar lentigo induces a lichenoid inflammatory-cell infiltrate to become a lichen planus-like keratosis is not yet understood.

4. Allergic Contact Dermatitis *vs.* Irritant Contact Dermatitis

Allergic Contact Dermatitis

1. No erosions or ulcerations usually

2. Lower portion of epidermis affected early

3. Marked spongiosis (intercellular edema) leading to intraepidermal spongiotic vesicles

4. Slight ballooning (intracellular edema)

5. No necrotic keratinocytes

6. Lymphocytes or eosinophils in foci of spongiosis

7. Superficial perivascular lympho-histiocytic infiltrate with varying number of eosinophils

Irritant Contact Dermatitis

1. Erosions or ulcerations may occur

2. Upper portion of epidermis affected early

3. Slight spongiosis early

4. Marked ballooning leading to intraepidermal vesicles

5. Necrotic keratinocytes in variable numbers ranging from necrosis of individual keratinocytes to necrosis of the entire epidermis

6. Neutrophils in foci of ballooning and necrosis

7. Superficial perivascular lympho-histiocytic infiltrate with varying number of neutrophils

Allergic Contact Dermatitis

Irritant Contact Dermatitis

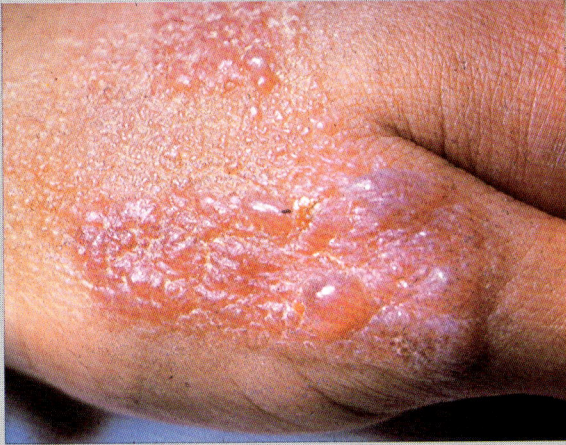

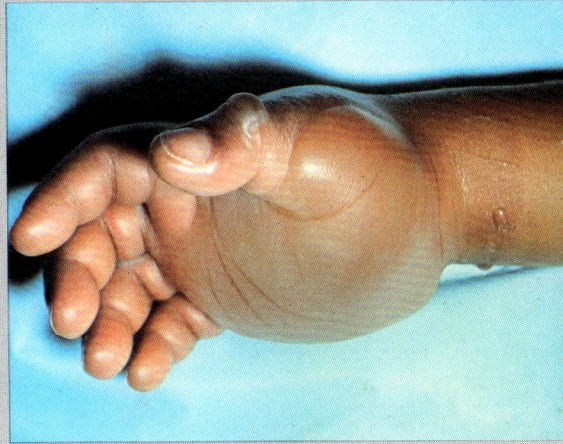

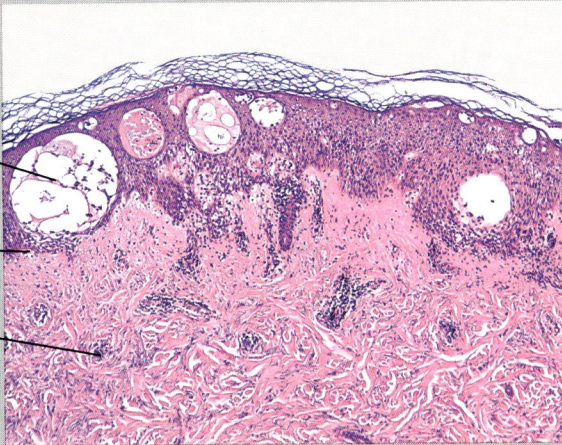

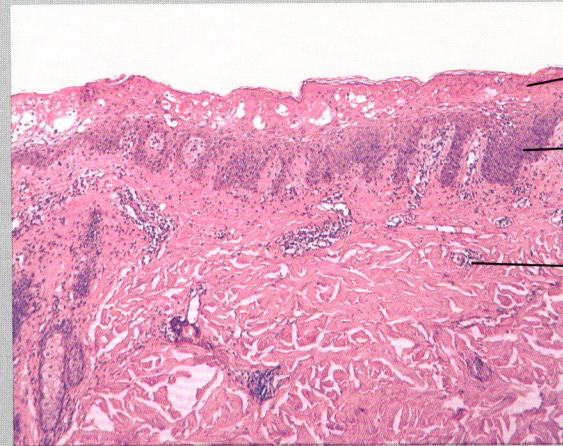

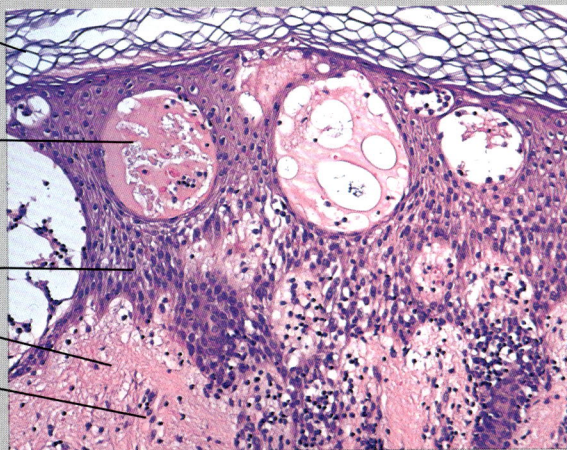

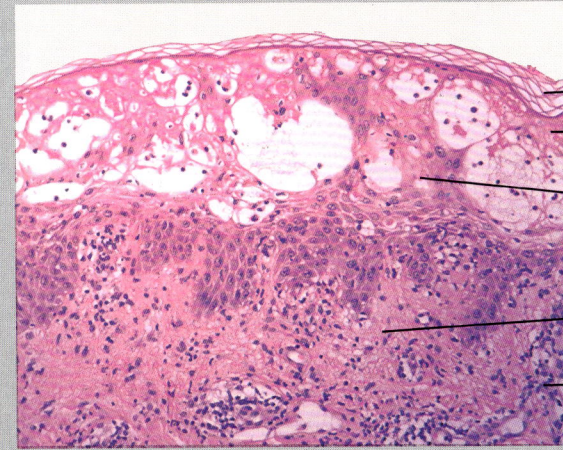

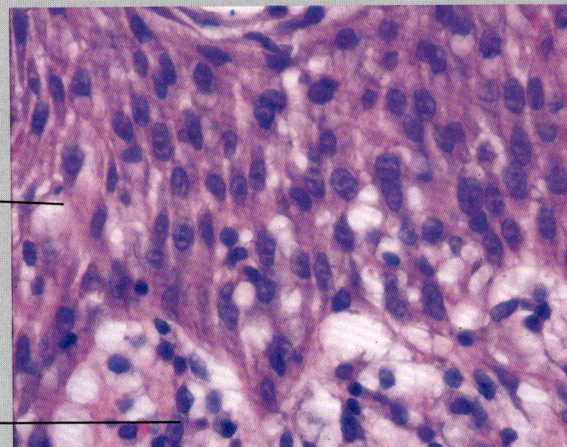

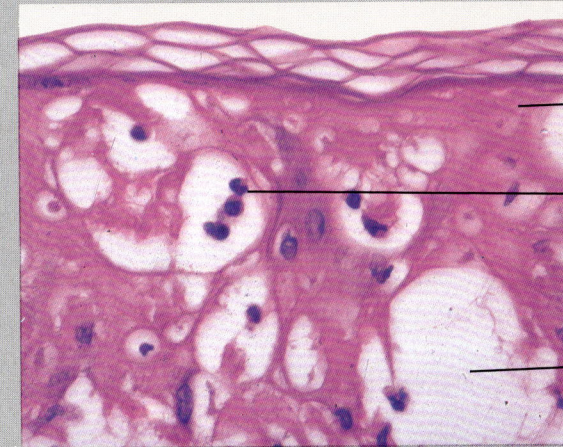

spongiotic
vesicle

slightly
hyperplastic
epidermis

perivascular
infiltrate

necrotic
epidermis

slightly
hyper-
plastic
epidermis

sparse
perivascular
infiltrate

basket-
weave
cornified
layer

vesicle
secondary to
spongiosis

spongiosis

edema

mixed-cell
infiltrate
with
eosinophils

basket-weave
cornified
layer

necrotic
epidermis

ballooning

edema

mixed-cell
infiltrate
with
neutrophils

spongiosis

lymphocytes

necrotic
epidermis

neutrophil

vesicle
secondary
to
ballooning

ACUTE allergic contact dermatitis and acute irritant contact dermatitis are both intraepidermal vesicular dermatitides that appear after exposure to different kinds of contactants, namely, allergens in the one and irritant substances in the other.

Histologically, allergic and irritant contact dermatitis have in common intra- and intercellular edema, edema of the papillary dermis, and superficial perivascular mixed inflammatory-cell infiltrates. Both may also be associated with subepidermal vesiculation; in irritant contact dermatitis it is due either to rupture of intraepidermal ballooning vesicles or to massive epidermal necrosis with subsequent dermo-epidermal separation. In allergic contact dermatitis, it is secondary to either bursting of intraepidermal spongiotic vesicles or to massive edema of the papillary dermis.

Allergic contact dermatitis results from exposure of previously sensitized persons to contact allergens. It is a delayed type of hypersensitivity reaction in contrast to irritant contact dermatitis which is not a hypersensitivity reaction at all. Irritant contact dermatitis results from direct irritation to the skin by a variety of agents like strong acids and alkalis and to less irritating substances like croton oil and sodium lauryl sulfate.

Clinically, allergic contact dermatitis appears as edematous pink papules that soon become papulovesicles. That these are actually vesicles may be better appreciated by gentle palpation than by sight. With progression, the vesicles become clearly discernable and in severe cases, huge bullae may be striking. Histologically, by serially taken biopsies, the acute stage may be seen to eventuate into a subacute stage that shows epidermal hyperplasia in addition to spongiosis (spongiotic psoriasiform dermatitis), and still later into a chronic stage in which there is psoriasiform hyperplasia (psoriasiform dermatitis) and no spongiosis. In long-enduring lesions of allergic contact dermatitis, there are usually histologic evidences of persistent rubbing (i.e., lichen simplex chronicus) in the form of thickening of the papillary dermis by coarse collagen bundles arranged in vertical streaks.

The histologic differential diagnosis of acute allergic contact dermatitis involves consideration of acute nummular dermatitis, dyshidrotic dermatitis, id reactions, and vesicular dermatophytic infections, all of which may show the same histologic features in sections stained by hematoxylin and eosin. The presence of eosinophils within the infiltrate favors the diagnosis of contact or nummular dermatitis.

Photo-allergic contact dermatitis, such as to salicylanilides, and photo-allergic dermatitis, such as to systemically administered chlorpromazine, are similar histologically to allergic contact dermatitis, except that the inflammatory-cell infiltrate is usually both deep as well as superficial and a few necrotic keratinocytes may be found within the epidermis. Clinically, photo-allergic contact dermatitis and photo-allergic dermatitis are usually confined to regions of the skin that are ordinarily exposed to sunlight.

Irritant contact dermatitis may clinically range from slight erythema and scaling to severe blisters and ulcerations. Like allergic contact dermatitis, irritant contact dermatitis has a common photo-related counterpart, namely, phototoxic contact dermatitis caused by substances that become irritants only after photo-activation. Phototoxic dermatitis may result from systemically administered chemicals such as psoralens and phototoxic contact dermatitis may result from chemicals such as psoralens applied topically. The phototoxic lesions are similar to irritant contact dermatitis histologically and clinically, and again they occur only on sunlight-exposed areas.

Some contactants, such as turpentine, may be both sensitizing and irritating.

5. Dermatitis Herpetiformis
vs. Pemphigoid

Dermatitis Herpetiformis	*Pemphigoid*
1. Subepidermal blister containing mostly neutrophils; variable numbers of eosinophils	1. Subepidermal blister containing mostly eosinophils; variable numbers of neutrophils
2. Acantholytic cells, singly and in clumps, within the blister occasionally	2. No acantholytic cells within the blister
3. No spongiosis	3. Spongiosis with eosinophils at sides of blister often
4. Pattern of epidermal rete ridges and dermal papillae not usually preserved above and below the blister	4. Pattern of epidermal rete ridges and dermal papillae usually preserved above and below the blister
5. Abscesses of neutrophils, band forms of neutrophils, nuclear debris, basophilic collagen, and fibrin at tips of dermal papillae beneath and to the sides of the blister	5. No neutrophils or altered collagen at tips of dermal papillae; sometimes "abscesses" of eosinophils beneath blister in the dermal papillae
6. Slight to moderate edema of the papillary dermis	6. Marked edema of the papillary dermis
7. Superficial perivascular mixed-cell infiltrate of lymphocytes, histiocytes, neutrophils, and few eosinophils	7. Superficial perivascular mixed-cell infiltrate of lymphocytes, histiocytes, numerous eosinophils, and rare neutrophils and plasma cells

Dermatitis Herpetiformis

Pemphigoid

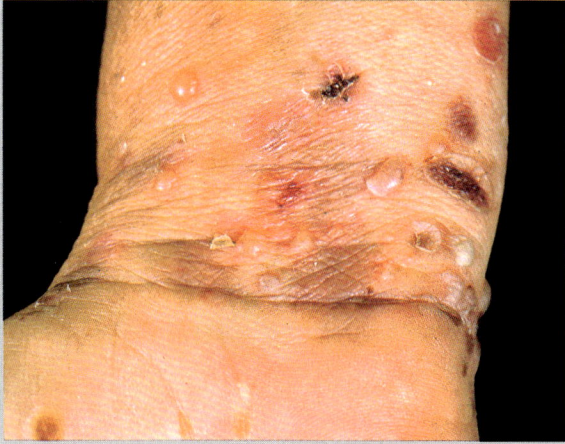
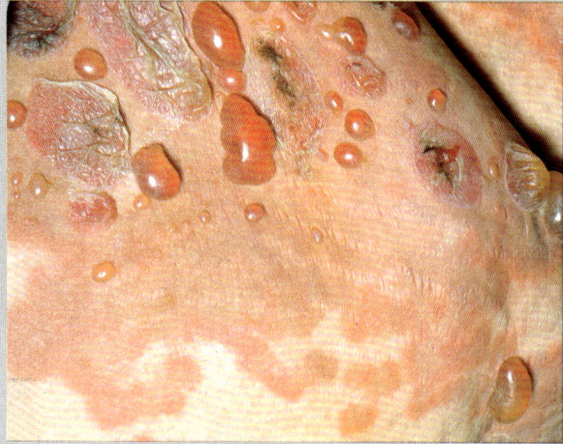

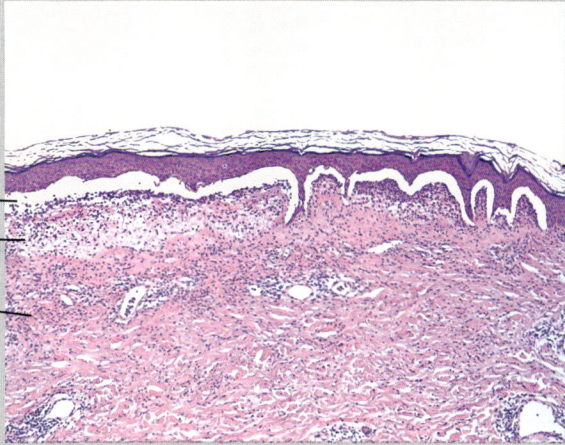

sub-epidermal blister

neutrophils and fibrin

mixed-cell infiltrate with neutrophils and eosinophils

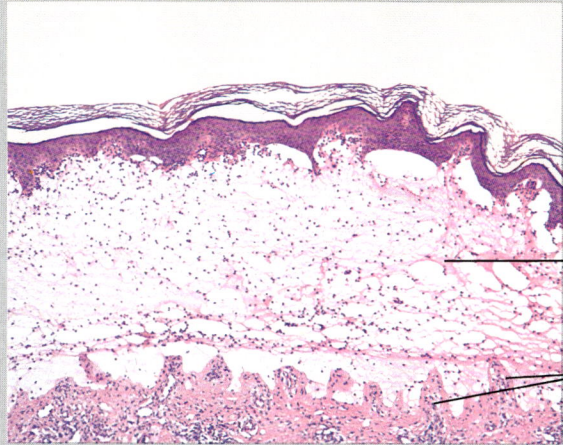

subepidermal blister with fibrin and eosinophils

dermal papillae preserved

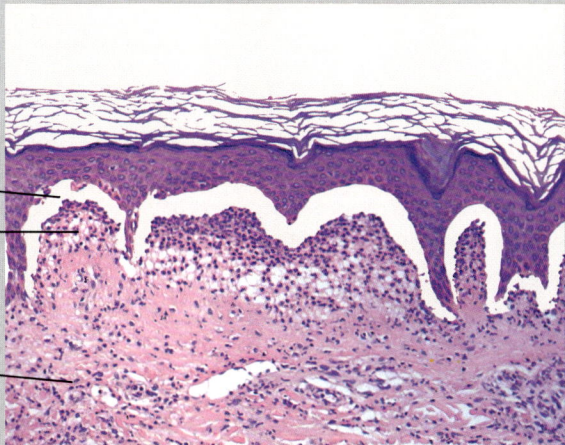

sub-epidermal blister

neutrophils at tip of papilla

neutrophils, eosinophils, and lymphocytes

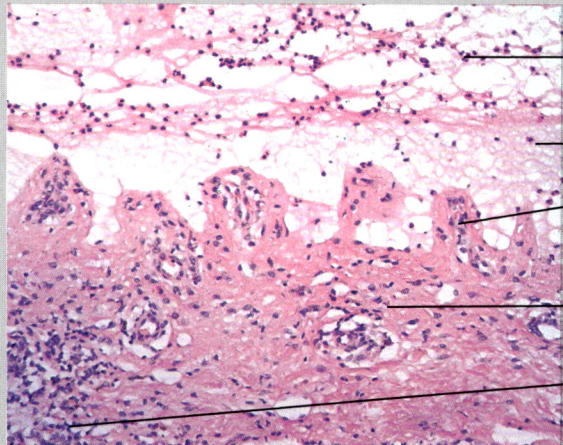

eosinophils

fibrin

papilla

interstitial infiltrate with eosinophils

lymphocytes and eosinophils

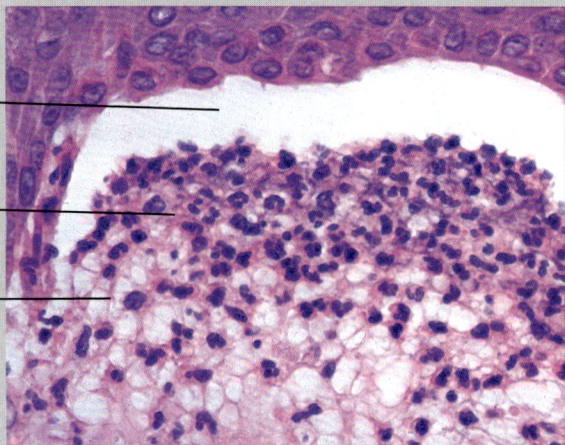

sub-epidermal blister

collection of neutrophils

fibrin

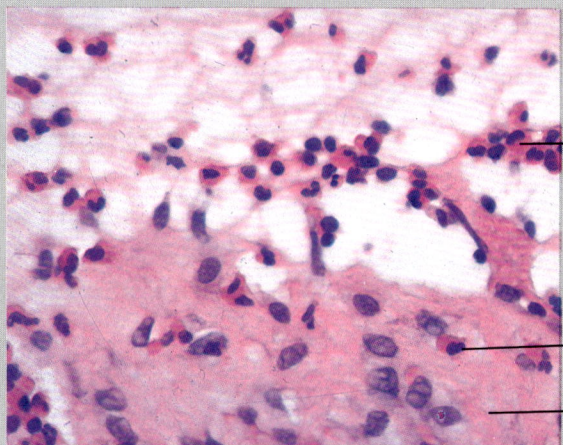

eosinophils

eosinophil

edema

DERMATITIS herpetiformis and pemphigoid share several features in common, namely, subepidermal vesiculation, edema of the dermal papillae, and mixed inflammatory-cell infiltrates containing some neutrophils and eosinophils.

The histologic changes enumerated above occur in the earliest blistering lesions of dermatitis herpetiformis and the cell-rich type of pemphigoid. A less common cell-poor type of pemphigoid has a sparse inflammatory-cell infiltrate, but in other respects resembles pemphigoid as described above.

As in all other inflammatory diseases in the skin there is an unfolding of pathologic changes that develop in time. In dermatitis herpetiformis (a disease of young adults), early edematous erythematous papules evolve into papulovesicles that become discrete vesicles, but rarely progress to bullae. Erosions and ulcerations are common features secondary to excoriations induced by severe pruritus. The lesions of dermatitis herpetiformis commonly involve the scalp and are symmetrically distributed over the scapulae, sacrum, buttocks, and extensor surfaces of the arms and legs. Pemphigoid (a disease of older persons) begins with widespread edematous erythematous papules and plaques that often have gyrate, arcuate, and annular configurations. Tense vesicles and, eventually, bullae arise on these bases. Excoriations of these pruritic lesions also result in erosions and ulcerations. Both dermatitis herpetiformis and pemphigoid resolve with hyperpigmentation.

Early edematous erythematous papules of dermatitis herpetiformis show upon biopsy:

1. Discrete vacuolar alteration and subepidermal clefts
2. Neutrophils and band forms sprinkled along and beneath the dermo-epidermal junction
3. Edema of the papillary dermis
4. Dilation of superficial capillaries
5. Sparse to moderately dense superficial perivascular lympho-histiocytic infiltrate with neutrophils

Early edematous erythematous papules of pemphigoid show:

1. Vacuolar alteration and scattered eosinophils along the dermo-epidermal interface
2. Eosinophils, singly and in clusters, within the epidermis, some in spongiotic foci
3. Edema of the papillary dermis

4. Superficial perivascular infiltrate of lymphocytes, histiocytes, eosinophils, and rare neutrophils

Late vesicular lesions of dermatitis herpetiformis are characterized by:

1. Confluence of tiny subepidermal vesicles
2. Dense collections of eosinophils and neutrophils within the dermal papillae
3. Edema of the papillary dermis
4. Moderately dense superficial perivascular mixed inflammatory-cell infiltrate of lymphocytes, histiocytes, eosinophils, and neutrophils
5. Varying degrees of epidermal necrosis

Late bullous lesions of pemphigoid have:

1. Focal or confluent epidermal necrosis above the blister
2. Superficial and mid-dermal mixed inflammatory-cell infiltrate of lymphocytes, histiocytes, and eosinophils with occasional neutrophils and plasma cells
3. Edema of the papillary dermis

It may be difficult to differentiate with certainty some late vesicular lesions of pemphigoid from those of dermatitis herpetiformis because both may show subepidermal vesiculation with numerous eosinophils in the upper part of the dermis. However, there are usually more neutrophils in dermatitis herpetiformis, especially in collections at the tips of the papillae to the sides of blister. It is advisable, therefore, to perform a biopsy on an early papule or papulovesicle, and if only a blister is available, the biopsy specimen should include it and the surrounding skin.

The histologic changes in dermatitis herpetiformis are similar if not identical, to those of chronic bullous disease of childhood and to linear IgA bullous dermatosis. Dermatitis herpetiformis also must be differentiated histologically from bullous systemic lupus erythematosus, cicatricial pemphigoid, and dermatitis herpetiformis-like drug eruptions. The histologic changes in pemphigoid are similar, if not identical, to those of herpes gestationis.

6. Erythema Multiforme
vs. Pityriasis Lichenoides et Varioliformis Acuta

Erythema Multiforme

1. In early lesions, basket weave patterned stratum corneum; in later lesions, slight parakeratosis

2. Epidermis not hyperplastic

3. In early lesions, numerous individual necrotic keratinocytes scattered within the epidermis

4. In late lesions, confluent necrosis throughout the full thickness of the epidermis

5. Neutrophils present only when epidermis is necrotic

6. Epithelium of adnexa (hair follicles and eccrine sweat ducts) involved by vacuolar alteration and necrotic keratinocytes commonly

7. Subepidermal vesiculation usually; intraepidermal vesiculation occasionally

8. Slight edema in the papillary dermis

9. Few extravasated erythrocytes in the papillary dermis

10. Sparse lympho-histiocytic infiltrate and vacuolar alteration obscure the dermo-epidermal junction

11. No lichenoid infiltrate of inflammatory cells in the papillary dermis

12. Sparse to moderately dense superficial perivascular lympho-histiocytic infiltrate

Pityriasis Lichenoides et Varioliformis Acuta (Mucha-Habermann Disease)

1. In early lesions, focal or confluent parakeratosis containing neutrophils; in later lesions, scale-crusts

2. Epidermis slightly hyperplastic occasionally

3. In early lesions, few individual necrotic cells scattered within the epidermis

4. In late lesions, well-circumscribed wedge-shaped necrosis especially in the upper half of the epidermis

5. Neutrophils within the epidermis (especially in parakeratotic zones and scale-crusts)

6. Involvement of epithelium of adnexa uncommon

7. Intraepidermal vesiculation usually; subepidermal vesiculation occasionally

8. Marked edema in the papillary dermis

9. Many extravasated erythrocytes in the papillary dermis and often within the epidermis

10. Moderately dense lympho-histiocytic infiltrate and vacuolar alteration obscure the dermo-epidermal junction

11. Lichenoid infiltrate of inflammatory cells in the papillary dermis often

12. Moderately dense superficial and deep perivascular and interstitial lympho-histiocytic infiltrate often in a V-shape pointing toward the subcutis (rarely merely superficial)

Erythema Multiforme

Pityriasis Lichenoides et Varioliformis Acuta (Mucha-Habermann Disease)

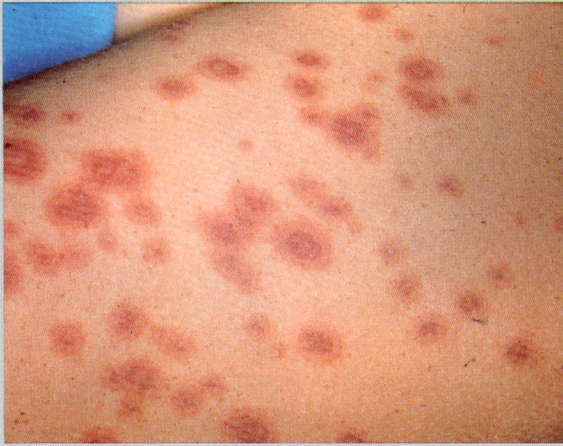

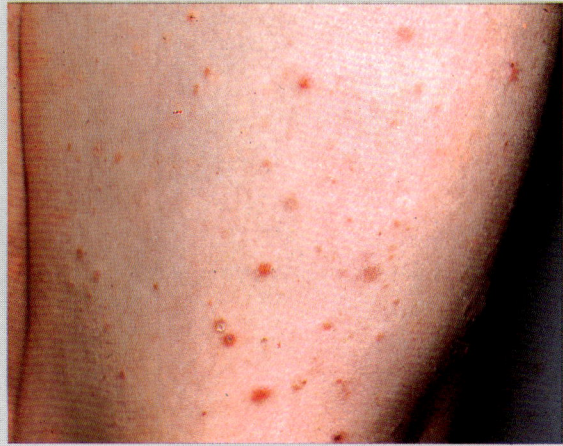

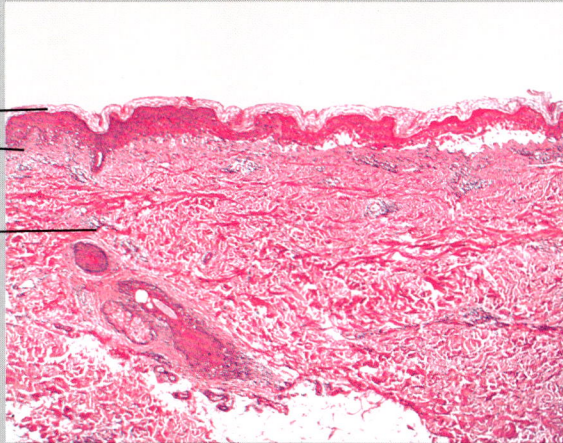

basket-weave cornified layer

sparse infiltrate at interface

sparse peri-vascular infiltrate

parakeratosis

interface obscured

superficial and deep perivascular infiltrate

lymphocytes in subcutis

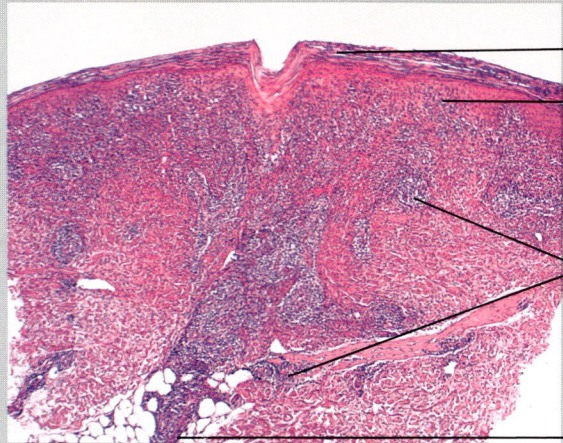

basket-weave cornified layer

necrotic keratinocyte

vacuolar alteration

few lymphocytes

parakeratosis

neutrophils

necrotic keratino-cytes

infiltrate obscuring dermo-epidermal junction

lymphocytes

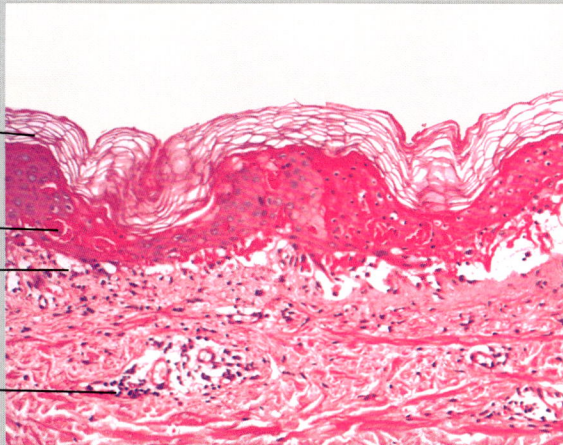

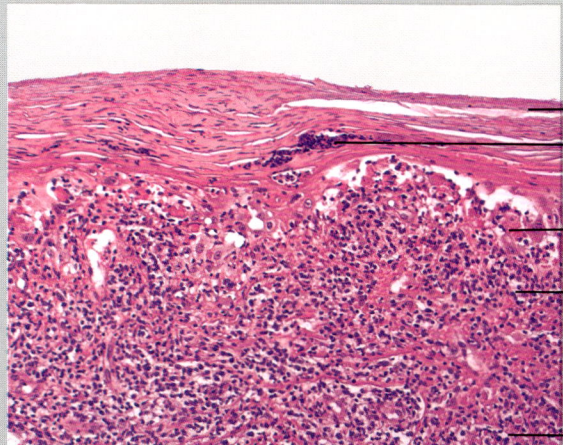

basket-weave cornified layer

ballooning

necrotic keratino-cytes

vacuolar alteration

parakeratosis

neutrophils

necrotic keratino-cytes

interface obscured by infiltrate

lymphocytes

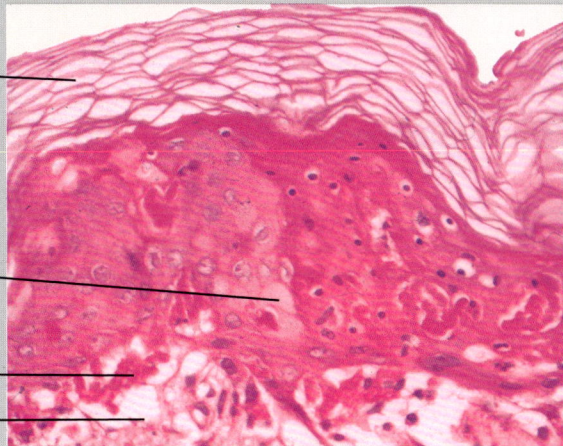

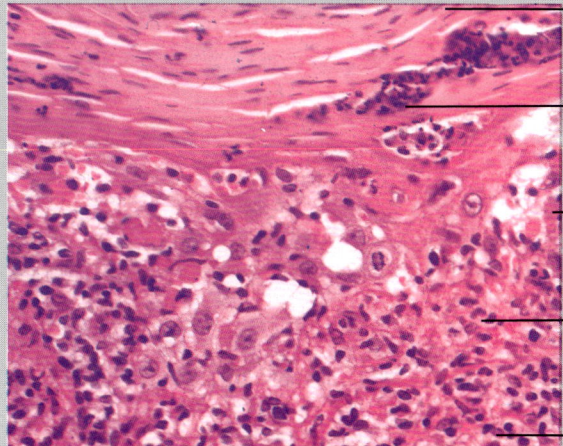

I<small>T</small> may be difficult or impossible to differentiate the histologic changes in the lower portion of the epidermis and at the dermo-epidermal interface of erythema multiforme from those of Mucha-Habermann disease. In both diseases there may be intra- and intercellular edema, individual dying keratinocytes, vacuolar alteration, and a sprinkling of lymphocytes and histiocytes. In most instances, however, the previously outlined differential features enable the pathologist to render a specific and precise diagnosis.

The early clinical lesions of erythema multiforme are edematous papules that soon become slightly purpuric plaques upon which blisters form. When a papule or plaque is ring-shaped with a central purpuric punctum, the lesion is termed herpes iris lesion (after Iris, the Greek goddess of the rainbow for whom the structure of the eye was also named), and when concentric rings develop, it is called a target lesion (after the marksman's target). The lesions of erythema multiforme have a predilection for acral skin parts and for mucous membranes.

The blisters of erythema multiforme usually develop beneath the epidermis, in part as a consequence of extensive vacuolar alteration, but blisters may also occur within the epidermis secondary to marked spongiosis and ballooning. The gray color of the blister roof reflects confluent epidermal necrosis.

Causes for erythema multiforme are not determinable with certainty in most cases; drugs and infectious agents (viruses, bacteria, and mycoplasmata) have been implicated. The process is usually short-lived, waning spontaneously and completely in a few weeks, or seemingly less if systemic corticosteroids are administered in sufficiently high dosage.

The histological differential diagnosis of erythema multiforme, besides Mucha-Habermann disease, includes fixed drug eruptions during acute phases and graft *vs.* host reactions during acute phases. These processes may have epidermal features indistinguishable from those of erythema multiforme. However, fixed drug eruptions, unlike erythema multiforme, usually show mixed inflammatory-cell infiltrates composed of many eosinophils and neutrophils, as well as of lymphocytes and histiocytes and the infiltrate is deep as well as superficial, and interstitial as well as perivascular. Some graft *vs.* host reactions are accompanied by lesions in the skin that closely resemble those of erythema multiforme histologically. The features which help to differentiate those graft *vs.* host reactions from erythema multiforme are parakeratosis and the presence occasionally of eosinophils within the infiltrate.

Clinically, Mucha-Habermann disease is a polymorphous eruption of widespread small lesions with no propensity for acral parts or mucous membranes. Its lesions are papules surmounted by brawny scales (pityriasis), flat-topped papules (lichenoid), purpuric, necrotic, and ulcerated papules, vesicles, and scars (varioliformis). The disease tends to occur in adolescents and young adults, to have a protracted course usually lasting for months, and to respond poorly or not at all to treatment in most instances.

Occasionally, some of the mononuclear cells in the infiltrate of Mucha-Habermann disease are atypical. This situation does not warrant the diagnosis of lymphomatoid papulosis, which is a different disease. The purpuric, vesicular, necrotic, and ulcerated lesions of Mucha-Habermann disease are sometimes misinterpreted clinically as representing vasculitis, but vasculitis is practically never seen histologically in those lesions.

7. Staphylococcal Scalded Skin Syndrome *vs.* Toxic Epidermal Necrolysis

Staphylococcal Scalded Skin Syndrome	*Toxic Epidermal Necrolysis (Severe Widespread Erythema Multiforme)*
1. Intraepidermal blister (approximately in the granular or upper spinous zones)	1. Subepidermal blister
2. Subcorneal pustules common	2. No subcorneal pustules
3. No significant number of necrotic epidermal cells	3. Necrotic keratinocytes scattered individually along the dermo-epidermal interface and throughout the epidermis in early lesions; confluent epidermal necrosis in later lesions
4. Acantholytic cells within the blister usually	4. No acantholytic cells
5. Moderately dense superficial perivascular mixed-cell infiltrate containing neutrophils	5. Scant superficial perivascular lympho-histiocytic infiltrate

Staphylococcal Scalded Skin Syndrome

Toxic Epidermal Necrolysis
(Severe Widespread Erythema Multiforme)

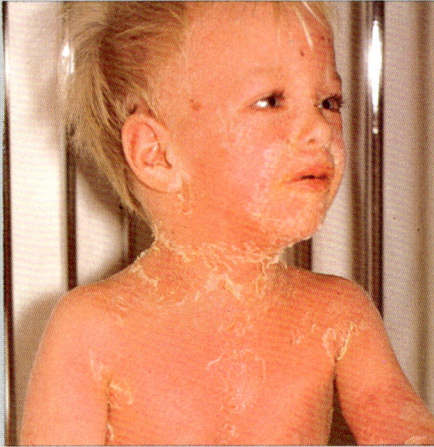

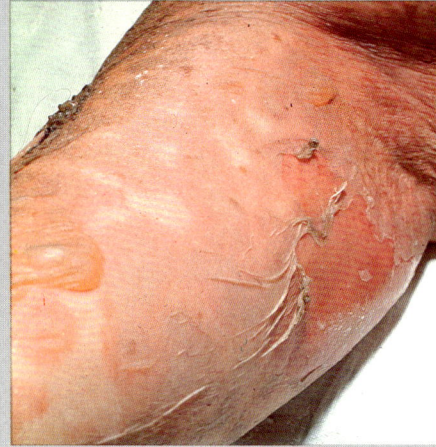

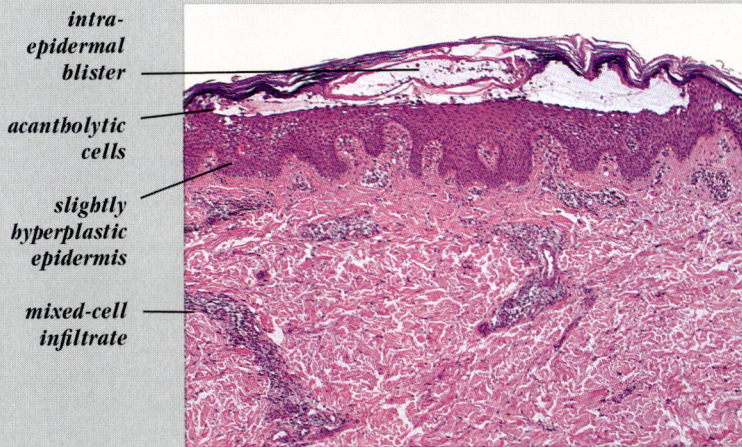

intra-
epidermal
blister

acantholytic
cells

slightly
hyperplastic
epidermis

mixed-cell
infiltrate

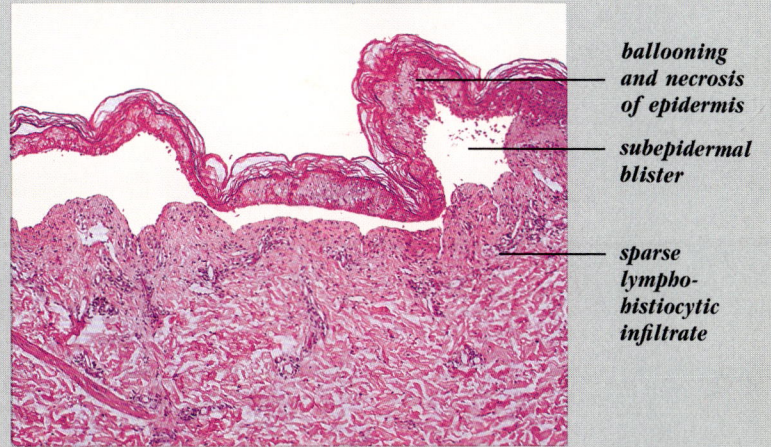

ballooning
and necrosis
of epidermis

subepidermal
blister

sparse
lympho-
histiocytic
infiltrate

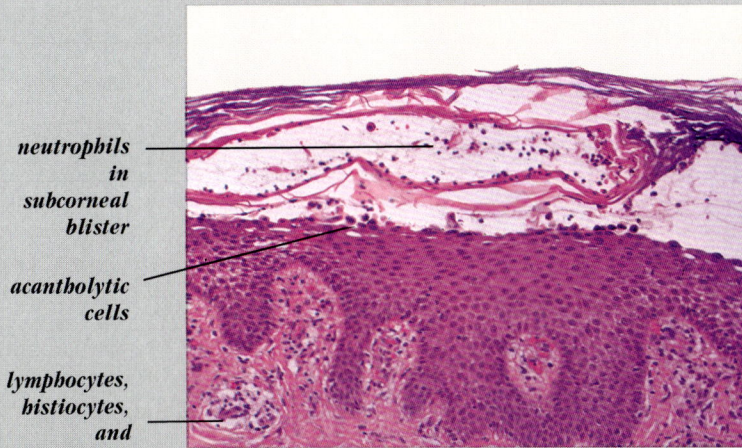

neutrophils
in
subcorneal
blister

acantholytic
cells

lymphocytes,
histiocytes,
and
neutrophils

cornified
layer

neutrophils

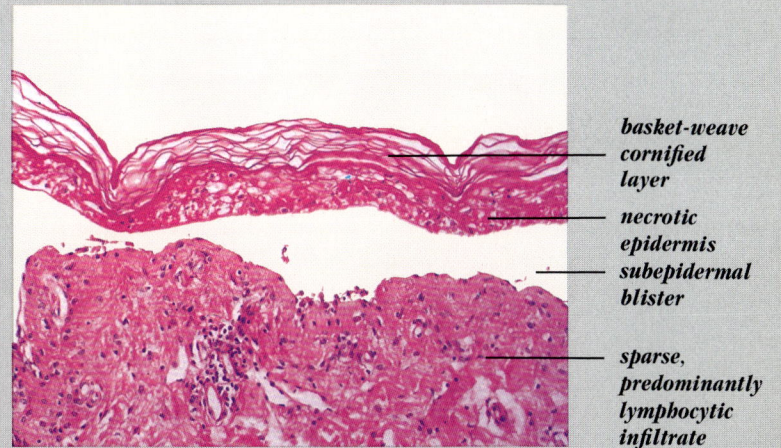

basket-weave
cornified
layer

necrotic
epidermis

subepidermal
blister

sparse,
predominantly
lymphocytic
infiltrate

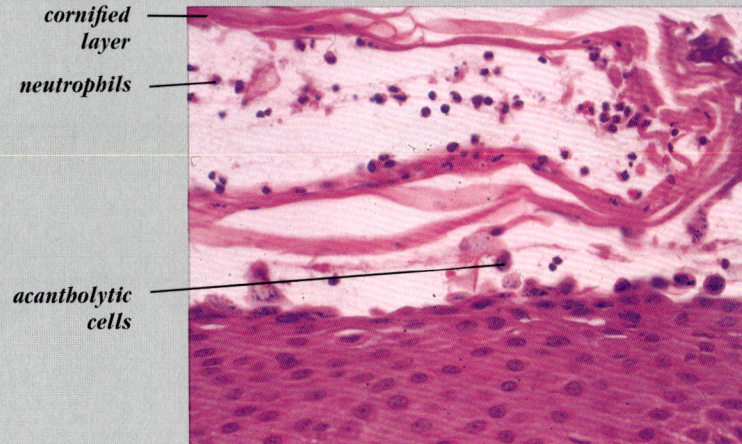

acantholytic
cells

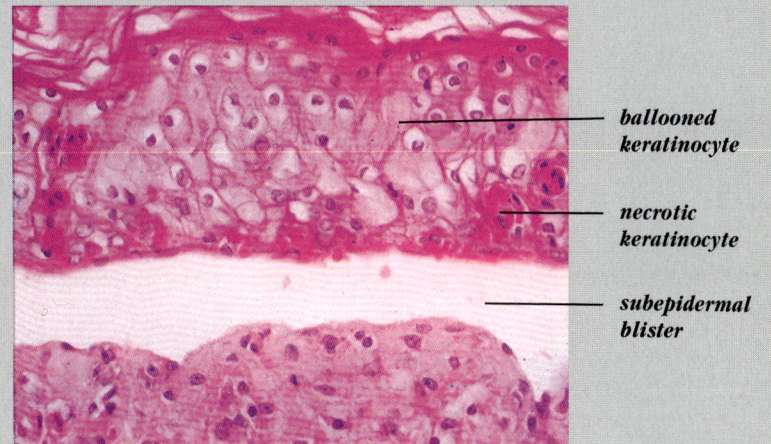

ballooned
keratinocyte

necrotic
keratinocyte

subepidermal
blister

TOXIC epidermal necrolysis and staphylococcal scalded skin syndrome are blistering dermatitides that, in the past, were often viewed as one disease because both resemble scalded skin clinically. In fact, they are completely different histologically, biologically, causally, and in response to therapy. So, too, Stevens-Johnson syndrome, pemphigus vulgaris, and extensive thermal burns may, at times, clinically resemble scalded skin, but each is a distinctive pathologic process.

We here use the term toxic epidermal necrolysis to refer strictly and specifically to a widespread subepidermal blistering disease that afflicts adults (children rarely), is usually idiopathic, but on occasion seems to be circumstantially related to administration of drugs or exposure to chemicals. An example of the latter is inhalation of fumes such as fumigants. Staphylococci are not cultured from the blisters or from the surrounding skin. Clinically, toxic epidermal necrolysis is characterized by sudden appearance of areas of redness and tenderness that evolve into large flaccid bullae. Mucous membranes are often affected too. Nikolsky's sign, i.e., induction of a lesion by firm oblique pressure, is readily elicitable. Because the blisters develop at the dermo-epidermal junction and are huge, excessive loss of fluids and electrolytes is a serious complication, as it is in severe burns. Indeed, toxic epidermal necrolysis should be managed like an extensive burn. Even with meticulous treatment and administration of corticosteroids, the mortality from the disease is about 25%.

Toxic epidermal necrolysis, in our opinion, is a severe widespread variant of erythema multiforme with which it has several clinical features ("iris" and "target" lesions and mucous membrane lesions may be present) and many histologic characteristics (superficial perivascular lympho-histiocytic infiltrate, vacuolar alteration, and necrotic keratinocytes) in common. Lyell initially grouped the staphylococcal scalded skin syndrome of children and severe widespread erythema multiforme in adults together under the title "toxic epidermal necrolysis." Toxic epidermal necrolysis is used by us as a synonym for a severe, often fatal, widespread form of erythema multiforme.

In contrast to toxic epidermal necrolysis, the staphylococcal scalded skin syndrome is an intraepidermal blistering disease that mainly affects children (adults rarely) and is caused, in every instance, by an epidermolytic toxin produced by a virally lysogenized staphylococcus. The presence of acantholytic cells in a blister high within the epidermis gives this condition histologic similarities to bullous impetigo and superficial forms of pemphigus (foliaceus and erythematosus). Unlike bullous impetigo, in which staphylococci are readily culturable from the blister field, no bacteria can be cultured from the blisters of staphylococcal scalded skin syndrome.

The staphylococcal scalded skin syndrome evolves in a clinical sequence that begins with erythematous macules on the face and neck and in the axillae and groin, progresses to extensive bulla formation and eventuates in "potato-chip" exfoliation. During the blistering phase, the Nikolsky sign may be elicited with ease. Unlike toxic epidermal necrolysis, the prognosis is very good; the condition responds promptly and completely to specific antibiotics.

Because the term "toxic epidermal necrolysis" means different things to different dermatologists, pathologists, and pediatricians, it might be preferable to avoid the term completely and simply to refer to the one disease as staphylococcal scalded skin syndrome and to the other as severe widespread erythema multiforme.

8. Pemphigus Vulgaris *vs.* Benign Familial Chronic Pemphigus

Pemphigus Vulgaris	Benign Familial Chronic Pemphigus (Hailey-Hailey Disease)
1. Epidermis above the suprabasal separation mostly intact	1. Epidermis above the suprabasal separation considerably altered by acantholysis
2. Few acantholytic cells above the suprabasal separation	2. Many acantholytic cells above the suprabasal separation
3. Acantholytic cells confined immediately above the basal layer	3. Acantholytic cells at least throughout the lower half of the epidermis in some rete ridges
4. No significant changes in the stratum corneum	4. Stratum corneum often altered by ortho- and parakeratosis, crusts, and scale-crusts
5. Epidermal hyperplasia rare	5. Epidermal hyperplasia usual
6. Suprabasal separation usually confluent within a 4 mm punch-biopsy specimen	6. Multiple, discrete suprabasal separations usually within a 4 mm punch-biopsy specimen
7. Epithelium of adnexa commonly affected by suprabasal separation and acantholytic cells	7. Epithelium of adnexa not commonly affected by suprabasal separation and acantholytic cells
8. Acantholytic cells almost always within suprabasal vesicles or bullae	8. Acantholytic cells sometimes discernible without suprabasal alteration
9. No dyskeratotic cells with the epidermis	9. Many dyskeratotic cells with pyknotic nuclei and eosinophilic cytoplasms within the epidermis often
10. No mitotic figures above the basal layer	10. Mitotic figures above the basal layer commonly
11. Eosinophils may be present in addition to lymphocytes and histiocytes in the dermis	11. Neutrophils may be present in addition to lymphocytes and histiocytes in the dermis

Pemphigus Vulgaris

Benign Familial Chronic Pemphigus
(Hailey-Hailey Disease)

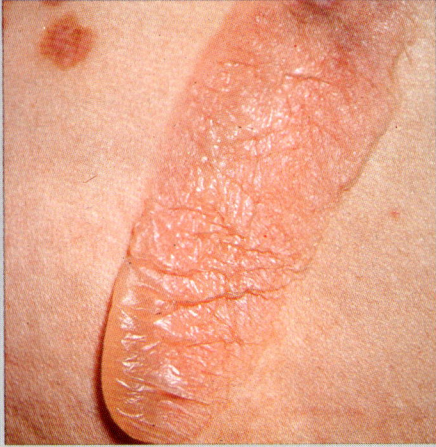

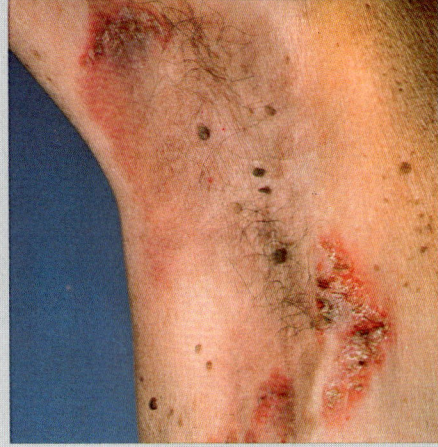

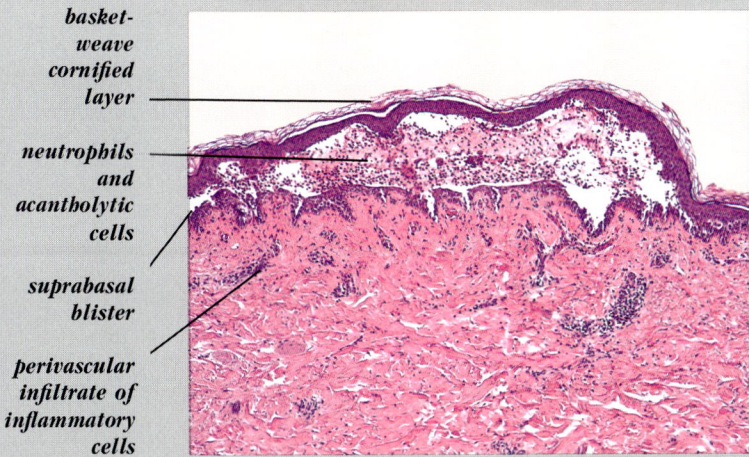

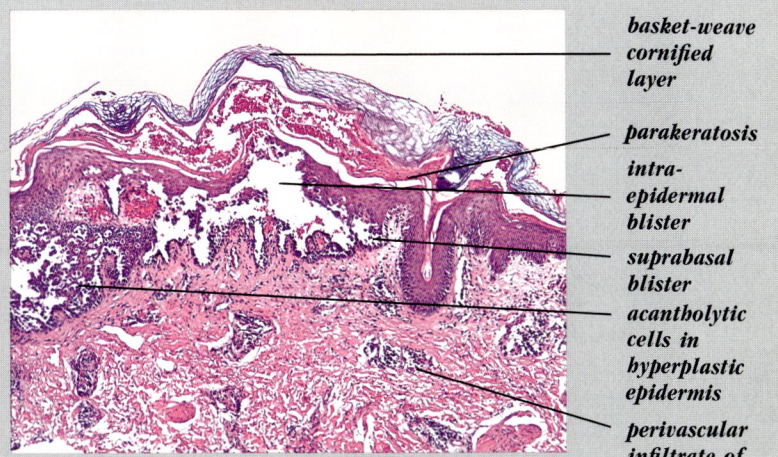

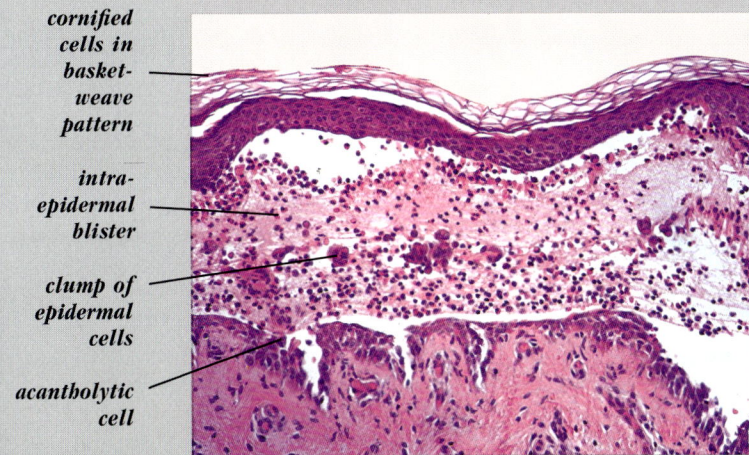

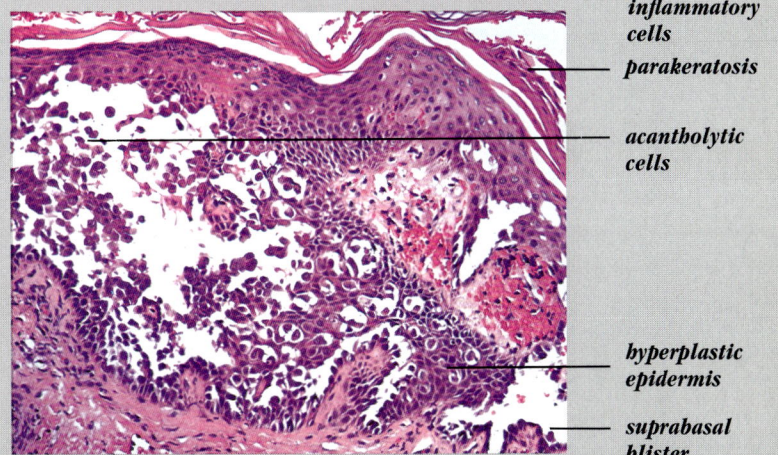

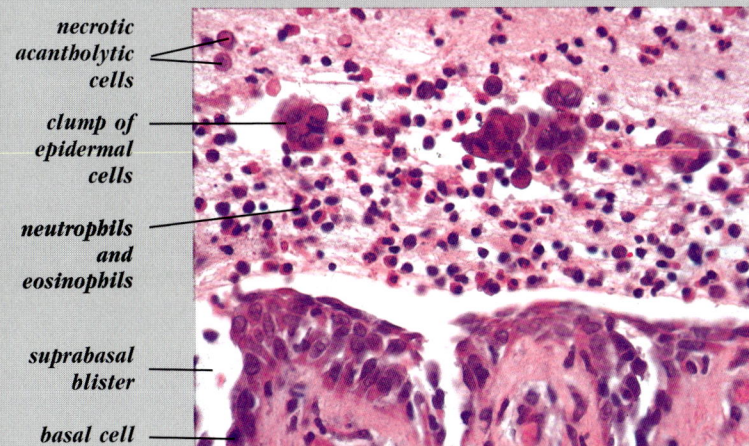

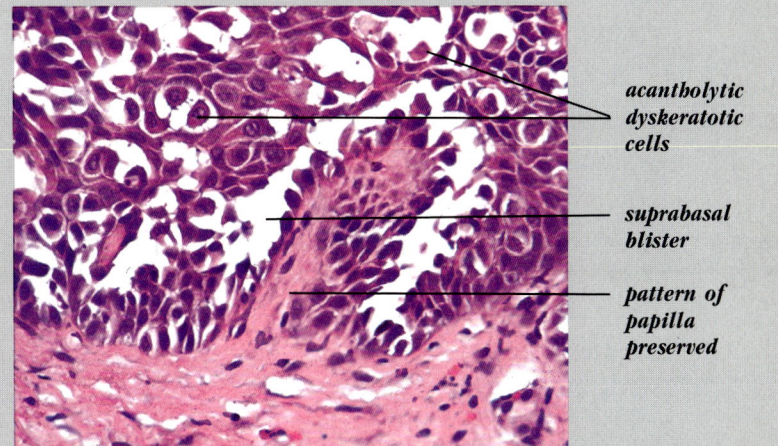

basket-weave cornified layer

neutrophils and acantholytic cells

suprabasal blister

perivascular infiltrate of inflammatory cells

basket-weave cornified layer

parakeratosis

intra-epidermal blister

suprabasal blister

acantholytic cells in hyperplastic epidermis

perivascular infiltrate of inflammatory cells

cornified cells in basket-weave pattern

intra-epidermal blister

clump of epidermal cells

acantholytic cell

parakeratosis

acantholytic cells

hyperplastic epidermis

suprabasal blister

necrotic acantholytic cells

clump of epidermal cells

neutrophils and eosinophils

suprabasal blister

basal cell

acantholytic dyskeratotic cells

suprabasal blister

pattern of papilla preserved

P EMPHIGUS vulgaris and familial benign chronic pemphigus are both acantholytic vesiculobullous dermatitides that in some instances may be exceedingly difficult to differentiate from each other. This is especially true when there are only a few acantholytic cells within apparently normal epidermis that has separated suprabasally. In these difficult cases, deeper sections through the specimen may reveal a focus of acantholytic cells that extends throughout much of the epidermis, a clue to the diagnosis of Hailey-Hailey disease. Such a focus may be confined to a single rete ridge. Again, deeper sections might show that epithelia of adnexa are significantly involved by the acantholytic process, a feature more commonly found in pemphigus vulgaris.

The typical clinical lesions of pemphigus vulgaris are flaccid bullae that arise on normal-appearing skin and mucous membranes. The blisters eventually break revealing a weeping surface that histologically can be seen to be covered by but a single layer of basal cells. The blisters of pemphigus vulgaris may be enlarged by downward pressure upon them and fresh blisters may often be induced by firm, oblique pressure on apparently normal skin (Nikolsky's sign). Uncomplicated lesions of pemphigus vulgaris heal without scarring.

The blisters of Hailey-Hailey disease vary from smooth-surfaced, flaccid vesicles and bullae to vesiculopustules and vegetating plaques. They occur predilectively in intertriginous regions and only rarely involve the mucosae. Scarring does not usually result. A familial history is commonly forthcoming.

Immunofluorescent studies, both direct and indirect, reveal intercellular deposition of antibodies and complement in most cases of pemphigus vulgaris, but not in cases of Hailey-Hailey disease.

Pemphigus vulgaris-like changes in the epidermis may be induced by penicillamine and, rarely, by other drugs. Histologic features of pemphigus vulgaris also may be encountered along with features of superficial pemphigus in some biopsy specimens from patients with pemphigus foliaceus, pemphigus erythematosus, and fogo selvagem. Histologic foci like those of pemphigus vulgaris are characteristic of one varient of transient acantholytic dermatosis (Grover's disease). Pemphigus vulgaris-like changes also may occur in the epidermis of severely anoxic limbs, particularly gangrenous ones. Lastly, pemphigus vulgaris-like foci may be found confined to one or a few epidermal rete ridges, analogous to isolated foci of acantholytic dyskeratosis, epidermolytic hyperkeratosis, and cornoid lamellation.

In the years following the original description of benign familial chronic pemphigus by the brothers Hailey, many pathologists considered the condition to be histologically indistinguishable from keratosis follicularis (Darier's disease). In fact, they are different diseases. Darier's disease is not a blistering disease at all, because vesicles and bullae are not seen on clinical inspection, and plasma is not seen in the epidermal clefts on histologic examination. Furthermore, Darier's disease differs histologically from Hailey-Hailey disease by having changes that are more focal, parakeratosis that is more prominent and dyskeratosis that is more extensive in the granular and cornified layers.

9. Keratosis Follicularis *vs.* Transient Acantholytic Dermatosis

Keratosis Follicularis *(Darier's Disease)*	**Transient Acantholytic Dermatosis** *(Grover's Disease)*
1. No evidence of excoriation usually	1. Erosions, ulcerations, and scale-crusts, i.e., evidences of excoriation present often
2. Focal vertical parakeratosis	2. Little parakeratosis as a rule (except in purely Darier type)
3. Intraepidermal clefts; no vesicles	3. Intraepidermal vesicles as well as clefts
4. No spongiosis	4. Spongiosis and acantholysis in the same focus (spongiotic type) often
5. No edema of the papillary dermis	5. Edema of the papillary dermis occasionally
6. No eosinophils in the dermis	6. Eosinophils in the superficial dermis often
7. Follicular infundibula may be involved	7. Follicular infundibula usually spared
8. Features of focal acantholytic dyskeratosis only	8. Features sometimes of pemphigus (superficial and deep types), familial benign chronic pemphigus (Hailey-Hailey disease), spongiosis with acantholysis, and focal acantholytic dyskeratosis in the same biopsy specimen
9. Usually several foci of acantholysis and dyskeratosis per 4 mm specimen	9. Usually only one or two foci of acantholysis and dyskeratosis per 4 mm specimen
10. Clefts and acantholytic cells obvious usually	10. Clefts and acantholytic cells, subtle often

Keratosis Follicularis
(Darier's Disease)

Transient Acantholytic Dermatosis
(Grover's Disease)

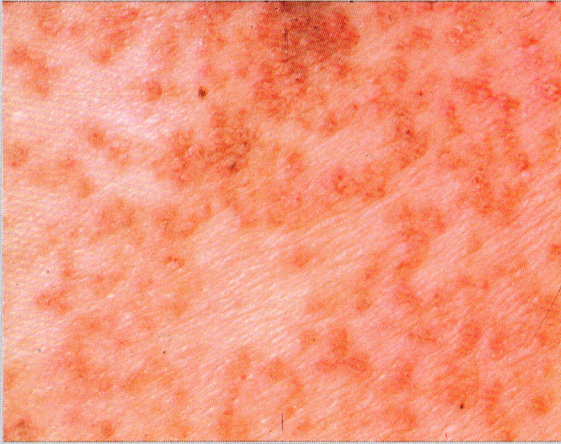

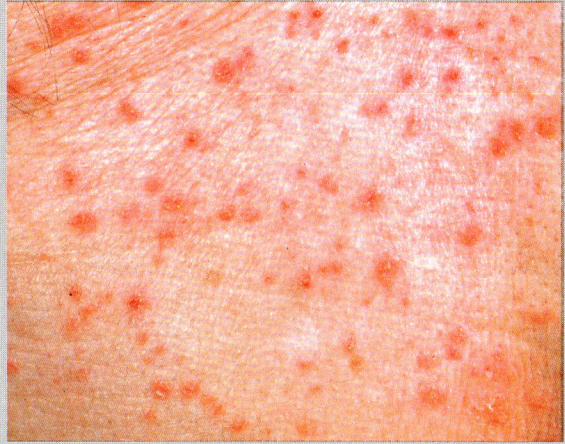

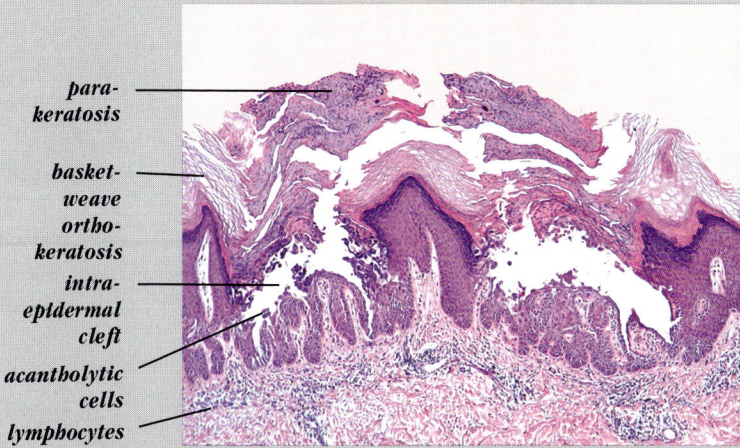

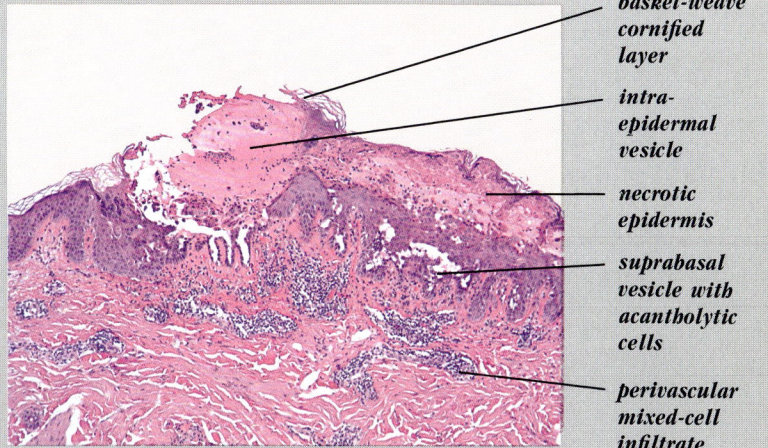

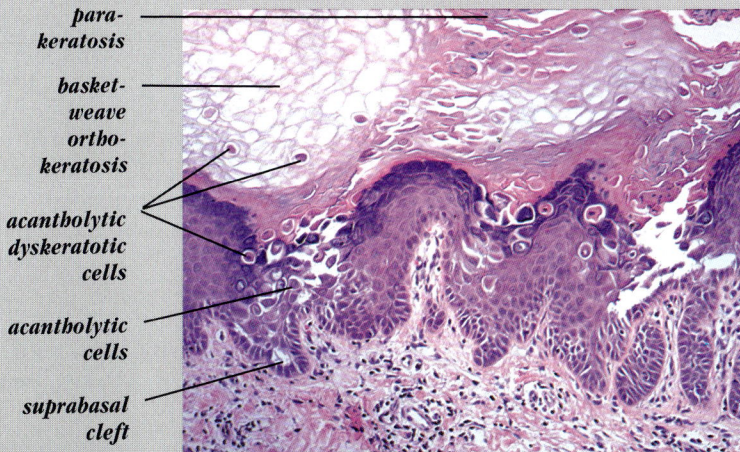

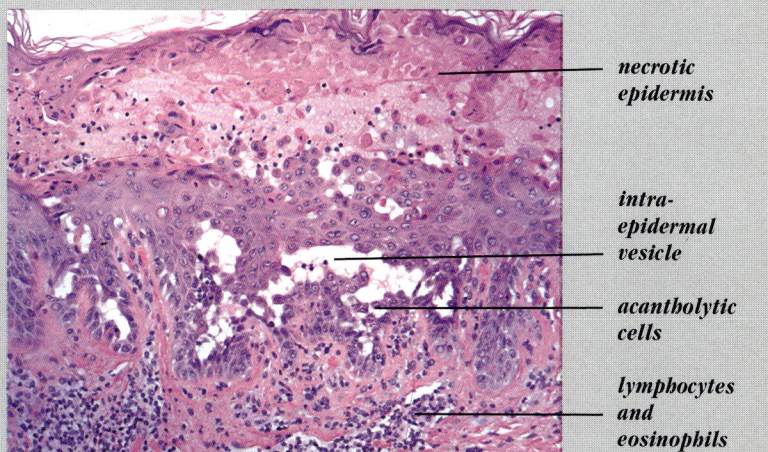

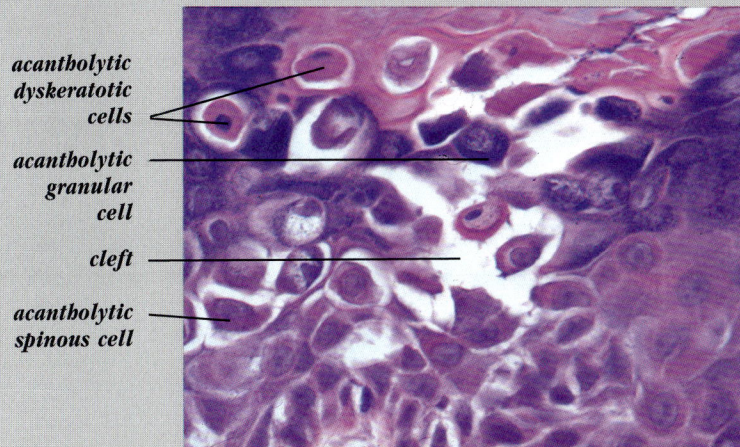

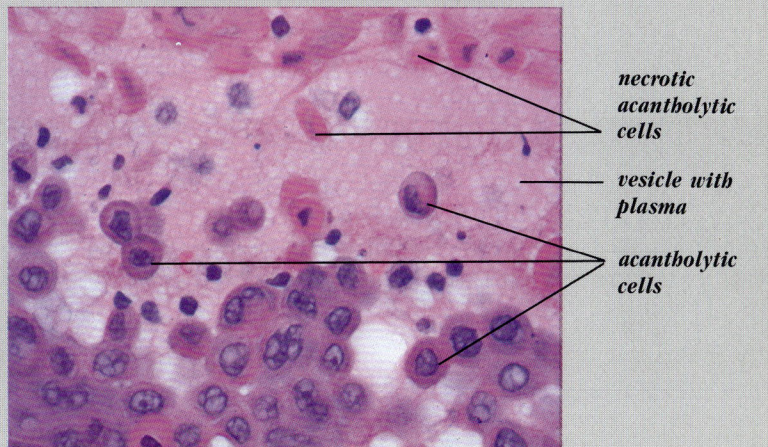

para-
keratosis

basket-
weave
ortho-
keratosis

intra-
epidermal
cleft

acantholytic
cells

lymphocytes

basket-weave
cornified
layer

intra-
epidermal
vesicle

necrotic
epidermis

suprabasal
vesicle with
acantholytic
cells

perivascular
mixed-cell
infiltrate

para-
keratosis

basket-
weave
ortho-
keratosis

acantholytic
dyskeratotic
cells

acantholytic
cells

suprabasal
cleft

necrotic
epidermis

intra-
epidermal
vesicle

acantholytic
cells

lymphocytes
and
eosinophils

acantholytic
dyskeratotic
cells

acantholytic
granular
cell

cleft

acantholytic
spinous cell

necrotic
acantholytic
cells

vesicle with
plasma

acantholytic
cells

DARIER'S disease and Grover's disease have these histologic features in common: foci of acantholysis and dyskeratosis within the epidermis and a superficial perivascular infiltrate of inflammatory cells within the dermis. One variant of Grover's disease may be indistinguishable histologically from Darier's disease and for that reason it is termed the Darier variant of Grover's disease.

Keratosis follicularis (Darier's disease) is a genodermatosis that is inherited as an autosomal-dominant condition. The lesions usually appear during the second decade of life as widespread, rough-surfaced, dirty brown, keratotic papules. On the skin there is some predilection for the "seborrheic areas" and the extensor surfaces, but Darier's disease may also affect the mucous membranes and the nails. The disease generally waxes and wanes throughout life and prior to the use of retinoids was usually refractory to treatment. Darier's disease does not show vesicles, histologically or clinically.

In contrast to Darier's disease, transient acantholytic dermatosis (Grover's disease) almost always occurs in adults over 40 years of age and especially those over 60. Except for the type of transient acantholytic dermatosis that resembles Darier's disease in which the discrete, gray, small papules are keratotic, the lesions of Grover's disease are smooth-surfaced papules and papulovesicles. They have a predilection for the V of the chest, trunk, flanks, and thighs. There is no involvement of mucous membranes or nails. The lesions, often pruritic, are evanescent and the condition usually disappears spontaneously within weeks or months. Rarely it persists for years. Histologically, Grover's disease is often vesicular rather than clefted.

Heretofore there were a few reports of evanescent cases of Darier's disease developing in adults. Almost certainly these represented examples of Grover's disease that resembled Darier's disease in histology.

The histologic features of focal acantholytic dyskeratosis are common, not only to classical Darier's disease and the variant of Grover's disease that resembles it, but to some epidermal nevi, solitary keratoses, infundibular cysts (warty dyskeratoma), and as an incidental finding confined to a single rete ridge or an infundibulum of a biopsy specimen that was taken for an unrelated pathological process.

There are four basic histologic patterns of acantholysis in Grover's disease. In addition to the variant that resembles Darier's disease, there are forms that are like those of pemphigus (superficial, i.e., foliaceus and erythematosus, and deep, i.e., vulgaris), familial benign chronic pemphigus (Hailey-Hailey disease), and spongiotic dermatitis. Acantholysis of some sort is the histologic mark of all these variants of Grover's disease. In some biopsy specimens, two or more of these patterns may be found concurrently.

Although Grover's disease usually may be differentiated from Darier's disease if the aforementioned criteria are employed, the Darier-like variant of Grover's disease may be histologically indistinguishable from authentic Darier's disease. In such instances, the two diseases still may be differentiated by the utilization of clinical criteria, namely, age of the patient, duration and distribution of the lesions, and the presence or absence of severe pruritus.

10. Discoid Lupus Erythematosus, Subacute Stage *vs.* Polymorphous Light Eruption

Discoid Lupus Erythematosus, Subacute Stage

1. Compact orthokeratosis of epidermis
2. Follicular infundibula plugged by orthokeratosis
3. Epidermis usually thinned; sometimes hyperplastic focally
4. Pattern of epidermal rete ridges and dermal papillae not preserved
5. Necrotic keratinocytes in the epidermis occasionally
6. No spongiosis
7. Vacuolar alteration at the dermo-epidermal junction
8. Basement membrane thickened at dermo-epidermal junction
9. Slight edema of the papillary dermis
10. Few extravasated erythrocytes
11. Melanophages and siderophages in papillary dermis
12. Stellate fibroblasts, some multinucleated, in the upper part of the dermis
13. Mucin, in varying amounts, in the reticular dermis usually
14. Moderately dense superficial and deep perivascular (including periadnexal) infiltrate of lymphocytes predominantly, but also of histiocytes and plasma cells occasionally

Polymorphous Light Eruption

1. Normal basket-weave cornified layer usually
2. No keratotic plugs in follicular infundibula
3. Epidermis normal usually
4. Pattern of epidermal rete ridges and dermal papillae preserved
5. No necrotic keratinocytes in the epidermis
6. Spongiosis rarely
7. No vacuolar alteration at the dermo-epidermal junction
8. Basement membrane not thickened
9. Marked edema of the papillary dermis; when severe, subepidermal vesiculation
10. Many extravasated erythrocytes when edema is massive
11. No melanophages or siderophages in papillary dermis as a rule
12. No stellate or multinucleated fibroblasts
13. No increased mucin in the dermis usually
14. Moderately dense superficial and deep perivascular predominantly lymphocytic infiltrate with some histiocytes, but no plasma cells

Discoid Lupus Erythematosus,
Subacute Stage

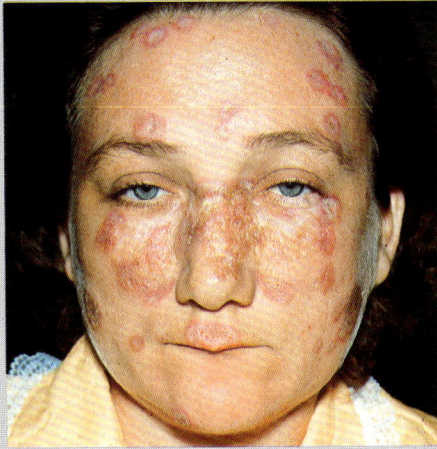

Polymorphous Light Eruption

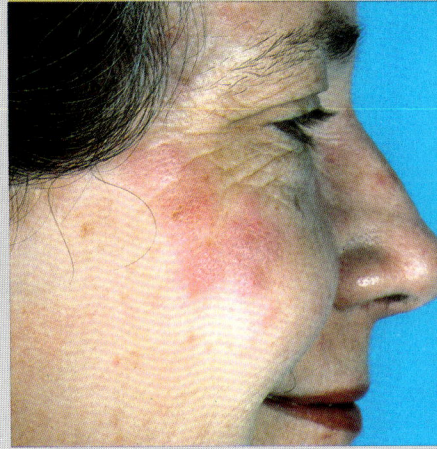

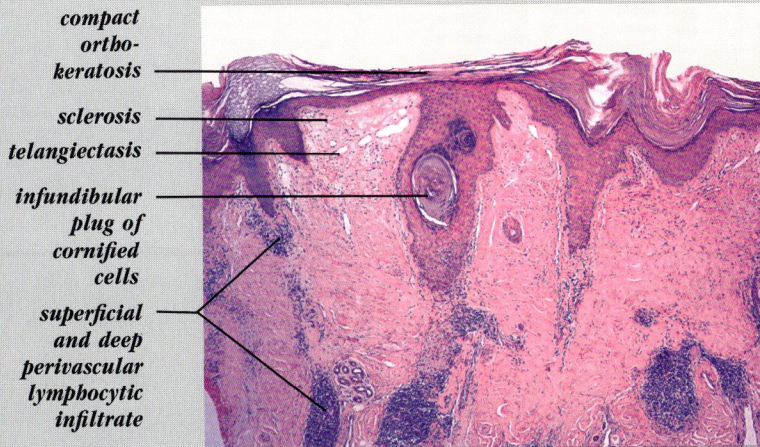

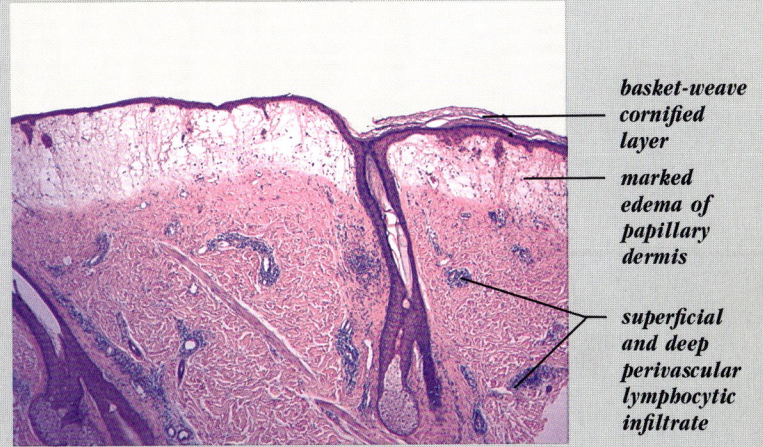

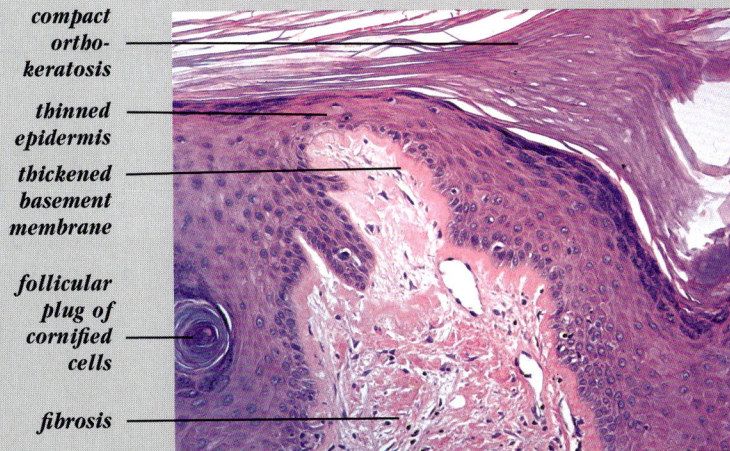

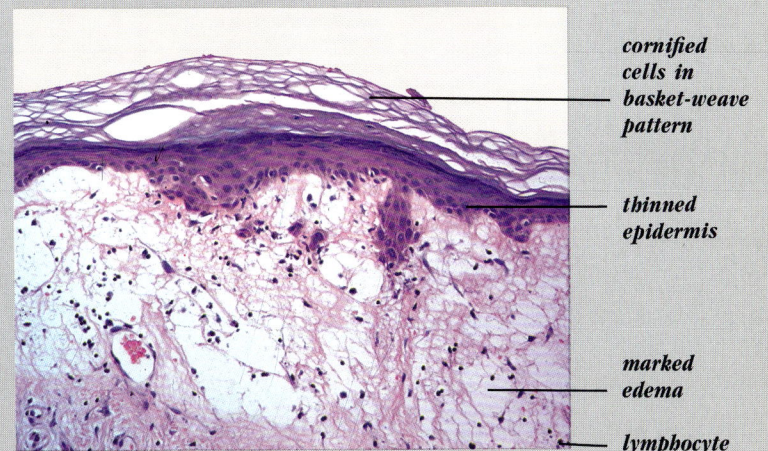

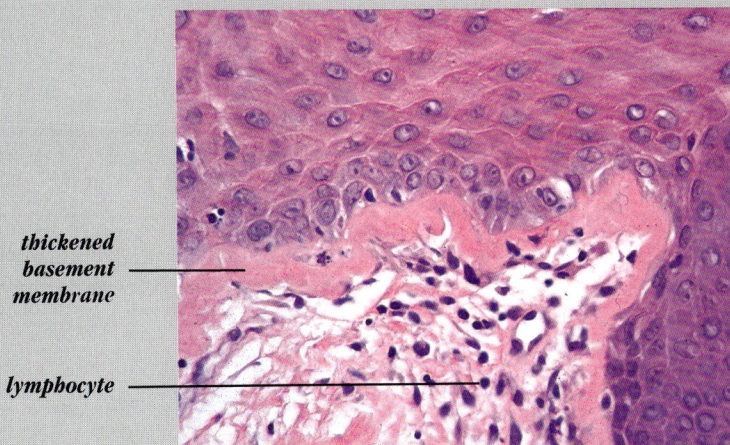

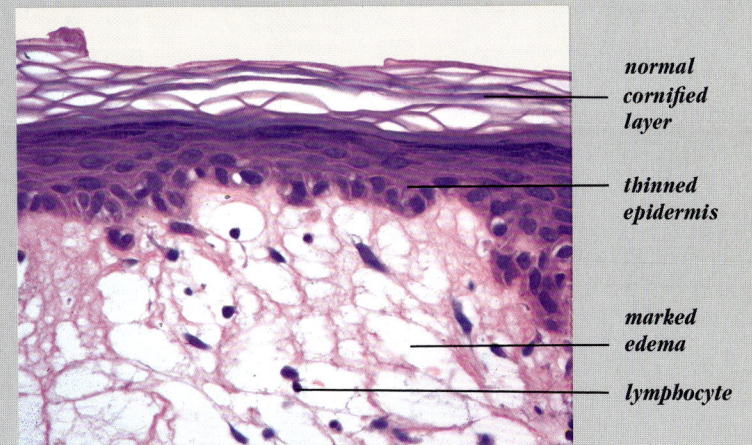

compact
ortho-
keratosis

sclerosis

telangiectasis

infundibular
plug of
cornified
cells

superficial
and deep
perivascular
lymphocytic
infiltrate

basket-weave
cornified
layer

marked
edema of
papillary
dermis

superficial
and deep
perivascular
lymphocytic
infiltrate

compact
ortho-
keratosis

thinned
epidermis

thickened
basement
membrane

follicular
plug of
cornified
cells

fibrosis

cornified
cells in
basket-weave
pattern

thinned
epidermis

marked
edema

lymphocyte

thickened
basement
membrane

lymphocyte

normal
cornified
layer

thinned
epidermis

marked
edema

lymphocyte

H ISTOLOGICALLY, subacute discoid lupus erythematosus and polymorphous light eruption have in common the presence of moderately dense predominantly lymphocytic infiltrates around the blood vessels of the superficial and deep vascular plexuses. Clinically, both of these diseases tend to occur on sun-exposed parts of the body and, in fact, polymorphous light eruption always is induced by sunlight and discoid lupus erythematosus often is.

Discoid lupus erythematosus is a specific skin disease that often proceeds through stages of redness, scaling (including keratotic follicular plugs), induration, hyper- and hypopigmentation, atrophy, and telangiectasia. These different clinical stages have equally precise histologic concomitants. Both the clinical and histologic features of discoid lupus erythematosus are as recognizable as those of psoriasis and lichen planus. However, the distinctive morphologic features of discoid lupus erythematosus, clinically and histologically, give no clue to whether the patient has concurrent disease of internal organs (systemic lupus erythematosus). As a rule, if the lesions of discoid lupus erythematosus are widespread, there is a greater likelihood that the patient has or will have systemic lupus erythematosus. Studies for antinuclear antibodies and L.E. preparations are far more reliable indicators of systemic lupus erythematosus than are histologic findings.

Lesions of discoid lupus erythematosus may be one manifestation of systemic lupus erythematosus (just as may leukocytoclastic [allergic] vasculitis, periungual telangiectases, and diffuse alopecia be manifestations of systemic lupus erythematosus), but in most instances patients with discoid lupus erythematosus never develop signs or symptoms of systemic lupus erythematosus. The clinical spectrum of discoid lupus erythematosus ranges from acute, reddish, scaly indurated lesions to chronic forms characterized by hypo- and/or hyperpigmentation, atrophic scars, and telangiectases. The histologic findings in this spectrum, as always, parallel the clinical changes. The histologic features of subacute discoid lupus erythematosus, as noted previously, are a combination of those found in acute and chronic discoid lupus erythematosus.

Acute discoid lupus erythematosus shows upon biopsy:

1. Predominantly lymphocytic infiltrate confined to the upper part of the dermis; occasional neutrophils in the papillary dermis; no or few melanophages
2. Telangiectases
3. Marked edema of the papillary dermis

4. Vacuolar alteration at the dermo-epidermal junction; if severe, sub-epidermal separation
5. Individual necrotic keratinocytes; occasionally confluent epidermal necrosis

There is no thickening of the basement membrane or dermal sclerosis in acute lesions of discoid lupus erythematosus.

Chronic discoid lupus erythematosus has these histologic features:

1. Sclerosis in the upper part of the dermis, sometimes obliterating epithelial structures of adnexa (when hair follicles are destroyed, permanent alopecia results)
2. Telangiectases
3. Increased numbers of melanophages in the upper part of the dermis
4. Vacuolar alteration, variable in extent
5. Marked thickening of the basement membrane at the junction between dermis and epidermis, between dermis and adnexal epithelium, and sometimes around telangiectatic superficial blood vessels
6. Relatively sparse lympho-histiocytic infiltrate in the lower and/or upper part of the dermis
7. Epidermal atrophy with occasional atypical keratinocytes (sometimes simulating solar keratosis)

Abundant acid mucopolysaccharides and dilated follicular infundibula plugged by compact orthokeratosis may be seen in chronic, as well as in subacute, discoid lupus erythematosus.

It may be difficult, and even impossible, to differentiate histologically between some lesions of discoid lupus erythematosus and dermatomyositis.

Polymorphous light eruption is characterized clinically by edematous erythematous smooth-surfaced papules that often coalesce to form plaques on sun-exposed skin. In rare instances, the edema becomes so severe that vesicles develop. All of the lesions of polymorphous light eruptions upon biopsy show variations on one histologic theme.

The histologic differential diagnosis of polymorphous light eruption, in addition to subacute discoid lupus erythematosus, includes lymphocytic infiltration (Jessner), gyrate erythema of the deep type, and the early inflammatory stage of scleroderma. If the subcutis and fascia are included in the biopsy specimen, scleroderma may be diagnosed with near certainty because of characteristic changes there.

Early and late lesions of polymorphous light eruption show little or no edema in the papillary dermis. Such lesions are virtually indistinguishable from the lymphocytic infiltrates just alluded to.

11. Reactions to Arthropod Assaults *vs.* Chronic Urticaria

Reactions to Arthropod Assaults	Chronic Urticaria
1. Scale-crusts over intraepidermal vesicles often	1. No scale-crusts
2. Well-circumscribed central spongiotic and ballooning vesicles within the epidermis often	2. No intraepidermal vesiculation
3. Marked edema of the papillary dermis	3. Slight edema of the papillary dermis
4. Subepidermal vesicles sometimes secondary to marked edema of the papillary dermis	4. No vesiculation
5. Many extravasated erythrocytes in the upper part of the dermis commonly	5. Few extravasated erythrocytes in the upper part of the dermis usually
6. Superficial and deep perivascular and interstitial, moderately dense, mixed inflammatory-cell infiltrate; rarely superficial only	6. Superficial, predominantly interstitial, sparse to moderately dense, mixed inflammatory-cell infiltrate; sometimes deep as well as superficial
7. Inflammatory-cell infiltrate in the dermis V-shaped with the point toward the subcutis	7. Infiltrate not V-shaped
8. Eosinophils, usually numerous, in addition to lymphocytes and histiocytes	8. Neutrophils and eosinophils in addition to lymphocytes and histiocytes
9. Inflammatory-cell infiltrate extends into the fat occasionally	9. Inflammatory-cell infiltrate confined to the dermis as a rule
10. Blood vessels often thick-walled with plump endothelial cells	10. Blood vessels dilated but not otherwise abnormal
11. Thrombi in capillaries and venules sometimes; vasculitis in the larger vessels of the deep dermis occasionally	11. No thrombi or vasculitis

Reactions to Arthropod Assaults

Chronic Urticaria

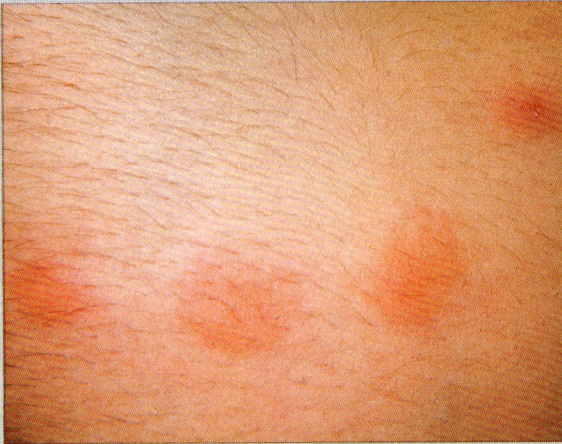

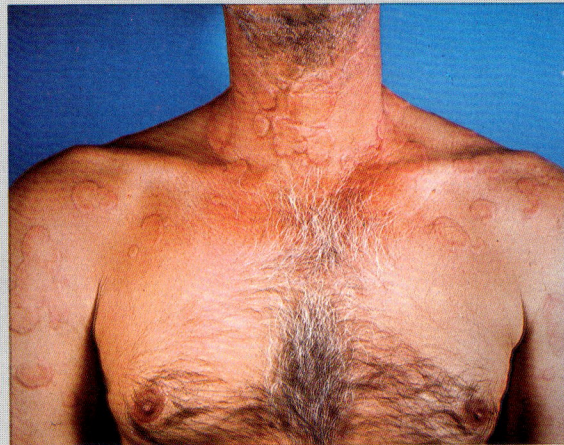

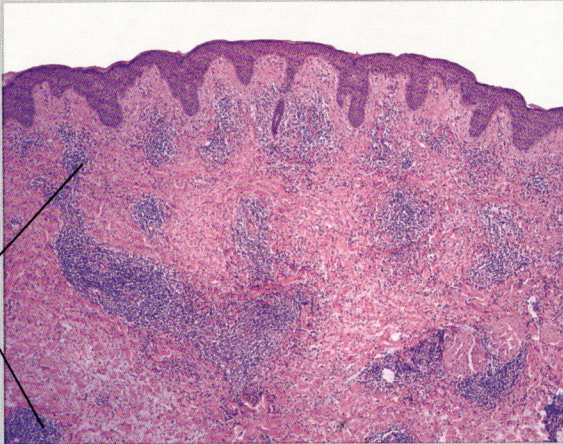

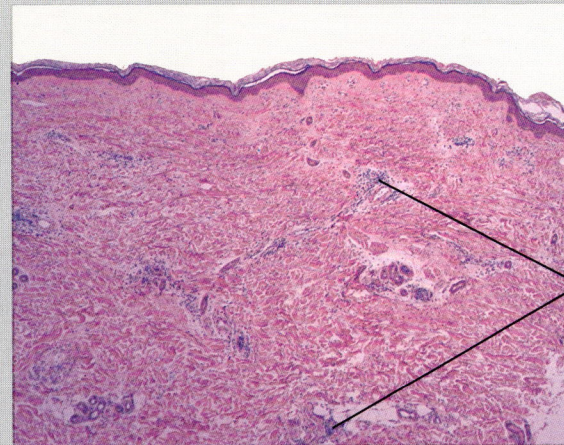

moderately
dense
superficial
and deep
perivascular
and
interstitial
infiltrate

sparse
superficial
and deep
perivascular
and
interstitial
infiltrate

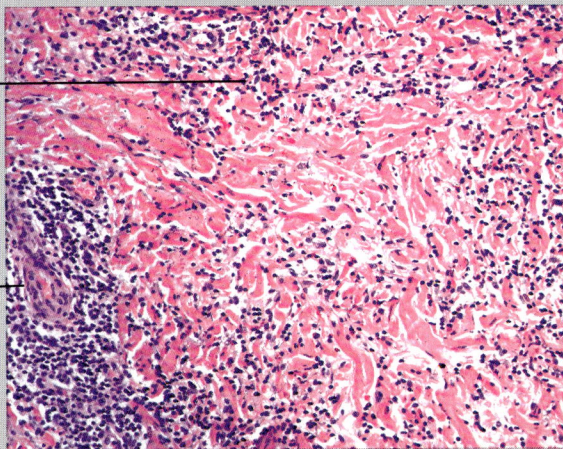

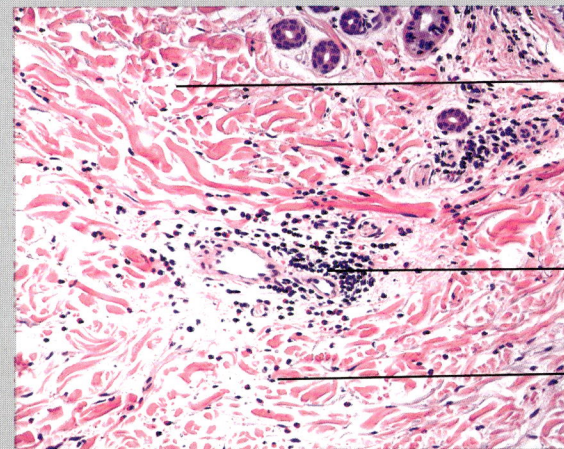

eosinophils
and
lymphocytes
between
collagen
bundles

edema

perivascular
infiltrate of
lymphocytes
mostly

lymphocytes
around
blood
vessels

interstitial
infiltrate of
neutrophils
and
eosinophils

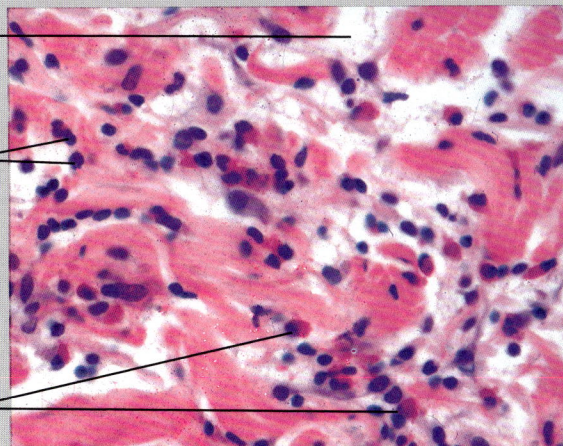

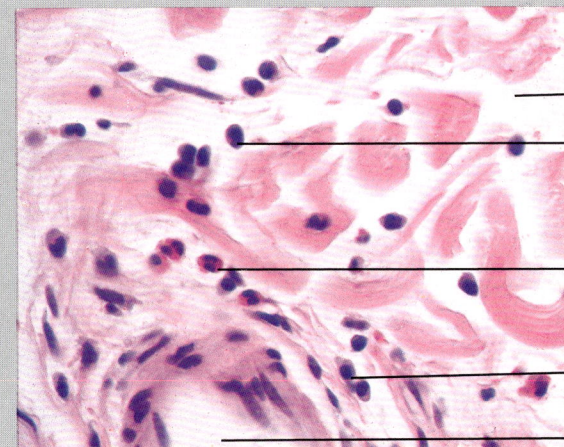

edema

edema

lymphocytes

neutrophil

eosinophil

mast cell

eosinophils

lumen of
venule

IN reactions to arthropod assaults and in lesions of chronic urticaria, the inflammatory-cell infiltrate is mixed, contains eosinophils and extravasated erythrocytes, and is accompanied by edema of the papillary dermis. However, the two conditions may be differentiated histologically by the features just enumerated, especially by the greater depth of the infiltrate in arthropod reactions and the usual preponderance of neutrophils in the infiltrate of chronic urticaria.

Reactions to arthropod assaults vary enormously in their histologic appearance depending upon the particular offending organism, the duration of the lesion at the time of biopsy, and the part of the lesion sampled (e.g., the center, which may be vesicular, or the periphery, which may be edematous). The usual histologic appearance of the entire lesion of a typical reaction to an arthropod assault is a superficial and deep perivascular and interstitial infiltrate of lymphocytes, histiocytes, and eosinophils, edema of the papillary dermis, and a central tense intraepidermal vesicle. However, there are subtle differences among some responses to arthropod assaults. For example, a sand-flea bite is associated with neutrophils rather than eosinophils; a bee sting in which the stinger has been left behind in the dermis may be associated with a foreign body granulomatous reaction; the mouth parts of a tick left in the dermis as the critter is pulled off may induce a pseudolymphomatous reaction replete with lymphoid follicles (germinal centers); and the nodular lesions of scabies are denser and deeper than the usual reactions to superficially housed mites and their products. Other metazoa may cause reactions in skin that are indistinguishable from those of arthropods, e.g., the larvae of creeping eruption, the cercariae of swimmer's itch, the nematocysts of the Portuguese man-of-war, the hairs of the puss caterpillar, and the spines of sea anemones and coral. When the dermal changes common to these various inducing agents are spotted, careful search should be undertaken in the cornified layer for the mite of scabies, in the spinous layer for cercariae, and in and above the basal layer for hookworm larvae.

Reactions to arthropod assaults are usually few and on non-covered parts, whereas the lesions of chronic urticaria are many and widespread. In most instances, no cause can be found for chronic urticaria. Rare causes are allergens, e.g., inhalants such as fumes, ingestants such as foods, injections such as drugs, and occult infections such as gastrointestinal parasites.

Clinically, the individual lesions of chronic urticaria may be morphologically indistinguishable from those of acute urticaria and of urticarial allergic eruptions such as those caused by drugs. All are edematous papules that may have pseudopods. Histologically, the lesions of acute and chronic urticaria seem to be different. The edematous papules of chronic urticaria mostly contain a perivascular and interstitial mixed inflammatory-cell infiltrate, whereas those of acute urticaria consist of but few inflammatory cells and those mostly lymphocytes around blood vessels. The histologic features of urticarial allergic eruptions are indistinguishable from those of chronic urticaria. Drugs are the commonest cause of urticarial allergic reactions.

It is somewhat artificial to designate lesions of urticaria that wax and wane for less than six weeks as "acute" urticaria, and those that continue to come and go for more than six weeks as "chronic" urticaria. For us, wheals that disappear entirely in about 24 to 48 hours, and whose cause the patient nearly always can identify, are those of acute urticaria. A condition of hives that lasts for longer than about 48 hours (but often for months and even years), and whose cause is not identifiable in time by either patient or physician, we consider chronic urticaria. Individual wheals of both acute and chronic forms of urticaria tend to be evanescent, lasting for only a matter of hours.

12. Allergic (Leukocytoclastic) Vasculitis *vs.* Septic Vasculitis

Allergic (Leukocytoclastic) Vasculitis	*Septic Vasculitis*
1. Erosion and ulceration rarely	1. Erosion and ulceration commonly
2. Epidermal damage (inter- and intracellular edema, intraepidermal vesicles and pustules, and necrosis) sometimes	2. Epidermal damage (inter- and intracellular edema, intraepidermal vesicles and pustules, and necrosis) usually
3. Neutrophils within the epidermis occasionally	3. Neutrophils within the epidermis usually
4. Necrosis of epithelial structures of adnexa rarely	4. Necrosis of epithelial adnexal structures frequently
5. Vasculitis involves venules and capillaries of the dermis and only occasionally of the subcutaneous fat	5. Vasculitis involves arterioles as well as venules and capillaries of the dermis and the subcutaneous fat
6. Deep plexus usually but not always involved	6. Deep as well as superficial plexus always involved
7. Thrombi rarely	7. Thrombi commonly
8. Fibrin in and around blood vessel walls commonly	8. Fibrin in blood vessel walls rarely
9. Nuclear debris (i.e., nuclear "dust", leukocytoclasis, fragmented nuclei of neutrophils) abundant	9. Little or no nuclear debris
10. Eosinophils commonly	10. Eosinophils rarely

Allergic (Leukocytoclastic) Vasculitis

Septic Vasculitis

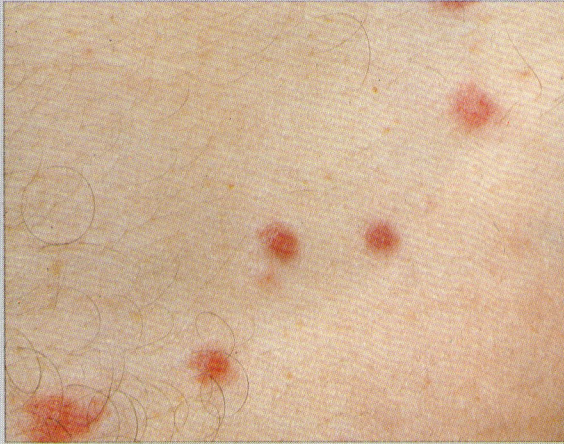

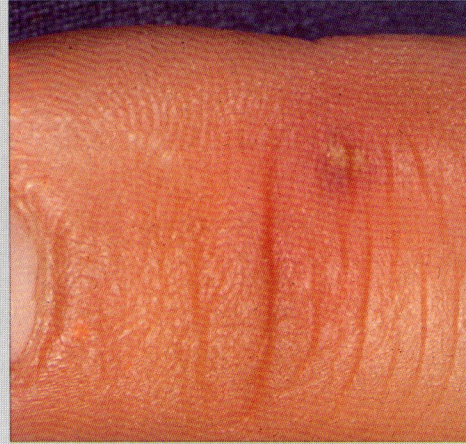

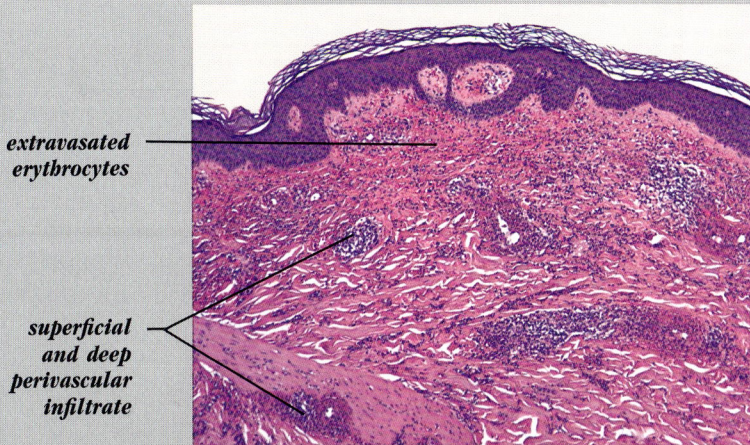

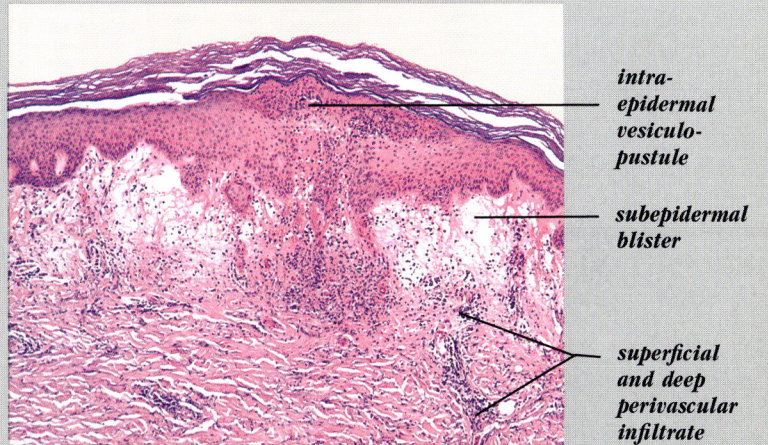

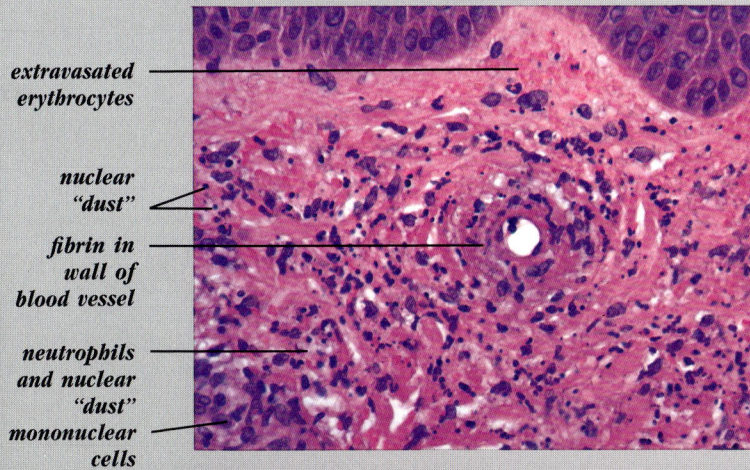

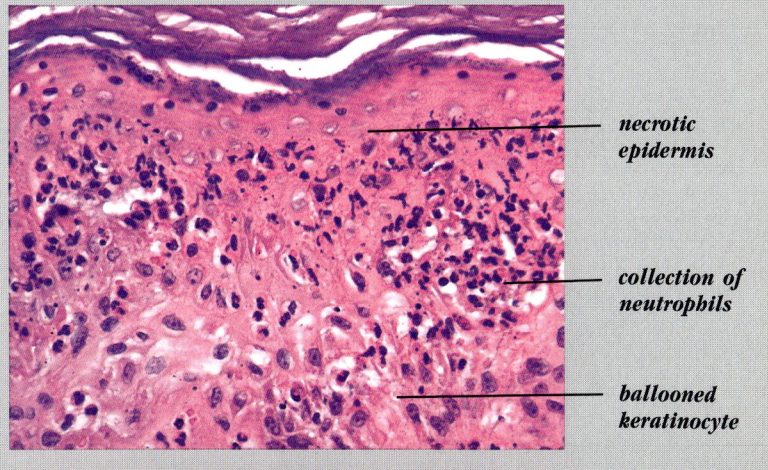

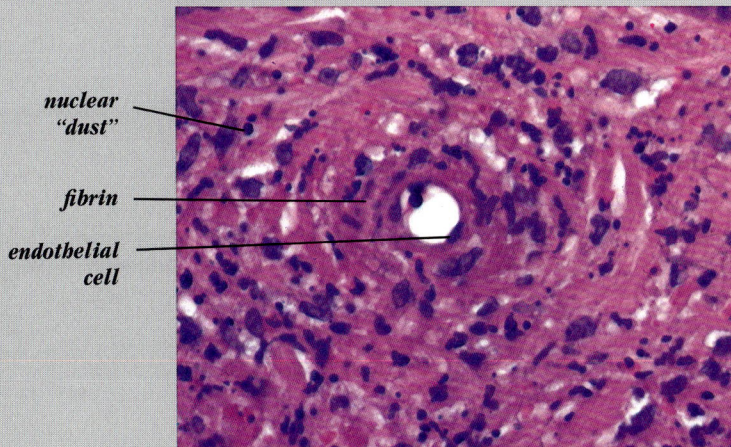

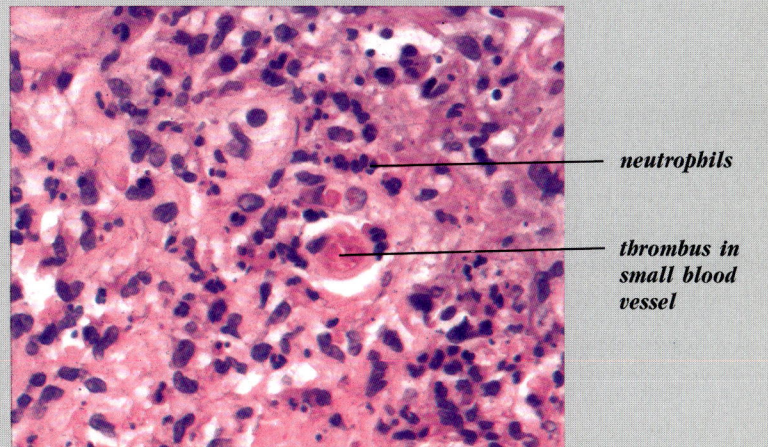

extravasated
erythrocytes

superficial
and deep
perivascular
infiltrate

intra-
epidermal
vesiculo-
pustule

subepidermal
blister

superficial
and deep
perivascular
infiltrate

extravasated
erythrocytes

nuclear
"dust"

fibrin in
wall of
blood vessel

neutrophils
and nuclear
"dust"
mononuclear
cells

necrotic
epidermis

collection of
neutrophils

ballooned
keratinocyte

nuclear
"dust"

fibrin

endothelial
cell

neutrophils

thrombus in
small blood
vessel

ALLERGIC (leukocytoclastic) vasculitis and septic vasculitis have several histologic features in common, namely, neutrophils within and around the walls of small dermal blood vessels, extravasated erythrocytes, and the tendency to necrosis of the epidermis.

Vasculitis is an inflammatory process that occurs partly within the walls of blood vessels and is attended by histologic evidences of damage to the walls of blood vessels in the form of deposits of fibrin, degeneration of collagen, and necrosis of endothelial cells. Thrombi may occlude the lumina of vessels so inflamed, and extravasation of erythrocytes is concurrent. The presence of inflammatory cells within the walls of small blood vessels is not in itself sufficient for a diagnosis of vasculitis, because the cells may simply be traversing the walls of blood vessels in their normal manner en route from the lumina to the surrounding tissue (diapedesis). It is for this reason that strict histologic criteria must guide differentiation of vasculitis from the much more common perivascular infiltrates of inflammatory cells.

Vasculitis may be classified according to the predominant inflammatory cell found (e.g., neutrophils, histiocytes in granulomas) and by the kind of blood vessel involved (e.g., artery, vein, arteriole, venule, capillary). Allergic vasculitis and septic vasculitis are examples of neutrophilic vasculitis that primarily affect the small blood vessels of the dermis. However, distinctive differences mark them. Nuclear "dust" and eosinophils are often abundant in and around the walls of venules and capillaries of allergic vasculitis, but not in septic vasculitis; thrombi develop more commonly in septic than in allergic vasculitis, and arterioles, as well as venules and capillaries, are involved in septic, but not allergic vasculitis. It is the usual finding of abundant nuclear debris that gave rise to the descriptive term "leukocytoclastic" ("clasis" from the Greek word meaning "burst"). There are also immunologic differences between these two vasculitides—deposits of immunoglobulins and complement are found in early lesions of leukocytoclastic vasculitis, but not in septic vasculitis.

Allergic vasculitis occurs in many conditions, e.g., drug reactions, systemic lupus erythematosus, rheumatoid arthritis, the Henoch-Schoenlein syndrome, cryoglobulinemia, Lucio's phenomenon (erythema necroticans), and in association with internal malignancies. A specific cause cannot be inferred from the histologic changes except in leprosy where foamy histiocytes (Virchow cells) are present. Leukocytoclastic vasculitis, irrespective of cause (often no probable cause is attributable), has the same appearance microscopically.

The clinical lesions of leukocytoclastic vasculitis, whatever their cause, are also similar in appearance. They usually begin as edematous papules that quickly progress to purpuric papules ("palpable purpura") and then may evolve into vesicles, bullae, pustules, or ulcers. The legs are sites of predilection, but no part of the skin is exempt from the possibility of such lesions. In some conditions, such as Henoch-Schoenlein syndrome, the skin lesions do not evolve beyond the stage of purpuric papules or nodules to vesicles or bullae. In lesions of granuloma faciale and of erythema elevatum diutinum, allergic vasculitis may persist for months and even years. These conditions are characterized by plaques and nodules rather than by edematous papules, vesicles, or ulcers.

Septic vasculitis may be caused by septicemias from gonococci, meningococci, pseudomonads, staphylococci, and spirochetes of syphilis ("lues maligna"). Skin lesions caused by each of these agents have features in common, namely, purpura (petechial and ecchymotic), vesiculopustules (often with gray roofs due to epidermal necrosis), hemorrhagic bullae, and, occasionally, ulceration. Chronic gonococcemia and chronic meningococcemia characteristically have only a few lesions that are confined to the extremities and acral parts. They are petechiae surrounded by a broad rim of erythema, necrotic vesiculopustules, and rarely, hemorrhagic bullae.

Because the septicemias of chronic gonococcemia and meningococcemia tend to be episodic and transient, many blood cultures are usually necessary to isolate the causative organisms.

The histologic changes of the septic vasculitides described above are seen typically in chronic gonococcemia and meningococcemia. The vasculitis associated with pseudomonad septicemia (echthyma gangrenosum), staphylococcal septicemia, and syphilitic septicemia ("lues maligna") have some features in common with gonococcemia and meningococcemia. However, there are significant differences such as the density of the inflammatory-cell infiltrate (e.g., sparse in pseudomonad septicemia, usually moderately dense in gonococcal septicemia), the number of organisms that can be detected in tissue sections (e.g., many pseudomonads, usually no gonococci), and the amount of tissue destruction (e.g., great in pseudomonad septicemia, slight in gonococcal).

In some instances it may be impossible to distinguish histologically between incipient or very early lesions of septic vasculitis and those of allergic vasculitis, especially in rare cases in which there are thrombi in allergic vasculitis and leukocytoclasis and fibrin in septic vasculitis. Early lesions of allergic vasculitis are usually devoid of fibrin. Such early lesions may show a predominance of intact neutrophils or, occasionally, a predominance of nuclear "dust". When nuclear "dust" predominates in a superficial or superficial and deep perivascular dermatitis, the diagnosis of leukocytoclastic vasculitis may be made with near certainty.

13. Granuloma Annulare
vs. Necrobiosis Lipoidica

Granuloma Annulare	*Necrobiosis Lipoidica*
1. No thinning of epidermis	1. Thinned epidermis with effacement of rete ridges
2. Superficial and deep perivascular predominantly lymphocytic infiltrate	2. Superficial and deep perivascular and subcutaneous infiltrate of plasma cells, lymphocytes, and histiocytes
3. Usually the upper part of the dermis is more involved than the lower part	3. Usually the lower part of the dermis (and the subcutis) is more involved than the upper part
4. Pathological changes focal with areas of intervening normal dermis within a 4 mm punch biopsy specimen	4. Pathological changes diffuse with no areas of intervening normal dermis within a 4 mm punch biopsy specimen
5. Discrete foci of histiocytes, some multinucleated, between collagen bundles and in palisaded array within the dermis (the upper part usually)	5. Scattered infiltrates of histiocytes, some multinucleated, between collagen bundles and in palisaded array within both the dermis (the lower part usually) and the subcutis
6. Histiocytes form a palisade around foci rich in acid mucopolysaccharides which cause separation of collagen bundles; slight degeneration of collagen	6. Histiocytes form a palisade around zones of degenerated collagen; little or no acid mucopolysaccharides in these zones
7. Mast cells increased in the mucinous focci	7. Mast cells not increased in number
8. No plasma cells as a rule; some rarely	8. Plasma cells numerous usually
9. No panniculitis except in the uncommon subcutaneous variant	9. Granulomatous septal panniculitis in early lesions usual
10. Resolves with near restoration of normal structure; no sclerosis	10. Resolves with sclerosis of the dermis and the subcutis

Granuloma Annulare

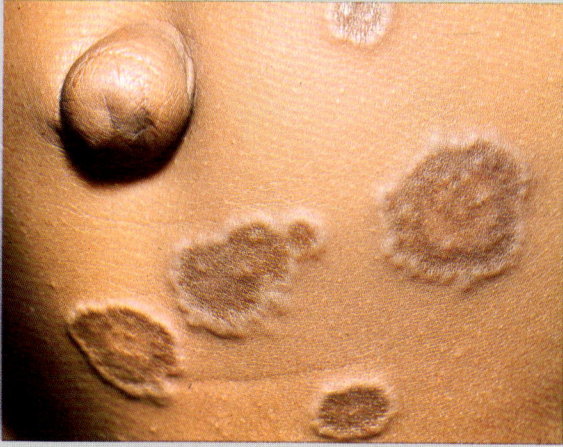

Necrobiosis Lipoidica

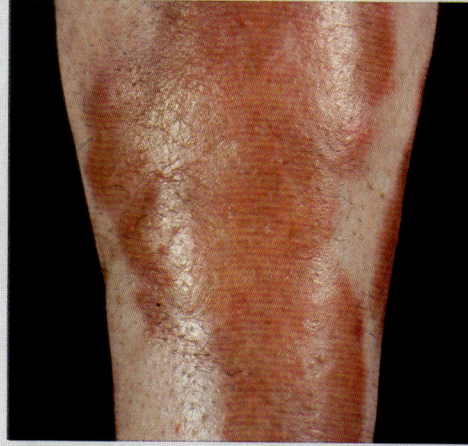

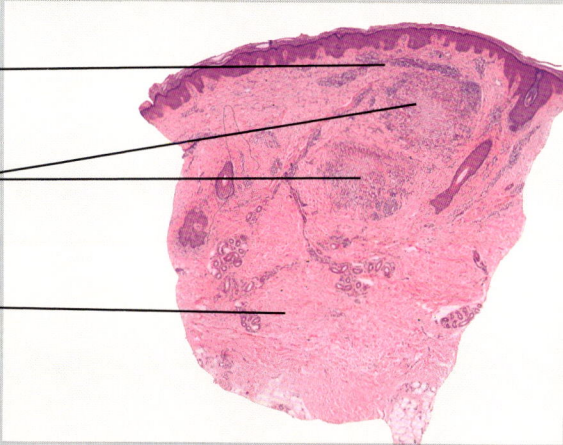

lymphocytes around blood vessels

two discrete foci of palisaded granulomas

normal reticular dermis

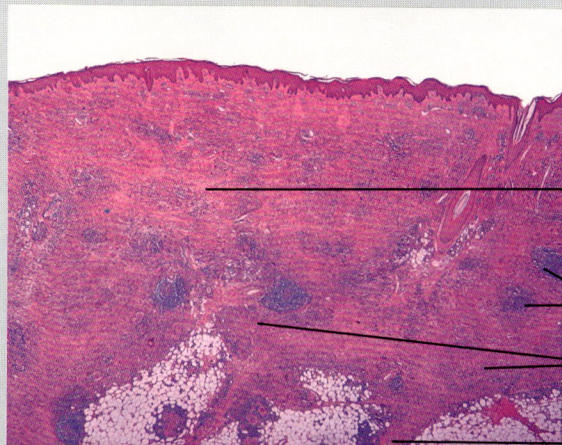

sclerosis in reticular dermis

lymphocytes and plasma cells around vessels

histiocytes in palisaded array

septal panniculitis

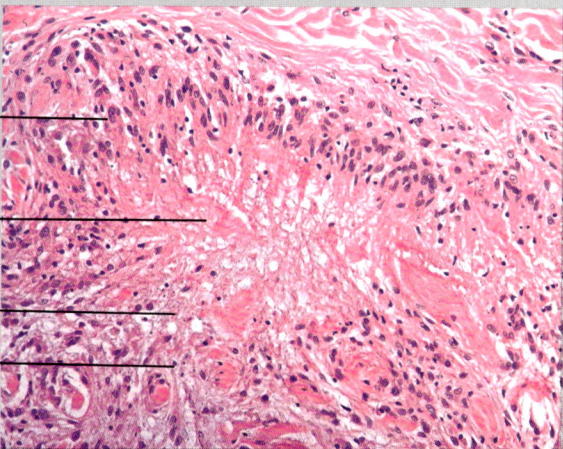

histiocytes in a palisade

degenerated collagen

mucin

nuclear "dust"

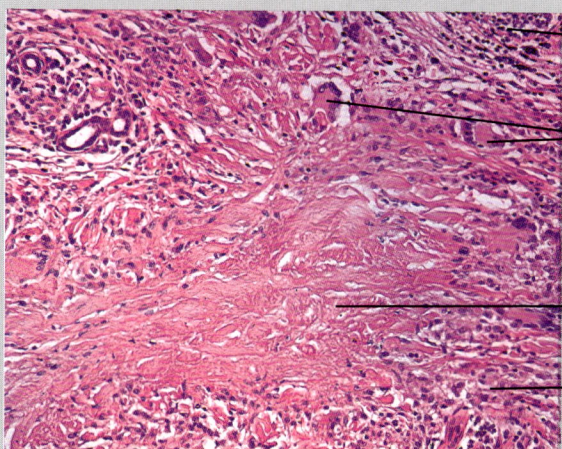

lymphocytes and plasma cells

multi-nucleated histiocytes

degenerated collagen

histiocytes in a palisade

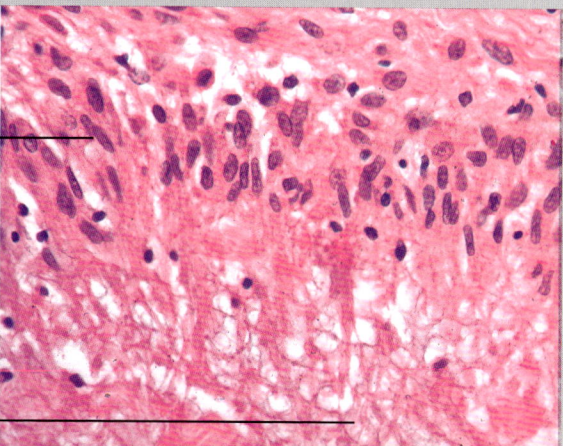

histiocytes in palisaded array

mucin

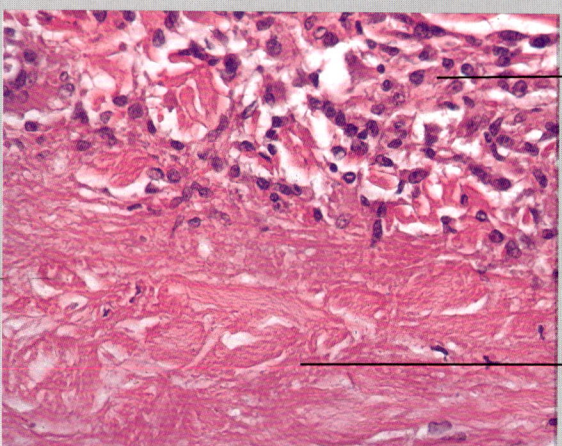

histiocytes in palisaded array

degenerated collagen

G RANULOMA annulare and necrobiosis lipoidica
are both characterized by palisaded granulomatous dermatitis, superficial
and deep perivascular mononuclear-cell infiltrates, and some degeneration
of collagen. Stains for elastic tissue reveal that elastic fibers are decreased or
absent from foci of degenerated collagen in both diseases.

The major histologic differences between granuloma annulare and necrobiosis lipoidica are that in granuloma annulare the granulomatous process is patchy, i.e., in several discrete foci amid otherwise normal dermis,
acid mucopolysaccharides are abundant, and the subcutaneous fat is usually spared. In necrobiosis lipoidica, the pathological process is diffuse, i.e.,
involves the entire dermis with no intervening normal areas, and there is
prominent degeneration of collagen, hardly any deposit of acid mucopolysaccharides and, almost always, involvement of the subcutis. Acid mucopolysaccharides are recognizable in reactions stained by hematoxylin and
eosin as granular and feathery slightly basophilic material.

In rare instances it is difficult, if not impossible, to differentiate granuloma annulare from necrobiosis lipoidica in sections stained by hematoxylin
and eosin. In these exceptional instances in which the biopsy specimen is
usually small and superficial, a stain for acid mucopolysaccharides, such as
the colloidal iron or alcian blue, may enable definitive diagnosis. In granuloma annulare, abundant acid mucopolysaccharides are usually demonstrable, whereas in necrobiosis lipoidica there is practically no increase of them.

In very early lesions of both diseases there is neutrophilic necrotizing
vasculitis with formation of thrombi. In granuloma annulare, a small necrotic blood vessel with fragmentation of inflammatory cell nuclei is generally found within the center of a palisade of histiocytes. In necrobiosis lipoidica, affected dermal vessels are found in the midst of degenerated collagen
in the deep reticular dermis and within the subcutis. The early neutrophilic vasculitis in necrobiosis lipoidica is often followed by a granulomatous vasculitis with eventual obliteration of affected small blood vessels.

There are several clinical presentations of granuloma annulare. The
most common is one or several rings of papules surrounding seemingly
normal or slightly hyperpigmented skin. Rarer are a widespread papular
form of discrete, tiny, smooth-surfaced papules, many of which have an
almost indiscernible central dell; a patch type composed of broad hyperpigmented zones at the periphery of which subtle papules coalesce to form a
gently elevated rim; and a subcutaneous form that occurs mainly in children
on the extremities. The deep lesions of the subcutaneous form are sometimes misinterpreted histologically as pseudo-rheumatoid nodules. Lastly,

there is a perforating type of granuloma annulare in which acid mucopolysaccharides and altered collagen from the papillary dermis are extruded through the epidermis upon the skin surface where they form tiny crusts atop discrete papules.

Necrobiosis lipoidica begins as a patch that becomes elevated as a reddish plaque and then, in years, evolves into an atrophic, yellowish, telangiectatic patch. Trauma, including biopsy, often results in indolent ulcers. The process is commonest in young diabetic women on the anterior aspect of the legs below the knees, but may develop anywhere in the skin. Necrobiosis lipoidica may occur in individuals without overt diabetes, but all patients with necrobiosis lipoidica should be studied and followed clinically to ensure that diabetes is not concurrent or in the offing.

14. Tuberculoid Leprosy

vs. Sarcoidosis

Tuberculoid Leprosy	*Sarcoidosis*
1. Elongated tubercles of epithelioid cells (oblong or sausage-shaped)	1. Rounded tubercles of epithelioid cells (occasionally elongated)
2. The tubercles tend to confluence rather than to be discrete	2. The tubercles tend to be discrete, rarely confluent
3. Granulomatous process predominantly in the lower dermis, rarely in upper dermis alone	3. Granulomatous process predominantly in the upper dermis, rarely in the lower dermis or subcutis
4. Moderately dense lymphocytic infiltration surrounds the tubercles	4. Sparse lymphocytic infiltrate surrounds the tubercles ("naked tubercles") usually
5. Inflammatory-cell infiltrate in and around cutaneous nerves in the deep reticular dermis	5. No inflammatory-cell infiltrate involving nerves usually
6. Cutaneous nerves often destroyed	6. Cutaneous nerves preserved
7. No fibrin within the tubercles	7. Fibrin within the tubercles often
8. Little or no fibrosis	8. Fibrosis in late lesions
9. Acid-fast bacilli demonstrable rarely	9. Never acid-fast bacilli
10. Asteroid bodies in histiocytes rarely	10. Asteroid bodies in histiocytes occasionally, especially multinucleated ones

Tuberculoid Leprosy

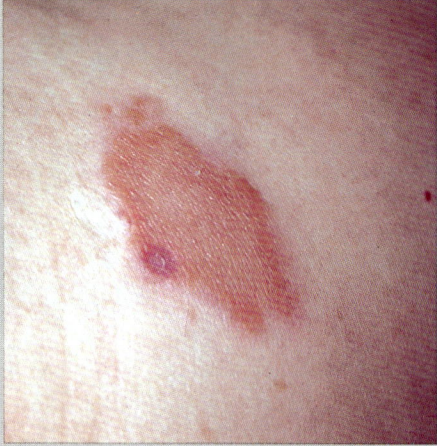

Sarcoidosis

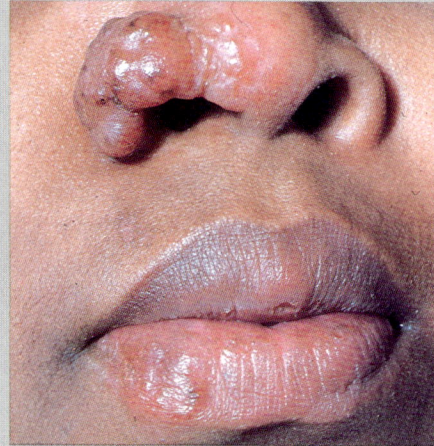

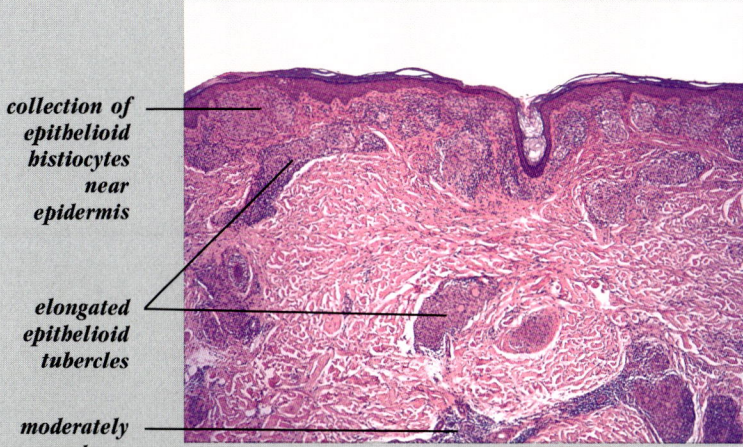

collection of
epithelioid
histiocytes
near
epidermis

elongated
epithelioid
tubercles

moderately
dense
infiltrate of
lymphocytes

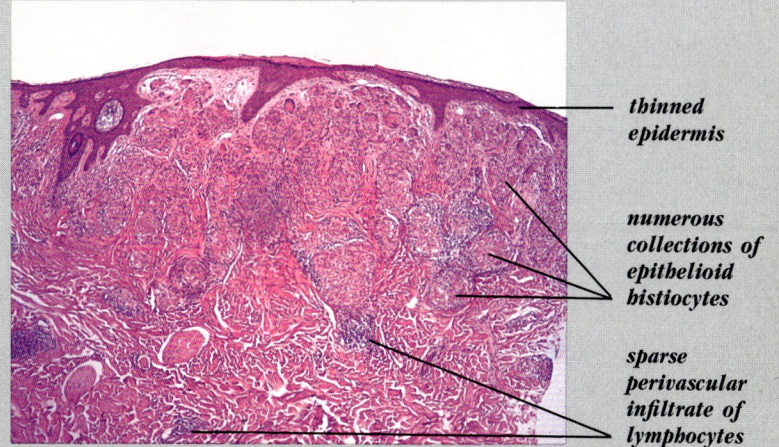

thinned
epidermis

numerous
collections of
epithelioid
histiocytes

sparse
perivascular
infiltrate of
lymphocytes

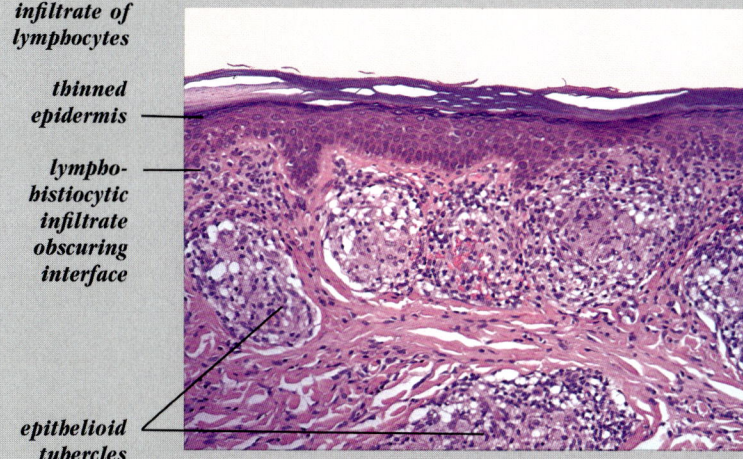

thinned
epidermis

lympho-
histiocytic
infiltrate
obscuring
interface

epithelioid
tubercles

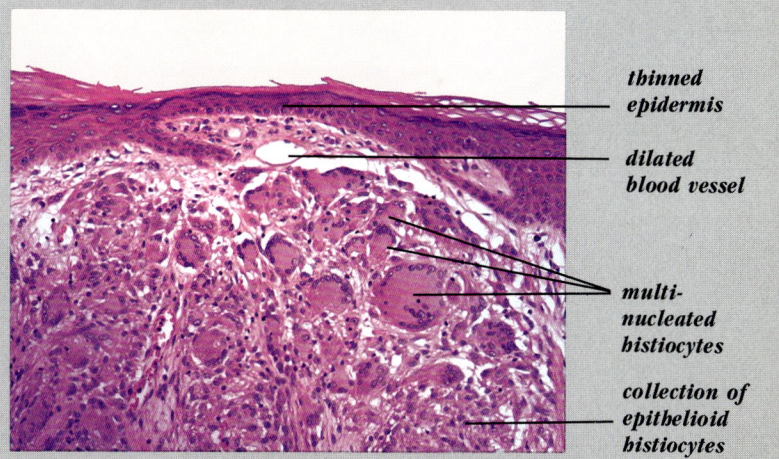

thinned
epidermis

dilated
blood vessel

multi-
nucleated
histiocytes

collection of
epithelioid
histiocytes

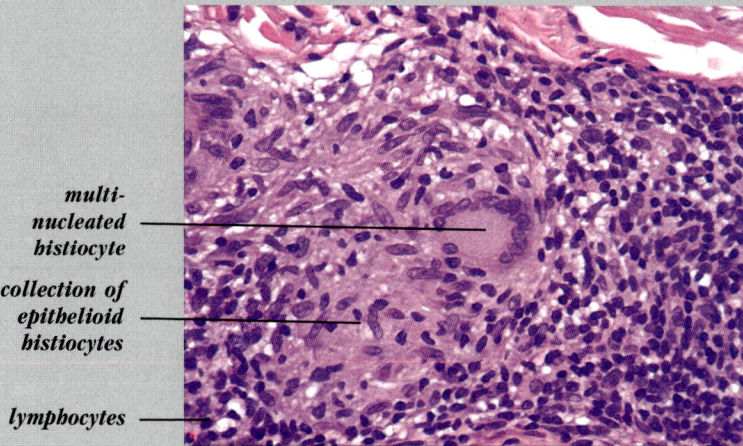

multi-
nucleated
histiocyte

collection of
epithelioid
histiocytes

lymphocytes

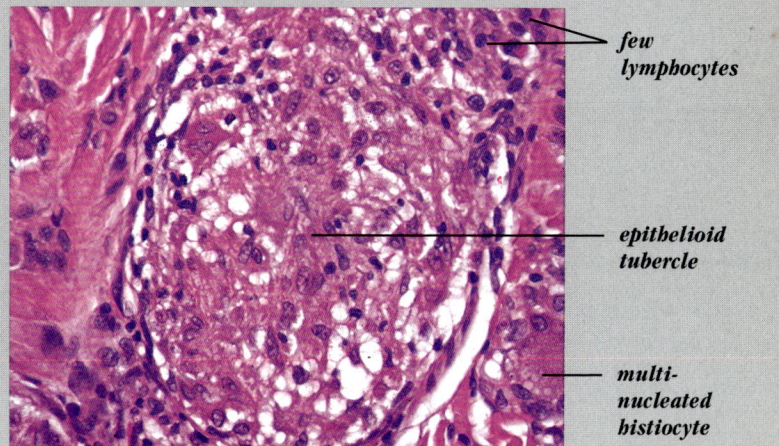

few
lymphocytes

epithelioid
tubercle

multi-
nucleated
histiocyte

T UBERCULOID leprosy and sarcoidosis are gran-
ulomatous dermatitides that resemble one another histologically because
both consist of tubercles of epithelioid cells in the dermis and sometimes the
subcutaneous fat. Despite these similarities, sarcoidosis may usually be differentiated from tuberculoid leprosy if the preceding criteria are sought and
found.

Tuberculoid leprosy is one of the two major expressions of leprosy, a
disease caused by an acid-fast bacillus (Mycobacterium leprae). Clinically,
tuberculoid leprosy is usually characterized by one or several discrete, hypopigmented anesthetic patches. Peripheral nerves may be palpably thickened
in patients with this form of the disease. Patients with tuberculoid leprosy
are capable of expressing delayed hypersensitivity, whereas those with sarcoidosis often are not. Rarely are bacilli demonstrable with the Fite stain.
However, with the assistance of the electron microscope, lepra bacilli may
be detected within histiocytes.

In contrast to tuberculoid leprosy, cutaneous sarcoidosis presents itself
clinically as multiple, firm, orange-brown papules, nodules, and plaques
that favor the face (especially the zones around the eyes, nose, and mouth),
but may be widespread. A rare form of sarcoidosis (Darier-Roussey type)
consists of granulomatous infiltrates in the subcutaneous fat. When lesions
of sarcoidosis manifest themselves in the skin, the likelihood is that other
organs are involved concurrently by this often systemic disease. The cause
for sarcoidosis is not yet known.

Other granulomatous dermatitides that may be indistinguishable histologically from idiopathic sarcoidosis are caused by silica, beryllium, and
zirconium. Silica is easily revealed in tissue sections examined by polarized
light. Microincineration and X-ray diffraction techniques are required to
detect beryllium. Zirconium may be identified by spectrographic analysis.

Papular lesions of rosacea may have granulomatous features that may
be confused with those of idiopathic sarcoidosis, especially because both
diseases have a predilection for the face. However, granulomatous rosacea
consists of poorly circumscribed epithelioid tubercules, marked edema and
telangiectases in the upper part of the dermis, and a perivascular and perifollicular mixed inflammatory-cell infiltrate. A suppurative folliculitis may
be present in addition to the granulomas in rosacea.

The histologic differential diagnosis of tuberculoid leprosy includes
lupus vulgaris and the relapsing form of leishmaniasis. Lupus vulgaris involves predominantly the upper portion of the dermis by well-circumscribed
epithelioid tubercles within which there may be necrosis. The inflamma-

tory-cell infiltrates do not involve small dermal nerves. The recidivans form of leishmaniasis more closely resembles lupus vulgaris than it does tuberculoid leprosy.

Sometimes, lesions of sarcoidosis may be accompanied by dense lymphocytic infiltrates in addition to epithelioid tubercles. In such instances, it may not be possible to differentiate sarcoidosis from tuberculoid leprosy, lupus vulgaris, and the recidivans form of leishmaniasis. Rarely, lesions of sarcoidosis may contain numerous plasma cells in addition to epithelioid tubercles, and such lesions must be differentiated from those of late secondary and tertiary syphilis.

15. Keloid *vs.*

Hypertrophic Scar

Keloid	*Hypertrophic Scar*
1. Lesions usually markedly elevated above the skin surface; little tendency to spontaneous regression	1. Lesions slightly elevated above the skin surface; later, flush or depressed as atrophic scars
2. No tendency to subepidermal clefting or vesiculation	2. Subepidermal clefting or vesiculation occasionally
3. Collagen in markedly thickened, homogenous bundles with small amounts of fibrillar form	3. Collagen in fibrillar form only and no markedly thickened bundles
4. Collagen brightly eosinophilic	4. Collagen slightly eosinophilic or amphophilic
5. Collagen bundles in haphazard array	5. Collagen fibers generally oriented parallel to the skin surface
6. Fibroblasts in haphazard pattern alongside thickened collagen bundles	6. Fibroblasts, like the collagen fibers, arranged parallel to the skin surface
7. Telangiectatic blood vessels oriented randomly	7. Telangiectatic blood vessels oriented perpendicular to the skin surface generally
8. Abundant mucin between collagen bundles often	8. Little mucin between collagen fibers except in early lesions when it may be abundant
9. Inflammatory-cell infiltrates especially around dilated blood vessels at peripheries of lesions	9. Inflammatory-cell infiltrates around dilated blood vessels throughout lesions

Keloid

Hypertrophic Scar

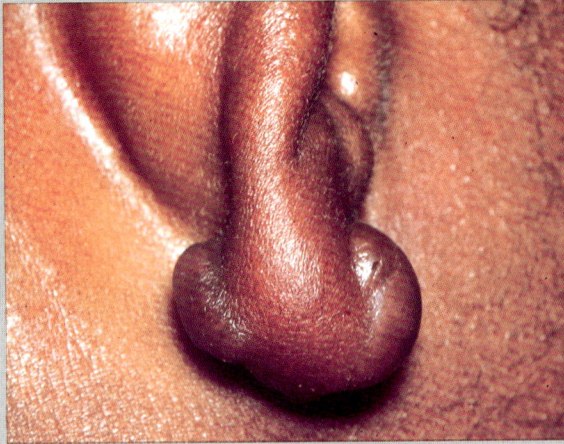

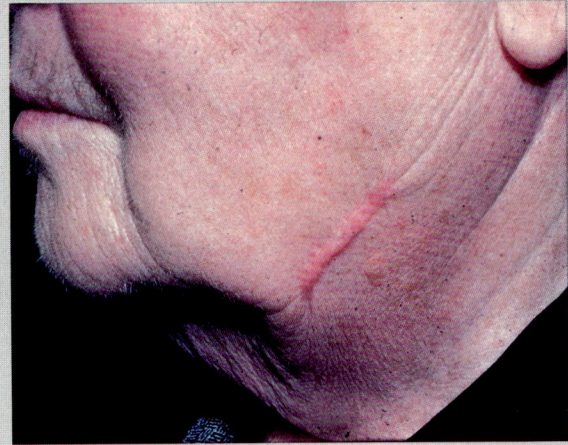

broad zone
of fibrosis

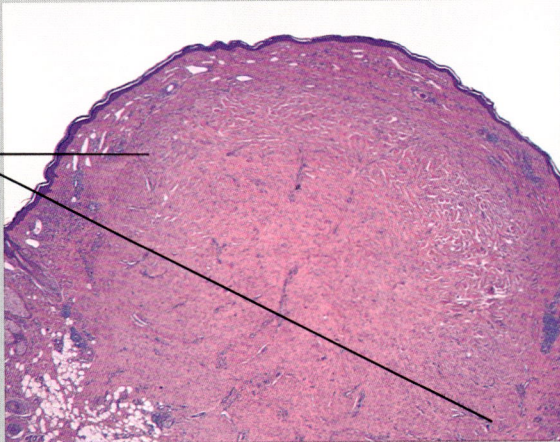

narrow zone
of fibrosis

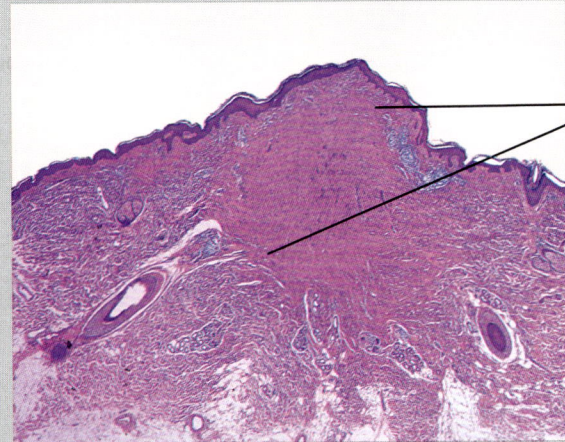

thinned
epidermis

thinned
epidermis

telangi-
ectases

fibrosis

lymphocytes
around
blood
vessels

lymphocytes
around blood
vessel

thickened
collagen
bundles in
haphazard
array

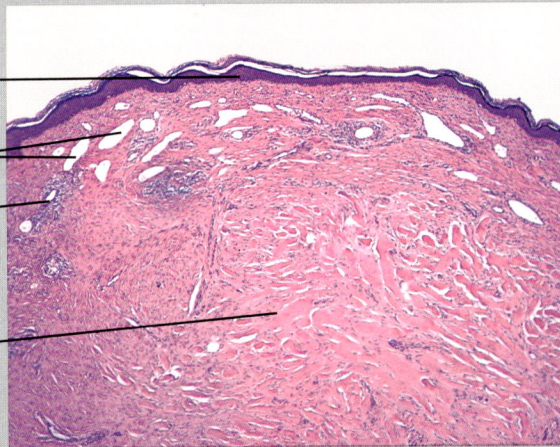

blood vessel
perpendicular
to skin
surface

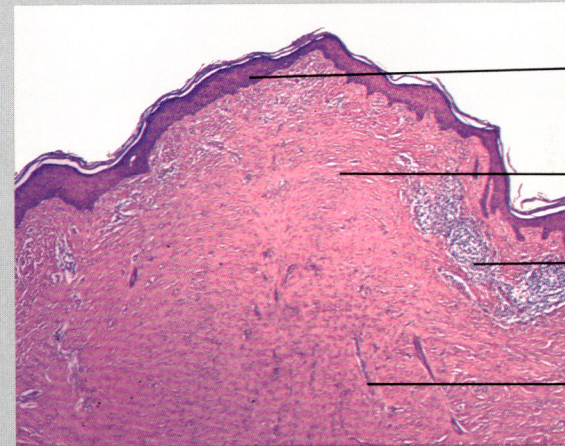

thickened
collagen
bundle
oriented
horizontally

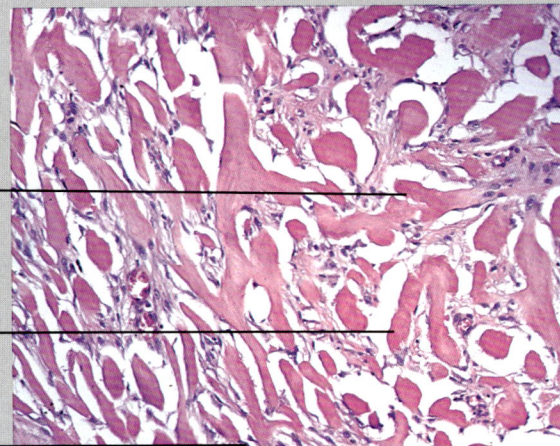

fibroblasts
parallel to
skin surface

blood vessels
perpendicular
to skin
surface

thickened
collagen
bundle
oriented
vertically

fibroblasts
parallel to
collagen
bundles

fibrillary
collagen
parallel to
skin surface

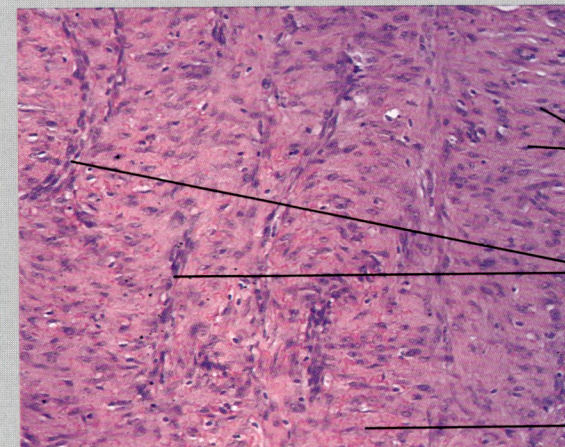

K ELOIDS and hypertrophic scars have many histologic features in common (e.g., fibroplasia, telangiectasis, inflammatory-cell infiltrates, mucin) and, in some instances, histologic features of keloids and hypertrophic scars may be found in the same specimen. When distinct keloidal features are present, the diagnosis, by convention, becomes keloid. On the other hand, when there are no broad bands of collagen and clinically there is strong tendency to spontaneous resolution, hypertrophic scar is the usual diagnosis made.

Keloids present themselves clinically as firm, bulbous nodules or markedly elevated plaques at sites of antecedent injury such as pierced earlobes, vaccinations, formal operations and accidental wounds, ruptured cysts of acne, and so on. They occur more frequently in people who are heavily pigmented, especially blacks.

Hypertrophic scars are usually linear lesions that follow traumas such as surgical incisions and accidental lacerations. These scars have no predilection for individuals of any particular pigmentation.

Both keloids and hypertrophic scars are types of fibrosing dermatitis, i.e., inflammatory reactions that resolve by unusual degrees of fibroplasia. The entire spectrum of inflammation from granulation tissue to sclerosis may be found in keloids and hypertrophic scars, depending upon when in their course the biopsy is obtained.

In early lesions of keloids, only abundant fibrillary collagen is present and no thickened, hyalinized collagen bundles in haphazard array. A clue to the diagnosis of keloids even at this early stage is the presence of this fibrillary collagen, like that of a scar in a lesion with a nodular configuration. In time, within such lesions, foci of markedly thickened, brightly eosinophilic-staining collagen bundles arranged randomly appear within the mass of fibrillary collagen. These thickened bundles of collagen in that particular setting are proof positive of a keloid. The recognition that histologically a lesion is a keloid has important implications for the patient in terms of the prevention of future keloids and the treatment of existing ones.

Thickened collagen bundles like those found in keloids also are seen episodically in otherwise typical lesions of dermatofibromas (dermatofibromas with keloidal features) and basal cell carcinomas (basal cell carcinomas with keloidal features). The factors that induce fibroblasts to manufacture the following types of collagen are not understood: thick collagen bundles in haphazard array, as in a keloid; fibrillary collagen, as in a scar; short, coarse collagen bundles in haphazard array, as in a dermatofibroma; thickened collagen bundles compactly arranged in parallel, as in scleroderma; lamellar collagen immediately beneath the epidermis in the papillary dermis, as in melanocytic hyperplasias of simple lentigo, junctional nevus, and malignant melanoma in situ; sclerotic collagen of homogeneous appearance, as in lichen sclerosus et atrophicus; and concentric lamellae of collagen around hair follicles, as in fibrous papules of the face and in lesions of adenoma sebaceum.

The cause is known, however, for the production by fibroblasts of coarse collagen fibers arranged in vertical streaks in a thickened papillary dermis. These coarse fibers in lichen simplex chronicus, prurigo nodularis, and picker's nodule are known to result from prolonged, persistent rubbing of the skin. The mechanisms whereby these characteristic changes occur have yet to be learned.

16. Lichen Sclerosus et Atrophicus *vs.* Scleroderma

Lichen Sclerosus et Atrophicus	Scleroderma
1. Marked laminated or compact orthokeratosis of the stratum corneum	1. Normal stratum corneum
2. Infundibula and acrosyringia plugged by orthokeratotic cells often	2. Adnexal ostia not plugged as a rule; may be plugged sometimes
3. Thinned epidermis with loss of the normal pattern between epidermal rete ridges and dermal papillae	3. Preservation of normal epidermis and pattern between epidermis and dermis
4. Epidermal melanin decreased uniformly	4. Epidermal melanin decreased and increased focally in some lesions
5. Vacuolar alteration at the dermo-epidermal junction	5. Little or no vacuolar alteration
6. Papillary dermis markedly thickened and homogenized	6. Papillary dermis relatively unaffected in most, but not all, lesions
7. Reticular dermis relatively unaffected	7. Reticular dermis thickened by bundles of sclerotic collagen arranged compactly and parallel to the skin surface
8. Moderately dense perivascular, predominantly lympho-histiocytic infiltrate with occasional plasma cells beneath thickened papillary dermis	8. Moderately dense superficial and deep perivascular and sometimes interstitial infiltrate of lymphocytes, histiocytes, plasma cells, and rarely eosinophils
9. Epithelial structures of adnexa mostly preserved	9. Epithelial structures of adnexa mostly destroyed
10. No involvement of the subcutaneous fat	10. Septal panniculitis and subsequent thickening and sclerosis of septa
11. No fasciitis	11. Fasciitis occasionally; process may extend into skeletal muscle and even into bone

Lichen Sclerosus et Atrophicus

Scleroderma

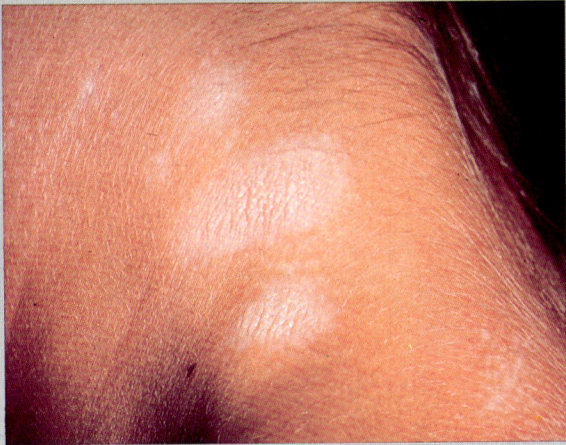
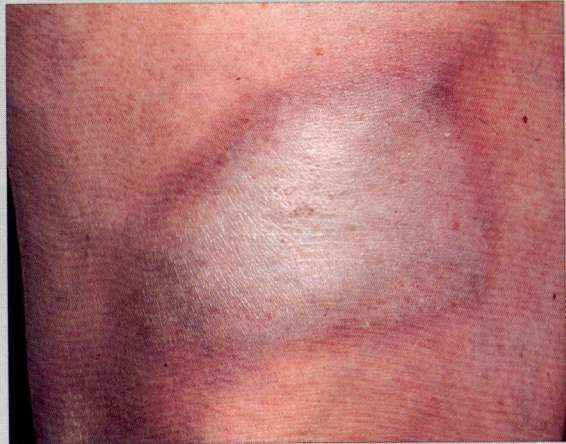

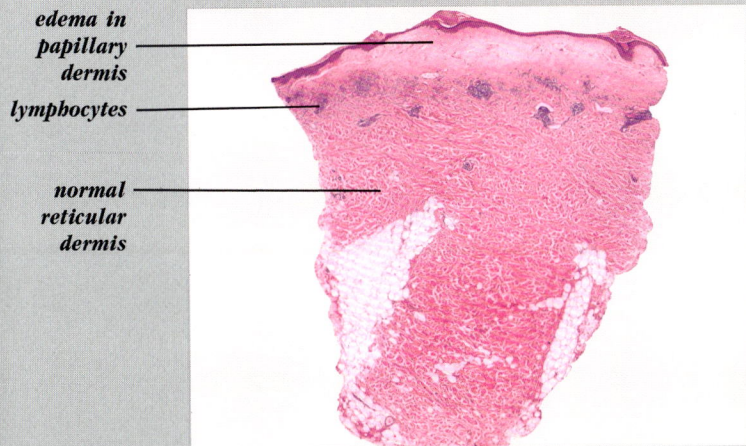

edema in papillary dermis

lymphocytes

normal reticular dermis

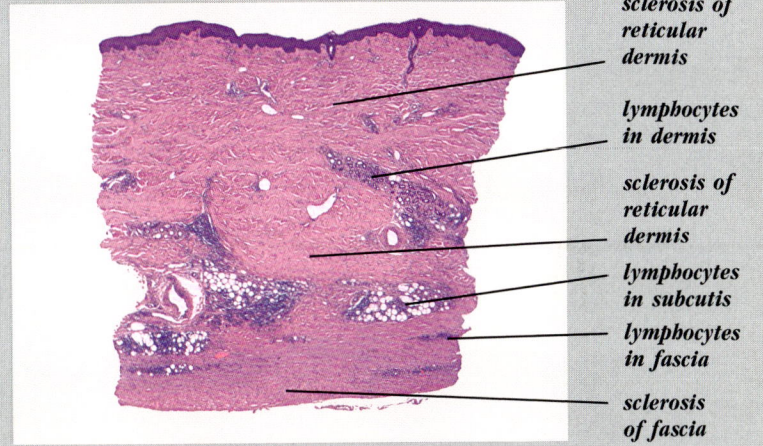

sclerosis of reticular dermis

lymphocytes in dermis

sclerosis of reticular dermis

lymphocytes in subcutis

lymphocytes in fascia

sclerosis of fascia

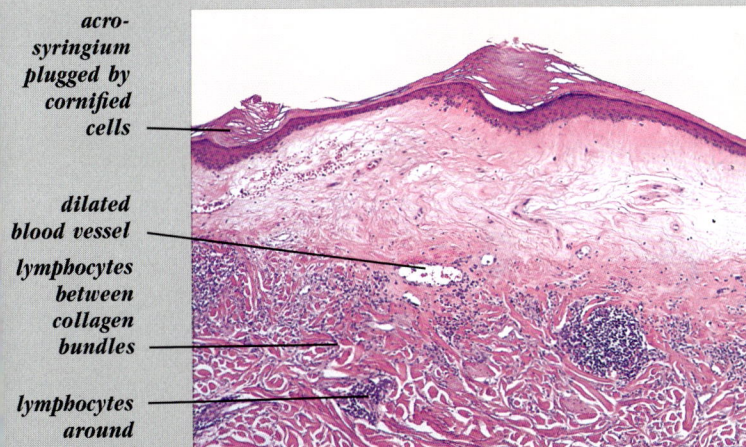

acro-syringium plugged by cornified cells

dilated blood vessel

lymphocytes between collagen bundles

lymphocytes around blood vessel

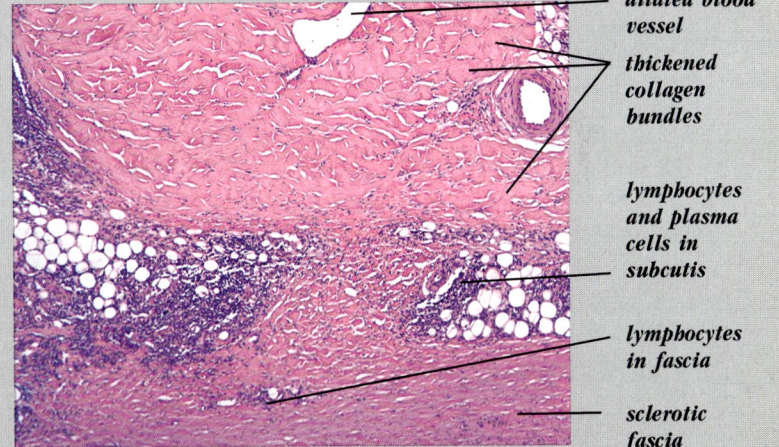

dilated blood vessel

thickened collagen bundles

lymphocytes and plasma cells in subcutis

lymphocytes in fascia

sclerotic fascia

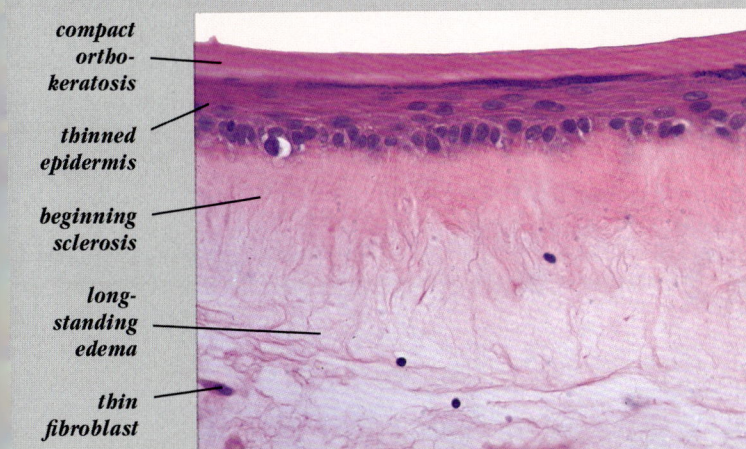

compact ortho-keratosis

thinned epidermis

beginning sclerosis

long-standing edema

thin fibroblast

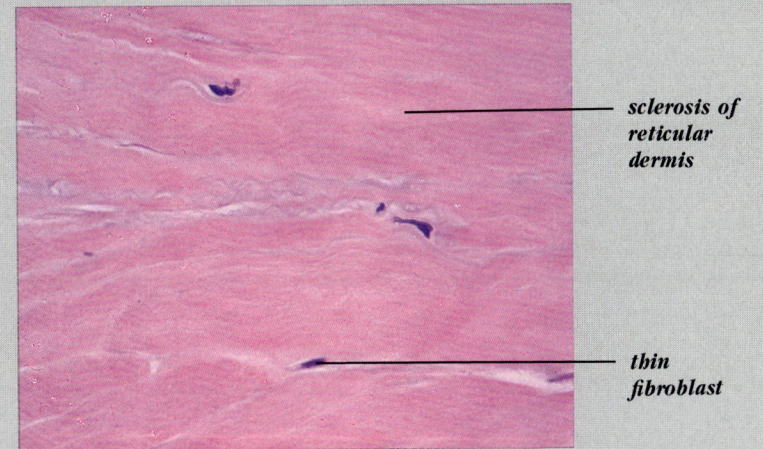

sclerosis of reticular dermis

thin fibroblast

ICHEN sclerosus et atrophicus and scleroderma are inflammatory processes that resolve with sclerosis. In lichen sclerosus et atrophicus the inflammatory changes are confined to the upper portion of the dermis, whereas in scleroderma the entire dermis, especially the lower half, the subcutis, and the fascia are involved.

The early histologic changes of lichen sclerosus et atrophicus include:

1. Prominent thickening of the papillary dermis by edema
2. Dense perivascular, often band-like, predominantly lymphocytic infiltrate beneath an edematous papillary dermis
3. Widely dilated blood vessels in the papillary dermis
4. Marked vacuolar alteration at the dermo-epidermal junction
5. Increased number of plump and stellate fibroblasts in the papillary dermis
6. Melanophages in the papillary dermis

The late histologic changes in lichen sclerosus et atrophicus are:

1. Prominent thickening of the papillary dermis by sclerosis
2. Few, thin fibroblasts
3. Telangiectases
4. Slight perivascular inflammatory-cell infiltrates beneath the sclerotic dermis
5. Vacuolar alteration at the dermo-epidermal junction, occasionally cleft formation, and rarely subepidermal blisters that may be hemorrhagic.

The early histologic changes of scleroderma are:

1. Moderately dense, perivascular and interstitial mixed inflammatory-cell infiltrates around the blood vessels of the superficial and deep plexuses, in the septa of the subcutaneous fat, especially at the junction of the septa and the lobules, and, sometimes, in the fascia
2. Slight homogenization of collagen bundles in the reticular dermis, septa of the subcutaneous fat, and fascia
3. Epithelial structures of adnexa preserved

The late histologic changes of scleroderma show:

1. Sclerosis of the entire dermis, especially the lower half, the subcutis, and the fascia; collagen bundles thickened and spaces between them narrowed

2. Slight or no perivascular inflammatory-cell infiltrate
3. Epithelial structures of adnexa mostly absent
4. Melanophages in the papillary dermis often

On occasion, histologic changes that resemble those of lichen sclerosus et atrophicus may be seen in lesions of morphea. Some have suggested that these represent examples of two diseases occurring together in the same specimen and others have suggested that lichen sclerosus et atrophicus and morphea are parts of a spectrum of one disease. At the moment, we interpret the histologic changes that resemble lichen sclerosus et atrophicus in otherwise typical lesions of morphea to be manifestations of scleroderma and not truly lichen sclerosus. Some early lesions of typical morphea are characterized histologically by extensive edema (even bullae) in the papillary dermis. That edema resolves slowly in months and is replaced by sclerotic collagen resembling the papillary dermis of lichen sclerosus et atrophicus.

Clinically, lichen sclerosus et atrophicus presents itself as whitish papules, plaques, and atrophic patches marked often by dilated follicular ostia filled with keratotic plugs. The typical patient is a middle-aged or older woman who complains of severe itching in the vulvar, perineal, and/or perianal areas. When the lesions have been persistently rubbed, the clinical and histologic features of lichen simplex chronicus may be found superimposed upon those of the underlying vulvar lichen sclerosus et atrophicus. Lichen sclerosus et atrophicus may involve the glans penis, where it has been termed balanitis xerotica obliterans and may also develop in children, where it is said to disappear spontaneously and completely on occasion.

The whiteness of the lesions of lichen sclerosus et atrophicus is caused by a combination of hyperkeratosis, loss of melanin from the epidermis, and sclerosis of the papillary dermis. The atrophy results from obliteration of the normal relationship between the dermal papillae and the epidermal rete ridges caused by sclerosis.

Clinically, the skin changes of scleroderma (i.e., guttate, morphea, linear, facial hemi-atrophy, diffuse fasciitis with eosinophilia), acrosclerosis, and diffuse sclerosis have features in common. All of these forms of scleroderma are characterized by cutaneous hardness caused by sclerosis in the dermis, the subcutis, and the fascia, and by pigmentary alterations that result from loss of epidermal melanin into dermal macrophages. The "salt and pepper" effect of intermingled spotty hypo- and hyperpigmentation results from contiguous foci of increased and decreased epidermal melanin. When subcutaneous fat and fascia are substantially replaced by sclerotic collagen, the skin in scleroderma has a "hide-bound" quality. Fasciitis with eosinophilia seems to be a peculiar deep form of scleroderma. The other forms of scleroderma may also show numerous eosinophils in the panniculus and the fascia.

17. Erythema Nodosum
vs. Nodular Vasculitis

Erythema Nodosum	*Nodular Vasculitis*
1. Never ulceration	1. Often ulceration
2. Sparse lympho-histiocytic infiltrates around dermal blood vessels	2. Dense, mixed inflammatory-cell infiltrates throughout the dermis
3. Involvement of septa in the subcutis principally	3. Involvement of fat lobules in the subcutis principally
4. Granulation tissue between septa and lobules of fat	4. Granulation tissue random within the lobules of fat
5. Granulomas in thickened fibrotic septa	5. Granulomas around foci of necrosis and suppuration in lobules
6. No vasculitis	6. Vasculitis of large vessel in subcutaneous fat
7. No significant necrosis of fat	7. Marked necrosis of fat
8. No suppuration	8. Suppuration
9. Few foam cells	9. Many foam cells
10. Eosinophils often	10. Eosinophils seldom

Erythema Nodosum

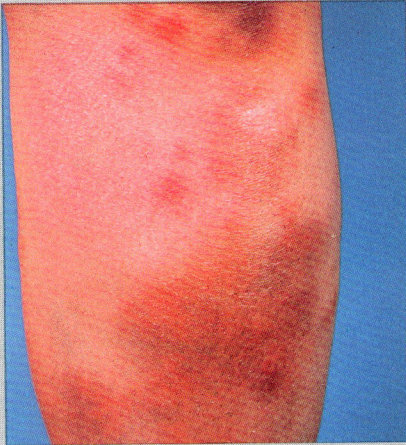

Nodular Vasculitis

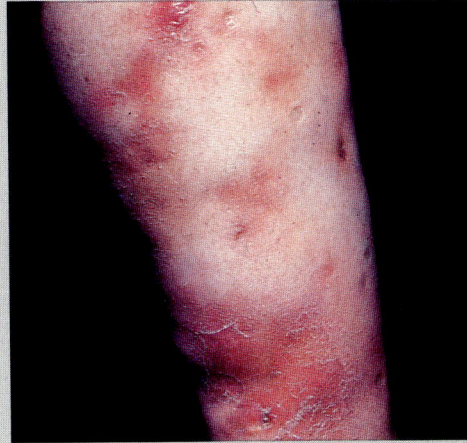

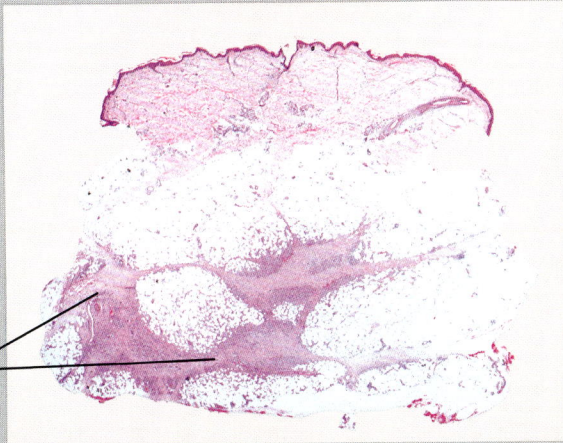

large-vessel
vasculitis

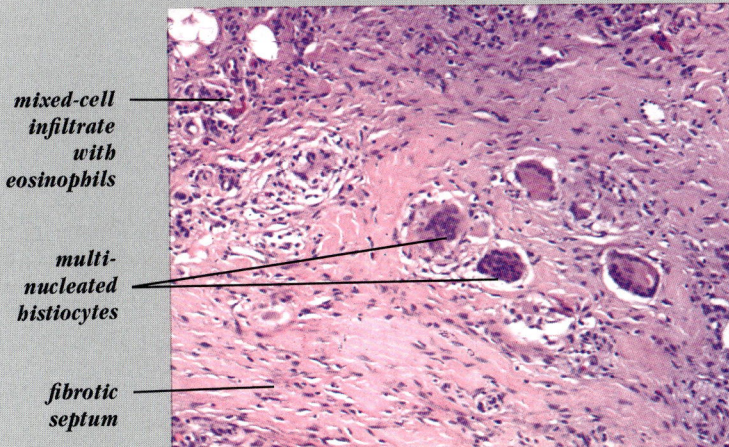

lobular
pannic-
ulitis

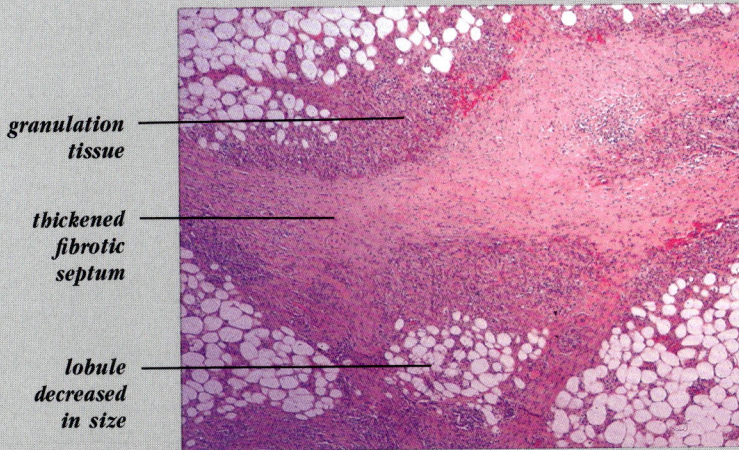

septal
pannic-
ulitis

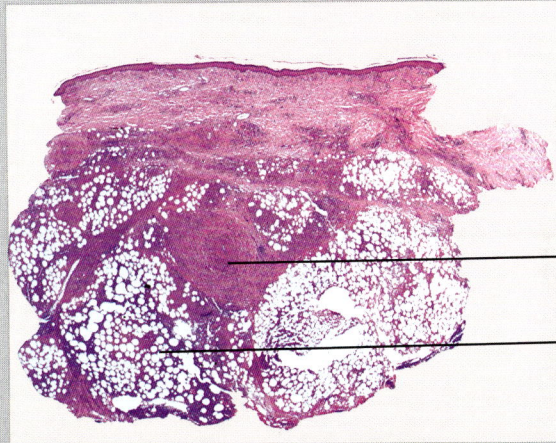

fat necrosis

mixed-cell
infiltrate
with
neutrophils

large-vessel
vasculitis

granulation
tissue

thickened
fibrotic
septum

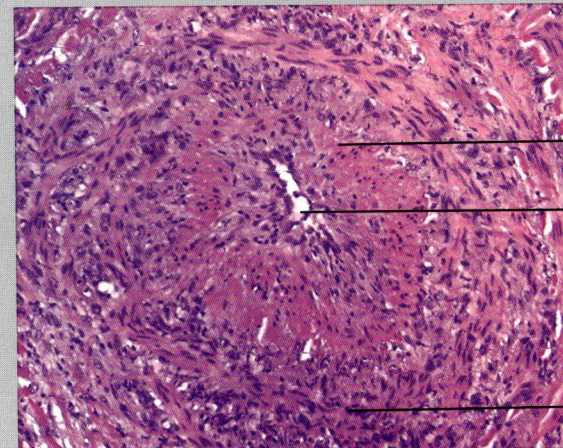

lobule
decreased
in size

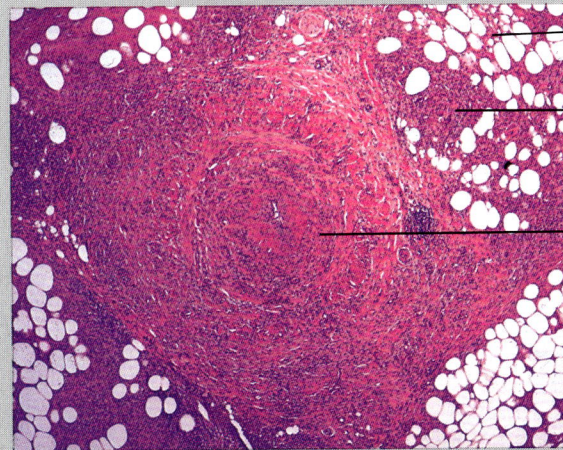

mixed-cell
infiltrate
with
eosinophils

multi-
nucleated
histiocytes

fibrotic
septum

thickened
intima

narrowed
lumen of
blood vessel

inflammatory
cells in
media

ERYTHEMA nodosum and nodular vasculitis are stereotypes of septal and lobular panniculitis respectively. When fully developed, erythema nodosum is a granulomatous septal panniculitis and nodular vasculitis a necrotizing, suppurative, granulomatous lobular panniculitis secondary to severe large blood vessel vasculitis. Because the damaged muscular blood vessel courses within a septum in the subcutis, nodular vasculitis involves some septa as well as some fat lobules, but the most extensive histologic changes, as viewed with the scanning objective of the microscope, are seen to be in the lobules. In erythema nodosum, when the inflammatory cells in the septa spill over into the peripheries of fat lobules, they induce granulation tissue and eventually fibrosis in the zones between septa and lobules. Thus, although erythema nodosum is fundamentally a septal process, as observed with the scanning objective, the peripheries of fat lobules may also be involved in the pathological process.

Erythema nodosum and nodular vasculitis, like most panniculitides, are not of short duration, but tend to last for weeks and even months. Individual lesions of nodular vasculitis may be especially longstanding. Depending upon when biopsies are taken, different histologic features will be found in the undisturbed progression of lesions.

Clinically, erythema nodosum and its more chronic variant, the subacute nodular migratory panniculitis (Vilanova and Pinol), begin as bright, red, shiny, warm, exquisitely tender patches or plaques that usually are distributed symmetrically on the extensor surfaces of the lower extremities of young women. Histologically, such early lesions show:

1. Edema in the fibrous septa of the subcutaneous fat
2. Neutrophils and occasional lymphocytes, histiocytes, and eosinophils within the septa and at the border of the fat lobules
3. Few necrotic fat cells

Later lesions of erythema nodosum are violet to brown, nontender nodules. Biopsy specimens of such lesions reveal:

1. Granulomas within fat septa that contain numerous multinucleated histiocytic giant cells
2. Fibrosis replacing granulation tissue in the zones between septa and lobules
3. Variable numbers of foam cells within lobules

Clinically, early lesions of nodular vasculitis are dull red, faintly tender, slightly elevated nodules that are distributed asymmetrically on the calves of thick-legged young and middle-aged women. Histologically, such lesions show:

1. Mixed-cellular infiltrates in a large muscular blood vessel running in a septum
2. Coagulation necrosis of fat and suppuration in lobules.

Later lesions of nodular vasculitis are characterized clinically by dusky nodules that ulcerate and heal with hyperpigmented and scaly scars. The histologic findings in such lesions are:

1. Ulceration
2. Focal necrosis, suppuration, granulation tissue, and granulomatous inflammation within lobules
3. Extensive fibrosis replacing the normal architecture of the subcutis

Because of the severe fat necrosis and granulomatous inflammation, nodular vasculitis was thought, in former times, to be a manifestation of tuberculosis and was named erythema induratum. Nowadays, tuberculous cause is rare (if it ever applied) and therefore we use the term nodular vasculitis as a general designation of the condition in point no matter what its cause.

The histologic distinctions between erythema nodosum and nodular vasculitis are readily apparent when a deep generous biopsy specimen delivered by scalpel is presented to the pathologist.

18. Alopecia of Discoid Lupus Erythematosus *vs.* Alopecia of Lichen Planus

Alopecia of Discoid Lupus Erythematosus

1. Epidermal atrophy usually

2. Vacuolar alteration at the junctions between epidermis and dermis and between follicular epithelium and dermis

3. Thickened basement membrane beneath epidermal and infundibular epithelium

4. Abundant acid mucopolysaccharides in upper half of dermis

5. Moderately dense predominantly lymphocytic infiltrates (with histiocytes and sometimes plasma cells) around the blood vessels of the superficial and deep plexuses

6. Patchy predominantly lymphocytic infiltrates along the length of the hair follicle

7. Fibrotic tracts at sites of extinct hair follicles as well as sclerosis in upper part of dermis

Alopecia of Lichen Planus (Lichen Planopilaris)

1. Normal epidermis usually; typical focal changes of lichen planus occasionally

2. Vacuolar alteration mostly at the junction of the follicular epithelium and the dermis

3. No thickened basement membrane

4. No increase of acid mucopolysaccharides in dermis

5. Moderately dense predominantly lymphocytic infiltrates (with histiocytes but no plasma cells) around the blood vessels of the superficial plexus

6. Band-like predominantly lymphocytic infiltrates along length of the hair follicle

7. Fibrotic tracts at sites of extinct hair follicles, but no significant dermal sclerosis

Alopecia of Discoid Lupus Erythematosus

Alopecia of Lichen Planus (Lichen Planopilaris)

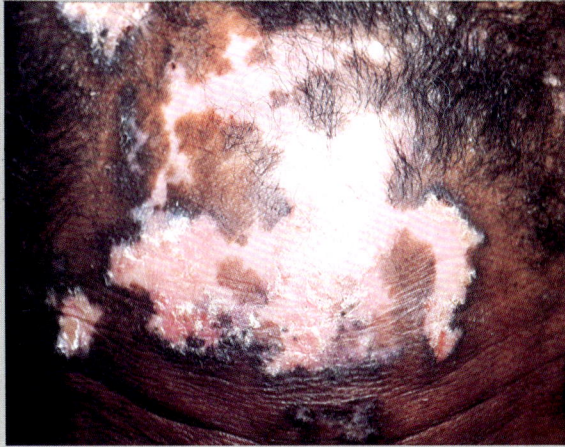

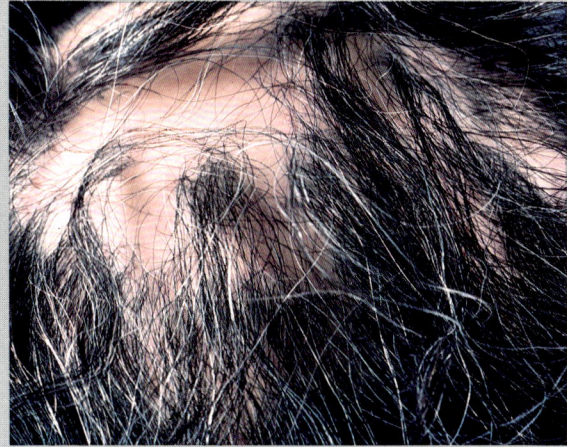

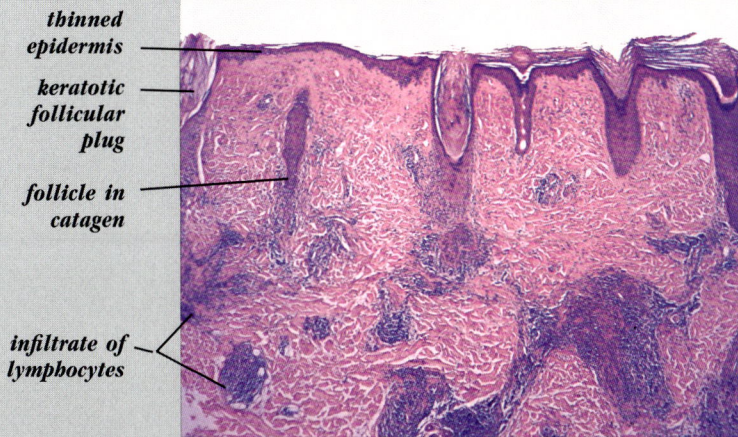

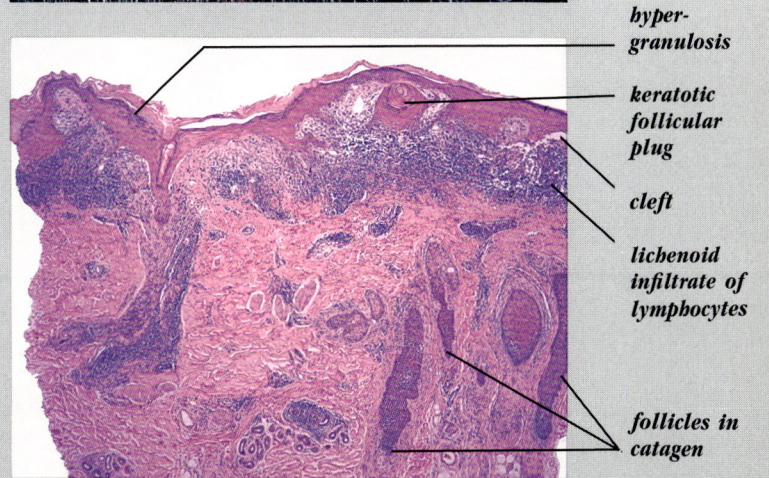

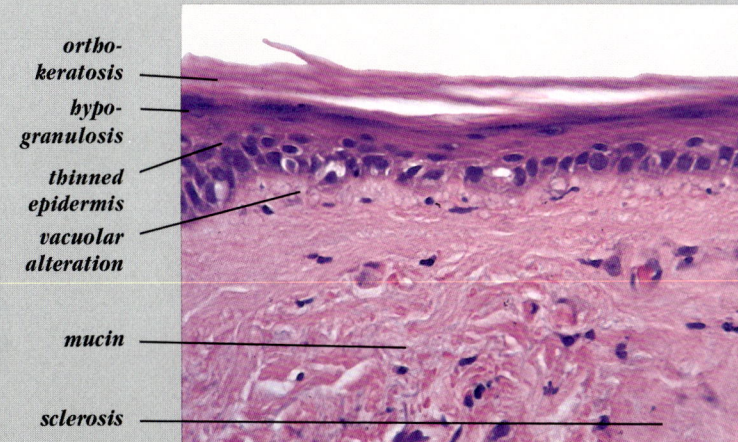

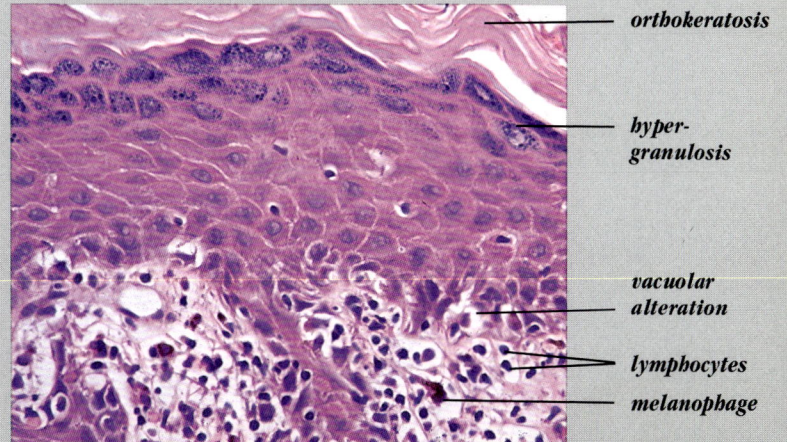

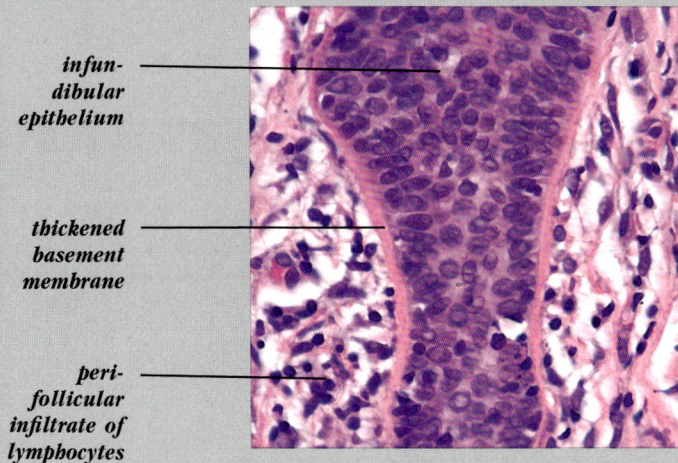

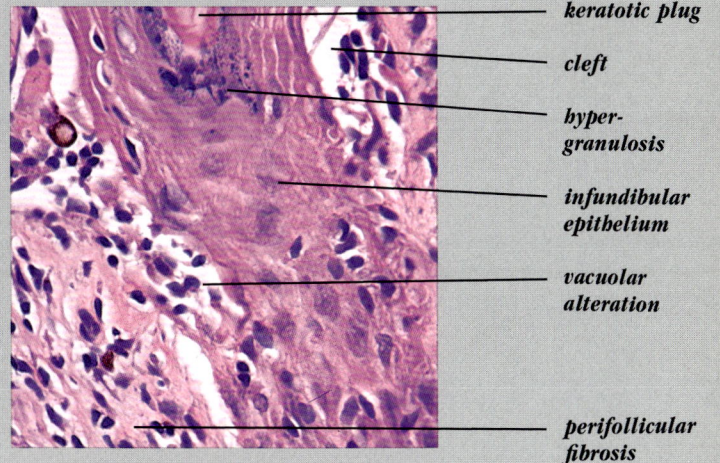

thinned epidermis

keratotic follicular plug

follicle in catagen

infiltrate of lymphocytes

hyper-granulosis

keratotic follicular plug

cleft

lichenoid infiltrate of lymphocytes

follicles in catagen

ortho-keratosis

hypo-granulosis

thinned epidermis

vacuolar alteration

mucin

sclerosis

orthokeratosis

hyper-granulosis

vacuolar alteration

lymphocytes

melanophage

infun-dibular epithelium

thickened basement membrane

peri-follicular infiltrate of lymphocytes

keratotic plug

cleft

hyper-granulosis

infundibular epithelium

vacuolar alteration

perifollicular fibrosis

T HE alopecias of discoid lupus erythematosus and of lichen planus share these histologic features: predominantly lymphocytic perivascular and perifollicular infiltrates, vacuolar alteration at junctions between follicular epithelium and the dermis, infundibular plugging by orthokeratotic corneocytes, and fibrotic tracts along the paths of extinct hair follicles.

The crucial features for histologic differentiation of the alopecia of discoid lupus erythematosus from that of lichen planus are found at the dermo-epidermal interface. In chronic lesions of discoid lupus erythematosus, there are vacuolar alteration and a thickened basement membrane beneath a thinned epidermis, whereas in lesions of lichen planopilaris the epidermal-dermal junction is often completely normal. Occasionally, the typical changes of lichen planus may be seen, namely irregular epidermal hyperplasia and a lichenoid infiltrate that obscures the dermo-epidermal junction at which vacuolar alteration occurs. In short, the alopecia of chronic discoid lupus erythematosus is always associated with involvement of both the epidermal and follicular epithelia, whereas that of lichen planus often spares the epidermis.

In discoid lupus erythematosus, studies by direct immunofluorescence show granular deposits of immunoglobulins and complement at the dermo-epidermal junction, whereas such is not the case in lichen planopilaris.

Clinically, the lesions of discoid lupus erythematosus go through stages of redness, scaling (with keratotic follicular plugs), and induration, and eventually to atrophic scars, wherewith alopecia may also supervene. The centers of the scars are usually hypopigmented and telangiectatic, but their peripheries are hyperpigmented. Keratotic plugs may be present in the hairless follicles. Alopecic lesions of discoid lupus erythematosus usually occur on the face and scalp. They may be associated with discoid lesions elsewhere on the skin.

In contrast, the lesions of lichen planopilaris begin as violaceous papules that soon become keratotic. With time, they evolve into atrophic scars that are devoid of hairs. Keratotic follicular skin lesions of lichen planopilaris, as well as mucous membrane and nail changes of lichen planus, may accompany the scarring alopecia.

Pseudopelade (i.e., pseudo alopecia areata) refers to the end stage of scarring alopecias. The most common cause of this condition, whose lesions have been likened clinically to "footprints in the snow" is the alopecia of lichen planus. However, similar alopecic lesions may be seen as a consequence of chronic discoid lupus erythematosus.

The term "scarring" alopecia is somewhat misleading because, at first blush, it would seem to imply the presence of a histologic scar. That truly may be the case in alopecias that result from ulcerations caused by physical or chemical injuries. But permanent "scarring" alopecias may occur in the absence of true histologic scars, for example, in scleroderma as a result of sclerosis in the dermis and in the subcutaneous fat, in lichen planopilaris as a result of fibrotic tracts at sites of extinct hair follicles, and even in alopecia areata as a result of whorls of sclerotic collagen at sites where formerly there were papillae of hair follicles. In short, there are several different kinds of "scarring" alopecia.

19. Alopecia Areata

vs. Trichotillomania

Alopecia Areata	Trichotillomania
1. Slight to moderately dense lympho-histiocytic infiltrate around the blood vessels of the superficial and deep plexuses	1. Practically no inflammatory-cell infiltrate around the dermal blood vessels
2. Predominantly lymphocytic infiltrate in hair papillae and fibrous sheaths surrounding hair bulbs in early lesions	2. No significant inflammatory-cell infiltrates around hair follicles, except granulomatous when follicle has ruptured
3. Increased numbers of mast cells and linearly arranged dilated capillaries at sites of what were formerly papillae of follicles	3. No increase in number of mast cells or blood vessels at sites of former hair papillae
4. More telogen than catagen follicles usually	4. More catagen than telogen follicles usually
5. Few intervening anagen follicles	5. Several intervening anagen follicles
6. No everted tricholemmal sheaths	6. Everted tricholemmal sheaths occasionally
7. No trichomalacia	7. Trichomalacia (pleated hair shafts containing irregularly shaped clumps of melanin within infundibula of follicles) commonly
8. In old lesions, whorls of sclerotic collagen containing melanophages in the deep reticular dermis	8. No whorls of sclerosis in the dermis
9. No superimposition of lichen simplex chronicus	9. Lichen simplex chronicus sometimes superimposed in the form of compact orthokeratosis

Alopecia Areata

Trichotillomania

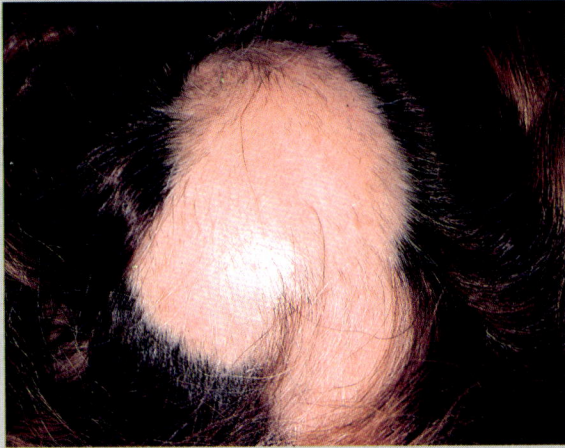

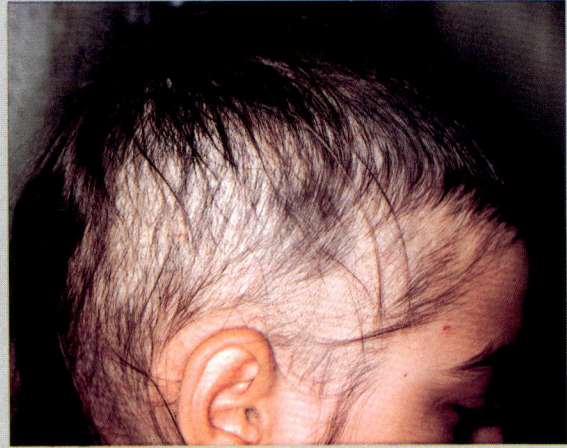

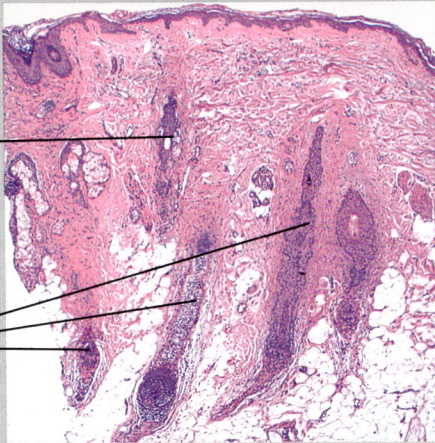

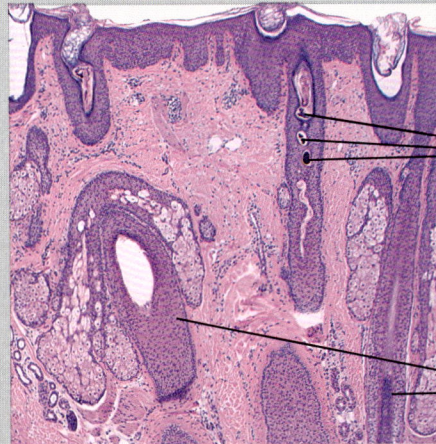

follicle in
telogen

follicles in
early
catagen

trichomalacia

follicles in
anagen

tricholemmal
sheath

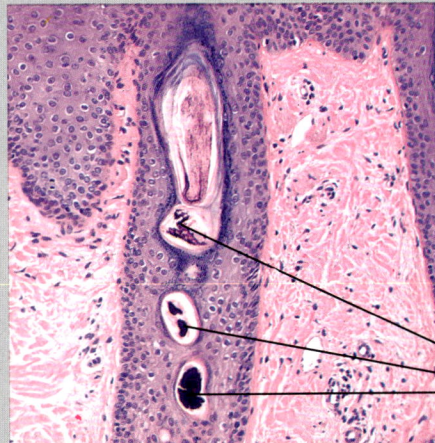

hair bulb

infiltrate of
lymphocytes

dilated
vessel in
fibrous tract

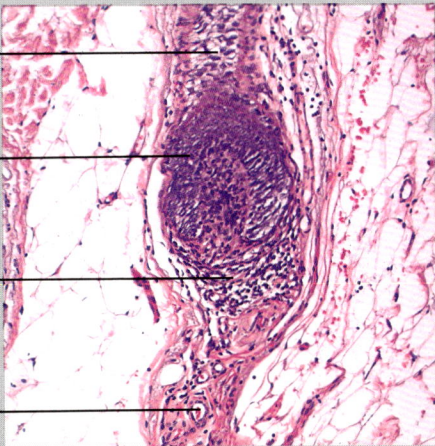

trichomalacia

hair bulb

papilla of
hair follicle

lymphocytes

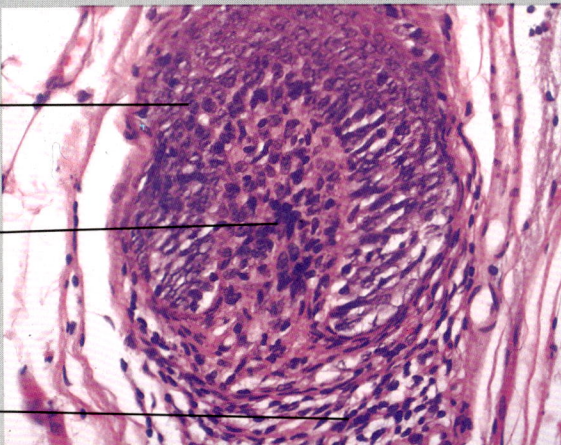

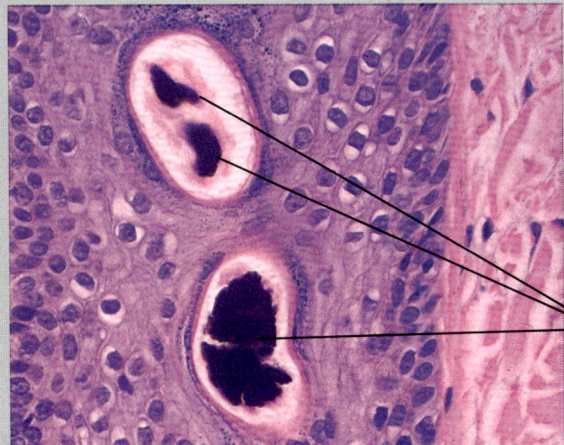

clumps of
melanin
in pleated
hair shaft
(trichomalacia)

ALOPECIA areata and trichotillomania have several histologic features in common, namely, sparse inflammatory-cell infiltrates in the dermis as a rule, some follicles in telogen (and often in catagen), and fibrous tracts at sites of extinct follicles.

Alopecia areata is an inflammatory disease of the perifollicular connective tissues, whereas trichotillomania is a factitious condition that results from persistent plucking or pulling of hairs.

Clinically, alopecia areata consists of sharply circumscribed, smooth, round to oval patches of skin devoid of hairs. It is especially frequent on the scalp and face. When the process involves the entire scalp, rather than simply discrete patches, the condition is termed alopecia totalis; when it affects the entire skin surface it is called alopecia universalis. The more widespread the condition and the longer its duration, the worse the prognosis for return of hair. Vitiligo and pitting of the nails are sometimes concomitants of alopecia areata and its variants.

Histologically, fibrous rather than fibrotic tracts form in the wake of catagen and telogen hairs in alopecia areata. The absence of scarring at the sites of extinct follicles presages, it is said, regrowth of hairs. In some cases of alopecia areata and of its variants, however, whorls of sclerotic collagen containing remnants of old hair bulbs, extinct papillae, and thickened "glassy" membranes, form in the deep reticular dermis. These are signs that the vital parts of the follicle, the matrix cells of the bulb and the papillae, are no longer functioning and will not regrow hairs.

Trichotillomania consists clinically of irregularly shaped, partially alopecic patches of hairs broken off at different lengths. The patches have a ragged appearance as a result of persistent manipulation, i.e., twisting and pulling of the hair shafts. If the patient can forego tugging at the hairs, the pelage may return to normal. However, longstanding trauma to the hair shafts may injure papillae sufficiently to result in permanent alopecia.

Trichomalacia, a cardinal sign of trichotillomania, results from persistent twisting of hair shafts with resultant fraying, breakage, and dispersal of melanin in variously sized clumps within bits of broken shafts. The number of follicles in the catagen or telogen stage of the hair cycle depends upon how soon after hairs were uprooted the biopsy was obtained (i.e., the nearer to the time that hairs were pulled out, the greater the number of follicles in catagen). Catagen follicles are identified histologically by the markedly thickened corrugated glassy membranes that envelop their lower portions.

The foregoing statements about the interpretation of histologic characteristics of alopecia areata and trichotillomania depend upon various factors, among them duration of the disease, site of biopsy, and the breadth and depth of biopsy.

A not uncommon concurrent feature of trichotillomania is the hyperkeratotic variant of lichen simplex chronicus. Unlike conventional lichen simplex chronicus consequent to prolonged and persistent rubbing of the skin on the trunk and extremities, characterized not only by epidermal hyperplasia but by coarse collagen fibers arranged in vertical streaks in the papillary dermis, hyperkeratotic lichen simplex chronicus on the scalp is characterized primarily by marked compact orthokeratosis that resembles the normal cornified layer on palms and soles.

In addition to the typical features of trichotillomania enumerated above, there are often features of hyperkeratotic lichen simplex chronicus, because the anxiety that prompts some patients to pluck hairs also causes them to rub their scalps vigorously for long periods. The hyperkeratotic variant of lichen simplex chronicus is also seen in pruritus vulvae and ani. On the lips and on the mucous membranes of the oral cavity, this hyperkeratotic variant is known as keratosis oris.

20. Follicular Cyst, Infundibular Type *vs.* Follicular Cyst, Isthmus-Catagen Type

Follicular Cyst, Infundibular Type	Follicular Cyst, Isthmus-Catagen Type
1. Cyst lining consists of stratified squamous epithelium that resembles that of the normal infundibulum of the hair follicle and the normal epidermis (i.e., the cells flatten as they mature; granular layer persists)	1. Cyst lining consists of stratified squamous epithelium that resembles that of the normal isthmus of the hair follicle and the inferior portion of the follicle in catagen (i.e., the cells become paler as they mature; granular layer disappears)
2. Lining epithelium does not project into the cyst cavity	2. Lining epithelium projects irregularly as scalloping into the cyst cavity
3. Cyst connects with the epidermis (if serial sections are cut)	3. Cyst does not connect with the epidermis usually
4. No calcification of cornified contents of cyst	4. Calcification of cornified contents of cyst commonly
5. Parakeratotic cells scattered within the cyst commonly	5. Few, if any, parakeratotic cells within the cyst usually and then only near the cyst lining
6. Normal pattern of the rete ridges and dermal papillae preserved around outer circumference of the cyst	6. No normal pattern of rete ridges and dermal papillae around circumference of the cyst
7. Melanin and melanocytes in the lining epithelium and melanin in the cornified cells	7. No melanin or melanocytes in lining epithelium
8. No cholesterol clefts within cysts	8. Cholesterol clefts within cysts commonly
9. Bacteria and yeasts within the cyst often	9. No bacteria or yeasts within the cyst usually
10. Sebaceous (bluish granular) material in the cyst contents	10. No sebaceous material in the contents
11. Cornified cells within the cyst in basket-weave and laminated pattern	11. Cornified cells within the cyst arranged compactly

Follicular Cyst, Infundibular Type   Follicular Cyst, Isthmus-Catagen Type

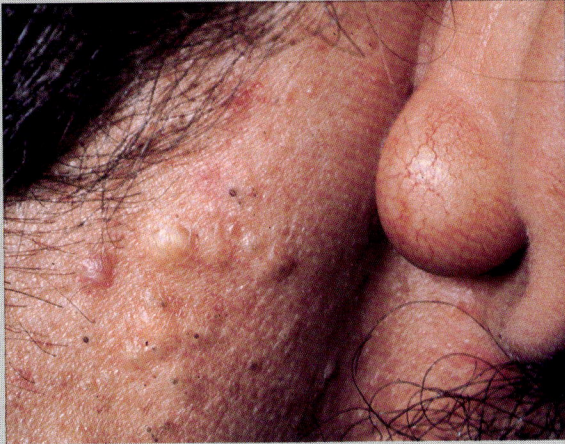

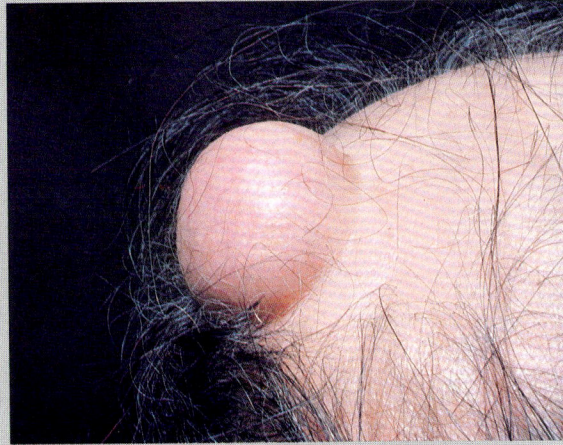

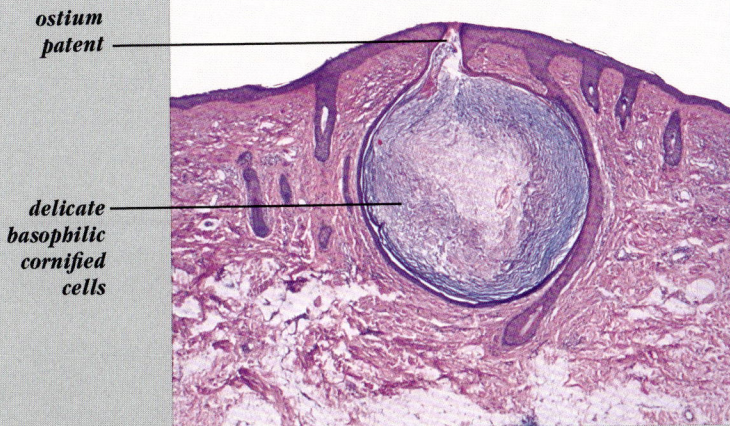

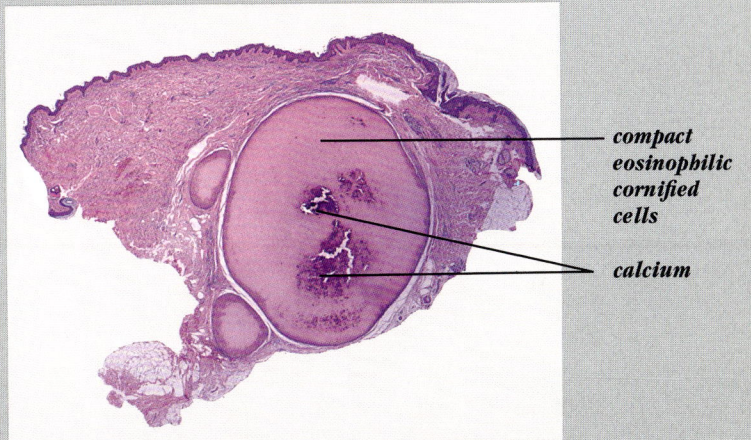

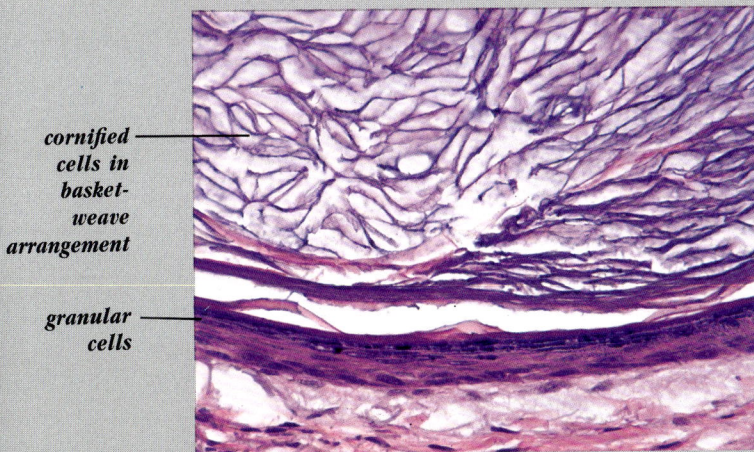

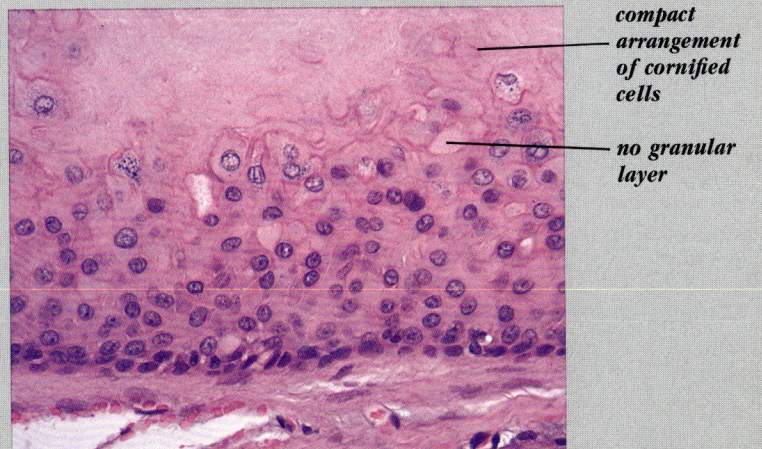

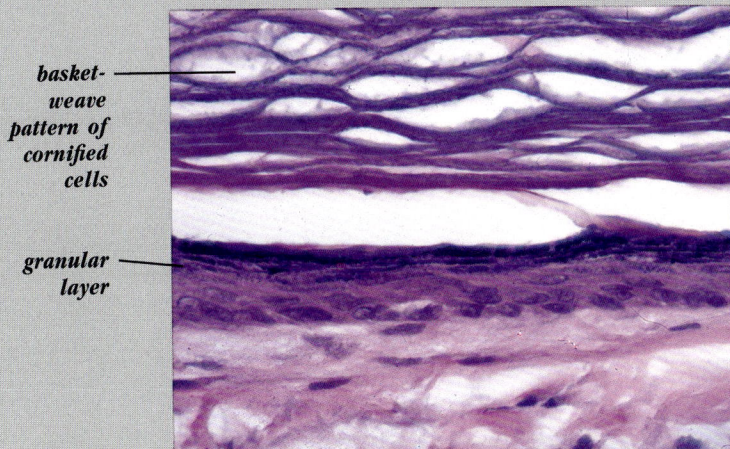

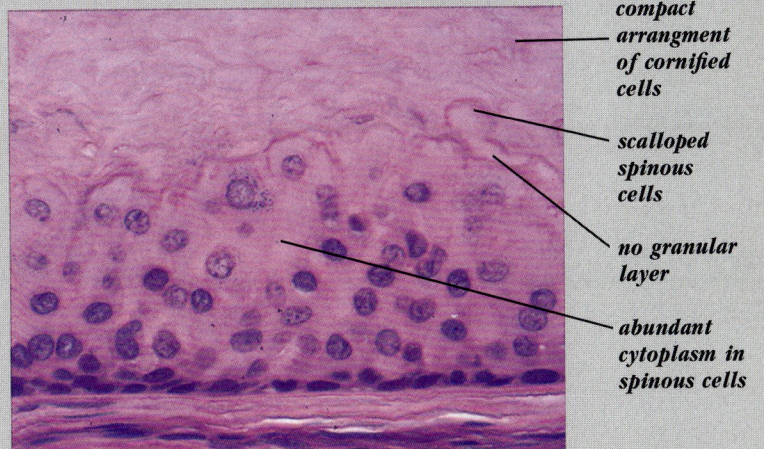

ostium
patent

delicate
basophilic
cornified
cells

compact
eosinophilic
cornified
cells

calcium

cornified
cells in
basket-
weave
arrangement

granular
cells

compact
arrangement
of cornified
cells

no granular
layer

basket-
weave
pattern of
cornified
cells

granular
layer

compact
arrangment
of cornified
cells

scalloped
spinous
cells

no granular
layer

abundant
cytoplasm in
spinous cells

THESE two common cysts of skin have several features in common, namely, both are lined by stratified squamous epithelium, are follicular in origin or differentiation, and contain cornified cells within their cavities.

We name cysts according to the nature of their lining and contents. Hair follicle cysts of the infundibular type have also been termed epidermoid or epidermal cysts, epidermal inclusion cysts, and retention cysts. Because these cysts usually develop from the epithelium of the infundibular portion of hair follicles and have a lining that is identical histologically to that of the infundibulum, we term them infundibular cysts. The epithelial lining of the infundibulum closely resembles the epidermis histologically, as one would expect from its origin and continuity; therefore, the term epidermoid cyst is also accurate morphologically. Milia are simply small infundibular cysts (rarely eccrine duct cysts).

Infundibular cysts develop especially on the face and trunk and are frequently noted to have a central comedo. They are slow-growing, round, and moderately firm. Upon gross sectioning, a rancid odor caused by the effect of bacteria upon the sebaceous material within them is emitted. Sebum enters infundibular cysts from the sebaceous gland via the sebaceous duct.

When rupture of infundibular cysts occurs, a foreign body reaction ensues in response to the cyst contents that are spewed into the dermis. Initially there is suppuration, followed by granulomatous inflammation, and finally by fibrosis.

Hair follicle cysts of the isthmus-catagen type have also been called tricholemmal cysts, wens, and, incorrectly, pilar cysts and sebaceous cysts. The lining of isthmus-catagen cysts is the same as that of the isthmus portion of the normal hair follicle and as that of the epithelium of the inferior portion of a normal catagen hair follicle. By such a system of nomenclature, steatocystoma multiplex can be conceived to be a sebaceous duct cyst; hidrocystoma, a sweat duct cyst; and calcifying epithelioma of Malherbe (pilomatrixoma), a combined infundibular-matrix cyst. "Pilar" means hair and therefore none of the follicular cysts are truly pilar cysts, although some of them, like steatocystoma multiplex and dermoid cysts, nearly always contain hairs.

Isthmus-catagen cysts, in contrast to infundibular cysts, usually develop on the scalp, are hard (probably partially due to calcification of the cyst contents), and rupture rarely.

A variant of isthmus-catagen cyst is the proliferating isthmus-catagen cyst, also known as proliferating tricholemmal cyst, proliferating pilar cyst, proliferating epidermoid cyst, pilar tumor of the scalp, and subepidermal acanthoma. Histologically, proliferating isthmus-catagen cysts show architectural disarray and cytologic atypia, thereby resembling squamous-cell carcinoma. In fact, formerly, a proliferating isthmus-catagen cyst was thought to be a carcinoma arising in a cyst. The histologic clue to the benign nature of proliferating isthmus-catagen cysts is their sharp circumscription.

Rarely, a hair follicle cyst may have a lining that in part resembles that of the infundibulum and in part the isthmus.

Finally, a word should be said of epidermoid cysts that occur on the palms and soles. Histologically, these cysts are identical to infundibular cysts, but in those locations cannot arise in pre-existing hair follicles. Whether epidermoid cysts on palms and soles are related to eccrine ducts or result from inclusions of epidermis into the dermis secondary to puncture wounds is not known.

21. Syringocystadenoma Papilliferum *vs.* Hidradenoma Papilliferum

Syringocystadenoma Papilliferum

1. Not truly cystic

2. Skin surface papillated

3. Surface of specimen covered by two types of epithelium; epidermal and apocrine

4. Bulbous papillated projections above the skin surface and into glandular epithelium-lined spaces in the dermis

5. Multiple sites of connection between glandular epithelium and surface epidermis

6. Increased numbers of apocrine glands deep in dermis often

7. Dense inflammatory-cell infiltrate of plasma cells mainly

8. Marked edema and telangiectases in stroma

9. Concurrent adnexal neoplasms and malformations (e.g., nevus sebaceus, apocrine hidrocystoma, solid hidradenoma, milia) in the same specimen

Hidradenoma Papilliferum

1. Truly cystic (space completely enclosed by epithelium)

2. Skin surface domed but smooth

3. Surface of specimen covered by epidermis only; cyst lined by apocrine epithelium

4. Numerous thin trabeculae lined by glandular epithelium within a large dermal cyst

5. One site of connection between glandular epithelium and surface epidermis usually; sometimes no apparent connection

6. No increased number of apocrine glands in dermis

7. Sparse inflammatory-cell infiltrate of lymphocytes mainly, but also of plasma cells and mast cells

8. Little edema and no telangiectases

9. No association with other neoplasms and malformations

Syringocystadenoma Papilliferum

Hidradenoma Papilliferum

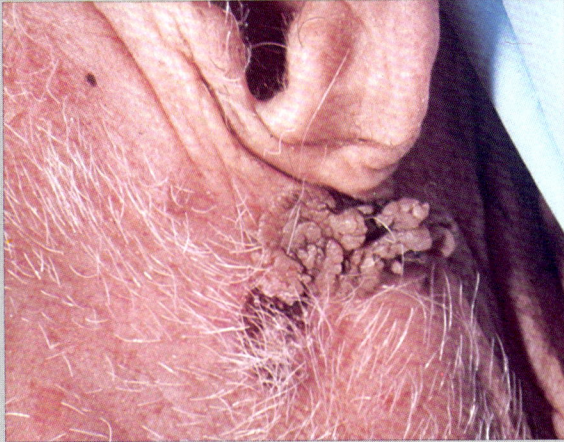

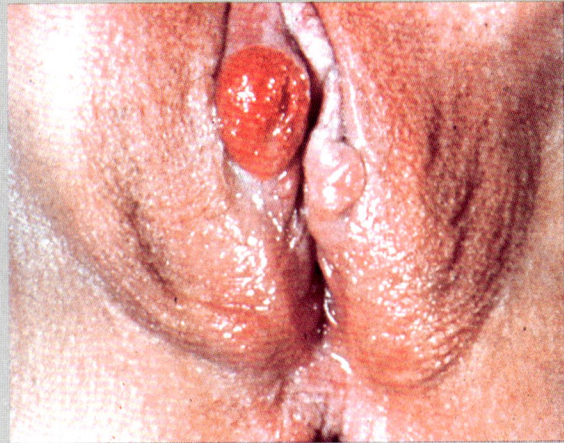

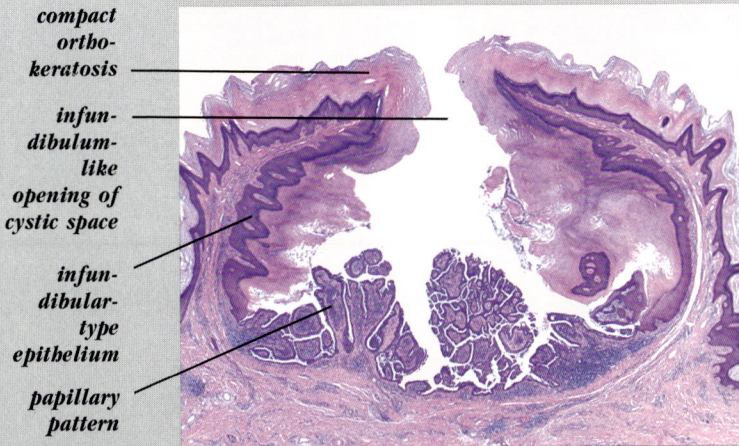

compact
ortho-
keratosis

infun-
dibulum-
like
opening of
cystic space

infun-
dibular-
type
epithelium

papillary
pattern

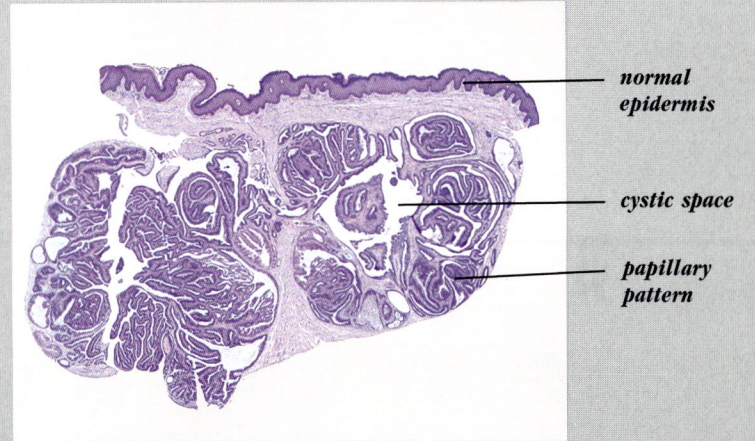

normal
epidermis

cystic space

papillary
pattern

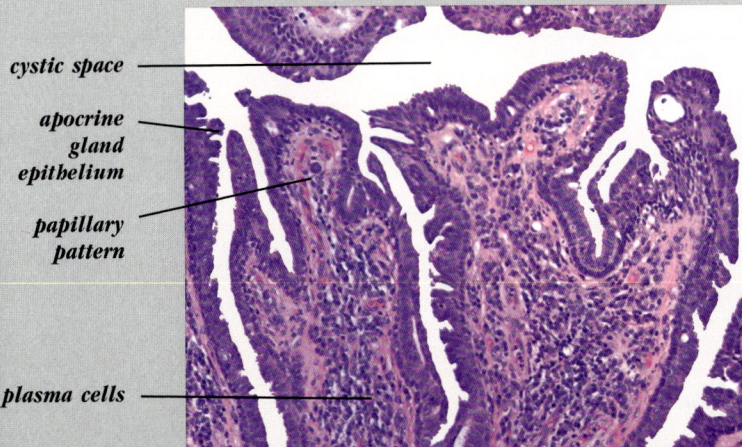

cystic space

apocrine
gland
epithelium

papillary
pattern

plasma cells

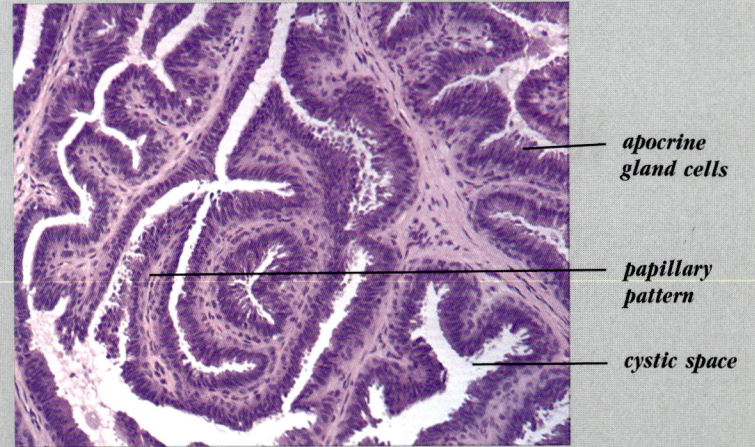

apocrine
gland cells

papillary
pattern

cystic space

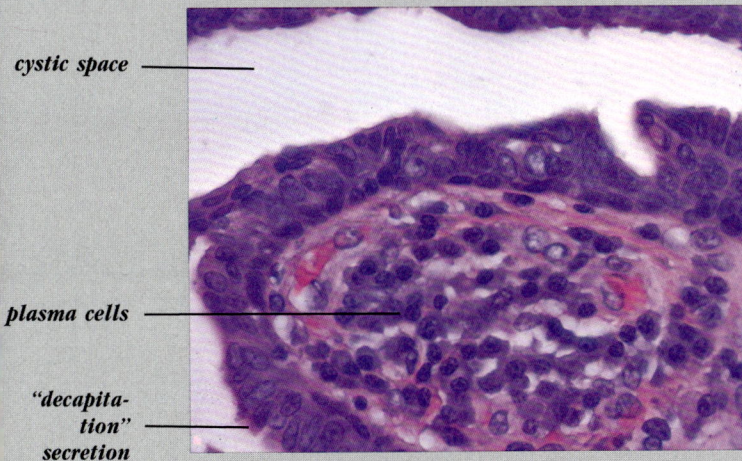

cystic space

plasma cells

"decapita-
tion"
secretion

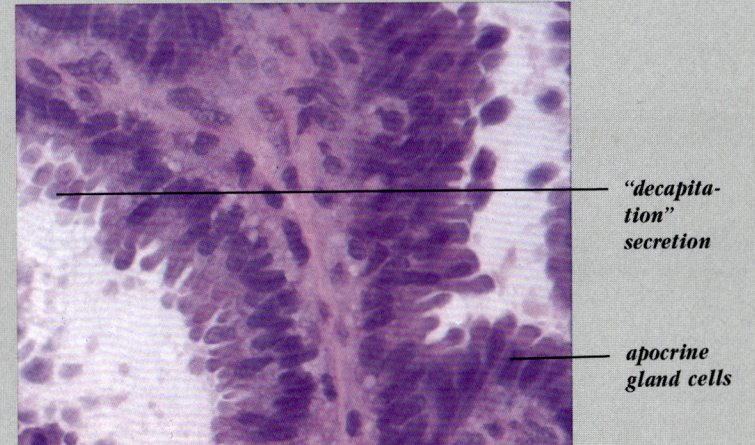

"decapita-
tion"
secretion

apocrine
gland cells

SYRINGOCYSTADENOMA papilliferum and hidradenoma papilliferum are both varieties of apocrine papillated cystadenomas, but they have very different clinical and histologic patterns.

Clinically, syringocystadenoma papilliferum occurs predominantly on the scalp as a crusted, often weeping, verrucous plaque. Occasionally, the malformation develops on the face and less frequently on the trunk or extremities. In contrast, hidradenoma papilliferum occurs almost always in women in the perineal and perianal areas, especially on the vulva, as a smooth-surfaced cystic nodule.

Histologically, the patterns of these two lesions are very different although both are lined by apocrine epithelium arranged in two layers, an inner columnar and an outer cuboidal layer showing the "decapitation secretion" typical of apocrine gland cells. Syringocystadenoma papilliferum has bulbous projections above the skin surface, whereas hidradenoma papilliferum consists of delicate trabeculae within a cyst that is wholly within the dermis.

Often in syringocystadenoma papilliferum the papillated cystadenoma seems to be continuous with widely dilated horn-filled follicular infundibula. When one considers that apocrine epithelium takes origin from follicular infundibulum in embryonic life, it should not be surprising that there is an association between apocrine epithelium and infundibular epithelium in the hamartomatous syringocystadenoma papilliferum.

Syringocystadenoma papilliferum is found sometimes in association with a lesion of nevus sebaceus of Jadassohn. Many authors contend that this association occurs in one of every three instances of syringocystadenoma papilliferum. Its incidence is considerably lower than this in our experience. Syringocystadenoma papilliferum is merely one of many hamartomas and benign and malignant neoplasms that may arise within nevus sebaceus, a condition marked by alterations of the dermis, the epidermis, and the epithelial structures of adnexa.

It is relatively easy clinically to suspect a syringocystadenoma papilliferum in association with a nevus sebaceus. The former lesion is often verrucous and reddish-brown, and its surface is moist as a consequence of secretions made by apocrine cells. In contrast, the latter lesion has a cobblestone-like surface and is yellowish and dry.

Syringocystadenoma papilliferum and hidradenoma papilliferum are the two most common cystadenomas in the skin that show apocrine differentiation. The other major cystadenomas in the skin show eccrine differentiation, namely, solid-cystic hidradenomas and mixed tumors of skin (chondroid syringomas). In order for apocrine cystadenomas to be diagnosed histologically with certainty and to be differentiated from eccrine cystadenomas, some epithelial cells must be seen to show evidence of "decapitation secretion." This is the sine qua non for establishing apocrine differentiation for hamartomas, cysts, neoplasms, and cystic neoplasms. Syringocystadenoma papilliferum and hidradenoma papilliferum practically never eventuate in apocrine carcinoma.

A few words should be written about an important cystadenoma with apocrine differentiation that is situated on the nipple. This lesion is known by a variety of names, among them nipple adenoma, subareolar papillomatosis, and erosive adenomatosis. This cystic adenoma of the nipple is a pseudo-malignancy because it has been misinterpreted histologically at times as a primary carcinoma of the breast. Such confusion has resulted in unnecessary mastectomy.

22. Ichthyosis Vulgaris
vs. X-linked Ichthyosis

Ichthyosis Vulgaris	X-linked Ichthyosis
1. Cornified layer slightly to moderately thickened	1. Cornified layer moderately to markedly thickened
2. Compact laminated orthokeratosis, often associated with plugging of infundibula (keratosis pilaris)	2. Compact laminated orthokeratosis, rarely associated with plugging of infundibula
3. Granular layer thinned (to one cell layer) or nearly absent	3. Granular layer normal (two to three cell layers) or slightly thickened
4. Thinned epidermis	4. Normal or slightly thickened epidermis
5. Thinned suprapapillary plates	5. Normal suprapapillary plates
6. Mitotic figures in the basal layer rare	6. Mitotic figures in the basal layer occasional
7. Interdigitations between epidermal rete ridges and dermal papillae shallow or flat	7. Pattern between epidermal rete ridges and dermal papillae normal

Ichthyosis Vulgaris

X-linked Ichthyosis

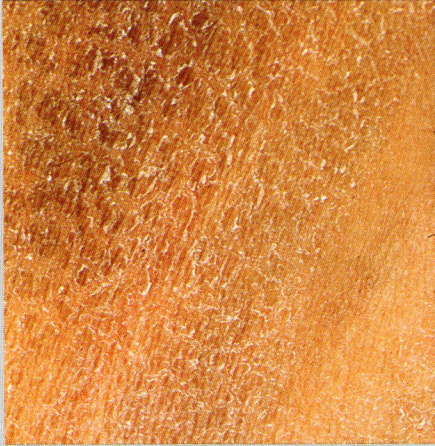

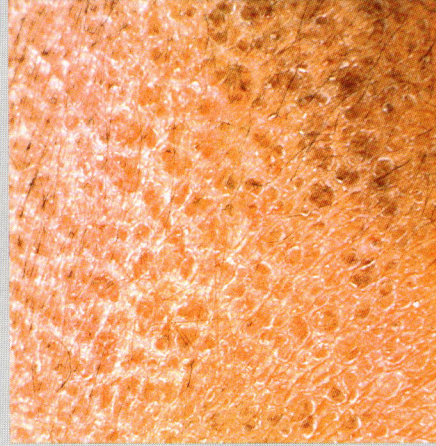

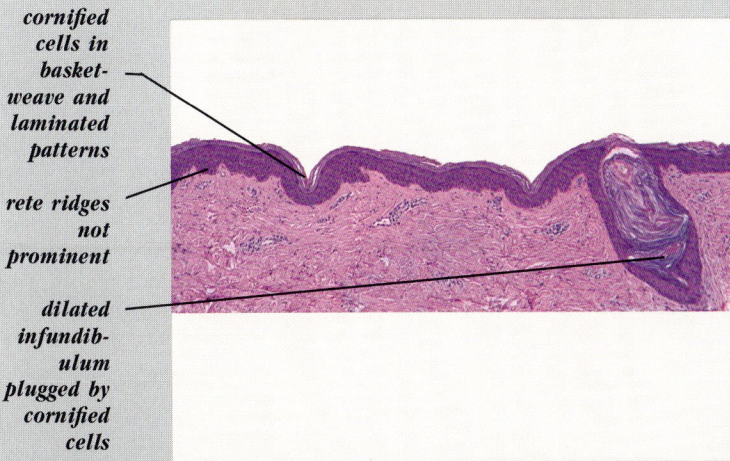

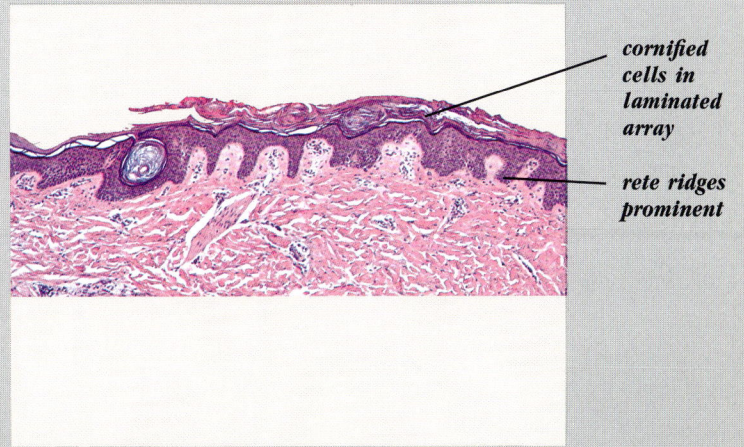

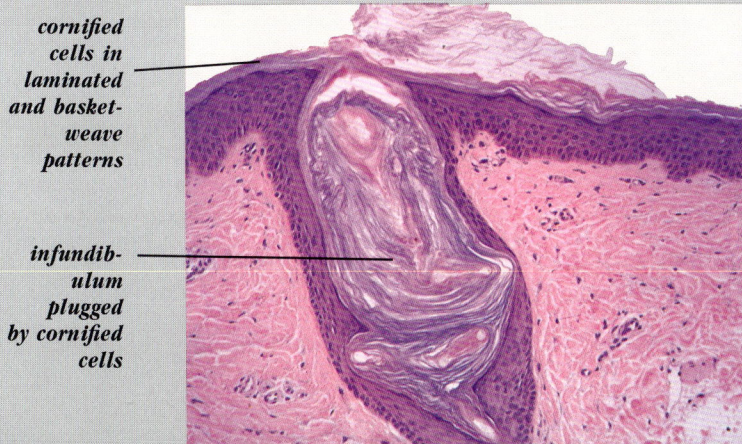

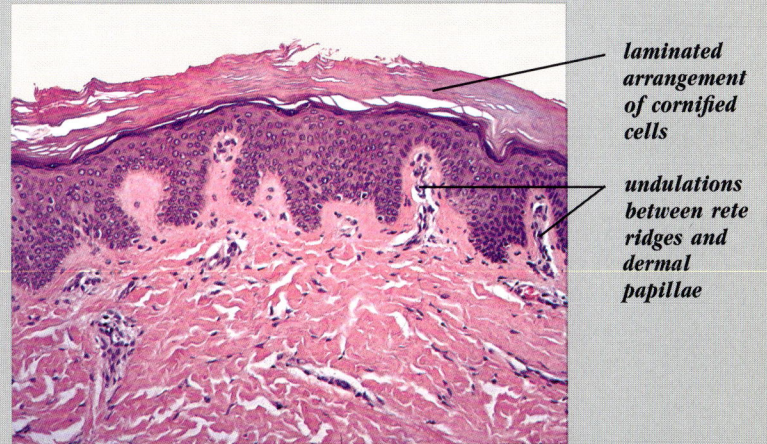

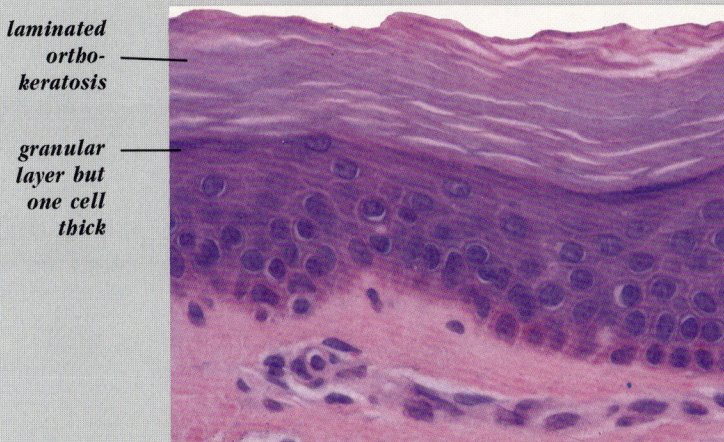

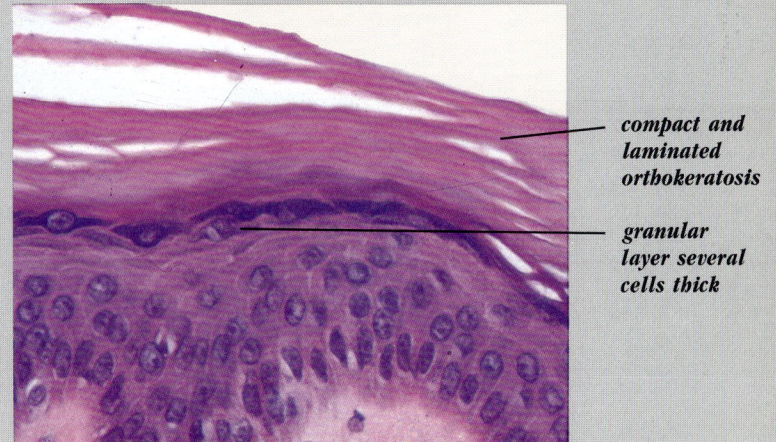

cornified
cells in
basket-
weave and
laminated
patterns

rete ridges
not
prominent

dilated
infundib-
ulum
plugged by
cornified
cells

cornified
cells in
laminated
array

rete ridges
prominent

cornified
cells in
laminated
and basket-
weave
patterns

infundib-
ulum
plugged
by cornified
cells

laminated
arrangement
of cornified
cells

undulations
between rete
ridges and
dermal
papillae

laminated
ortho-
keratosis

granular
layer but
one cell
thick

compact and
laminated
orthokeratosis

granular
layer several
cells thick

ICHTHYOSIS vulgaris and X-linked ichthyosis are truly ichthyotic conditions because the clinical appearance of their scales resembles those of fish (ichthos = Greek, fish, and -osis = Greek, a condition). As in all ichthyoses, the scales are thickest on the legs. The scales of both ichthyosis vulgaris and X-linked ichthyosis are seen histologically to consist of compact, laminated orthokeratosis. The epidermal turnover time in both conditions is about normal.

Ichthyosis vulgaris is an autosomal dominant condition which develops early in childhood. Affected individuals usually show widespread fine scaling of the skin, most marked on the extremities and trunk, but tending to spare the flexures. Common concomitants of ichthyosis vulgaris are atopic diathesis and propensity to keratosis pilaris. Youngsters with ichthyosis vulgaris have such severe accentuation of the normal skin markings on the palms and soles that the volar surfaces of their hands and feet tend to resemble those of elderly persons.

Ichthyosis vulgaris, as the name suggests, is more common than X-linked ichthyosis. The latter condition in its fullest expression affects males only; female heterozygotes may be slightly affected. Present at birth or shortly thereafter, X-linked ichthyosis tends to involve much of the body surface including the sides of the face, neck, and flexural areas. Unlike ichthyosis vulgaris, there are no abnormalities of the skin markings on the palms and soles. Corneal opacities, however, may be found in patients with X-linked ichthyosis and in female carriers of the disease.

A third truly ichthyotic condition is lamellar ichthyosis, also known as non-bullous congenital ichthyosiform erythroderma. Histologically, lamellar ichthyosis is characterized by:

1. Markedly thickened compact, laminated orthokeratosis (much thicker than that of either ichthyosis vulgaris or X-linked ichthyosis)
2. Hypergranulosis (a granular layer sometimes five to seven cell layers thick)
3. Psoriasiform hyperplasia
4. Increased numbers of mitotic figures within the basal layer of the epidermis (epidermopoesis is significantly increased in lamellar ichthyosis)
5. Sparse superficial perivascular infiltrate of lymphocytes and histiocytes

Lamellar ichthyosis is rarer than X-linked ichthyosis and much rarer than ichthyosis vulgaris. It is transmitted in autosomal recessive fashion and infants who have the condition are often born with skin that appears to be covered by a tight shiny envelope resembling collodion or a baked apple. When this shiny membrane disappears, erythroderma and large, plate-like scales supervene. The scaling is usually generalized and ectropion may develop.

A type of ichthyosis appears in adulthood as an acquired condition apparently as a consequence of underlying disease like Hodgkin's disease, carcinoma of the breast, and lepromatous leprosy. The individual scales of acquired ichthyosis have the clinical and histologic features of ichthyosis vulgaris.

Finally, bullous congenital ichthyosiform erythroderma is characterized histologically by epidermolytic hyperkeratosis and clinically by widespread verrucous hyperkeratosis. Intraepidermal blisters may develop in children with the disorder, perhaps in part as a result of superimposed bacterial infection of the skin. Bullous congenital ichthyosiform erythroderma is inherited as an autosomal dominant trait and is apparent at birth, but it is not true ichthyosis. Clinically, there is no resemblance of the hyperkeratosis to fish scales. Therefore, bullous congenital ichthyosiform erythroderma is best considered a widespread epidermal nevus and not a form of ichthyosis.

The term ichthyosis has also been incorrectly applied to ichthyosis hystrix, which is also a type of epidermal nevus, and to conditions like ichthyosis linearis circumflexa.

23. Epidermolytic Hyperkeratosis
vs. Plane Wart

Epidermolytic Hyperkeratosis	*Plane Wart (Verruca Plana)*
1. Laminated and/or compact orthokeratosis	1. Basket-weave orthokeratosis and/or parakeratosis
2. Prominent papillated (sometimes digitated) epidermal hyperplasia	2. Slight papillated epidermal hyperplasia
3. Moderately to markedly thickened epidermis, mainly of the spinous, granular, and cornified zones	3. Slightly thickened epidermis, mainly in the granular and cornified zones
4. Ill-defined, pale zones of various sizes around nuclei of keratinocytes in the lower half of the epidermis	4. Well-defined, clear spaces ("owl's eyes") of various sizes around nuclei of keratinocytes in the upper half of the epidermis
5. Keratinocytes lack distinct boundaries which gives the epidermis a reticulated appearance	5. Keratinocytes have distinct boundaries; no reticulated appearance to the epidermis
6. Increased number of large and small, irregularly shaped, basophilic keratohyaline-like bodies and eosinophilic trichohyaline-like bodies throughout the epidermis except for the basal layer	6. Large and small, irregularly shaped, basophilic keratohyaline-like bodies in the cells of the upper spinous and granular layers; no trichohyaline-like bodies
7. Increased numbers of mitotic figures in the lower portion of the epidermis	7. No increased number of mitotic figures in the epidermis
8. No arborization of the rete ridges at the periphery of the lesion	8. Slight arborization, i.e., inward turning of outermost elongated rete ridges or epithelial adnexa at the periphery of the lesions occasionally
9. Blood vessels in the papillary dermis not significantly dilated	9. Blood vessels in the papillary dermis dilated and tortuous

Epidermolytic Hyperkeratosis

Plane Wart (Verruca Plana)

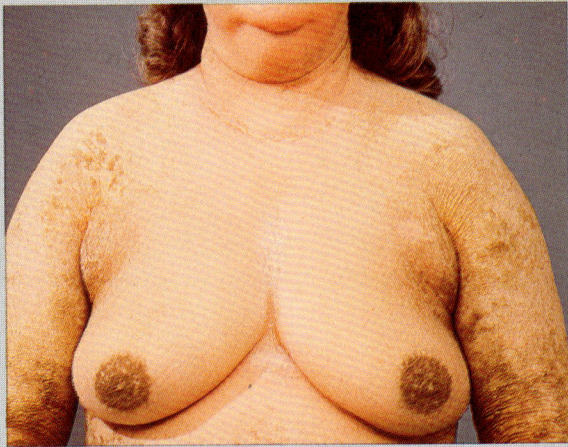

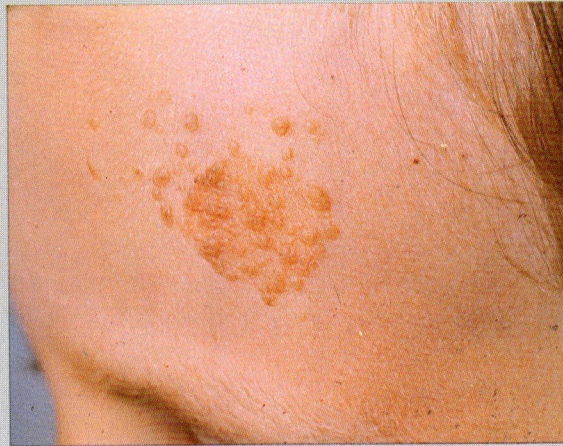

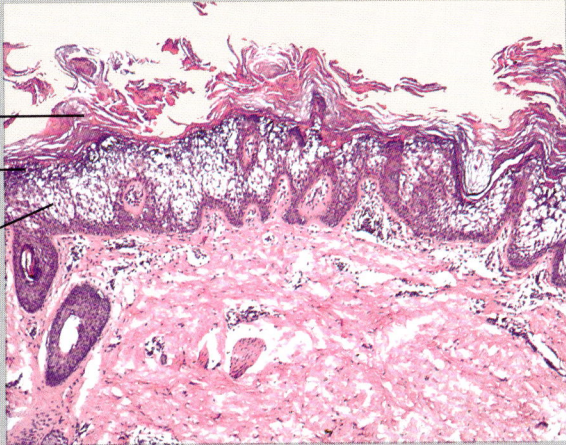

*ortho-
keratosis*

*hyper-
granulosis*

*"epidermo-
lysis"*

parakeratosis

*hyper-
granulosis*

*"owl's eye"
cells*

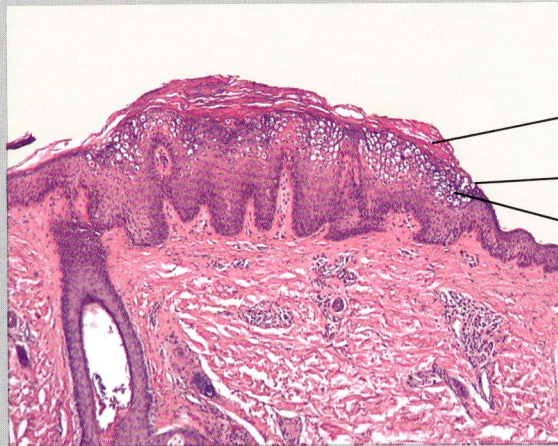

*ortho-
keratosis*

*eosinophilic
granule*

*basophilic
granule*

*"epidermo-
lysis"
throughout
epidermis*

parakeratosis

*cells with
"owl's eyes"
in upper
epidermis*

*basophilic
granules*

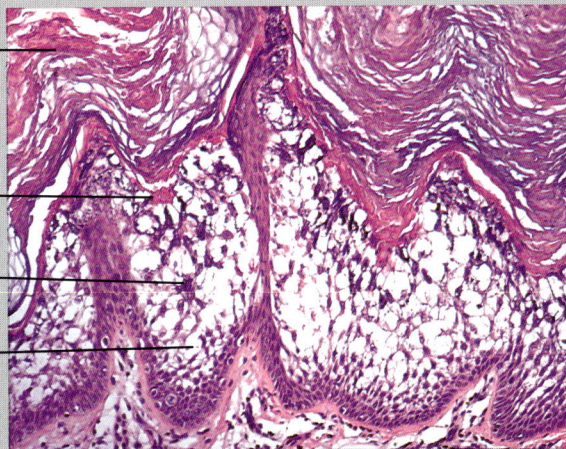

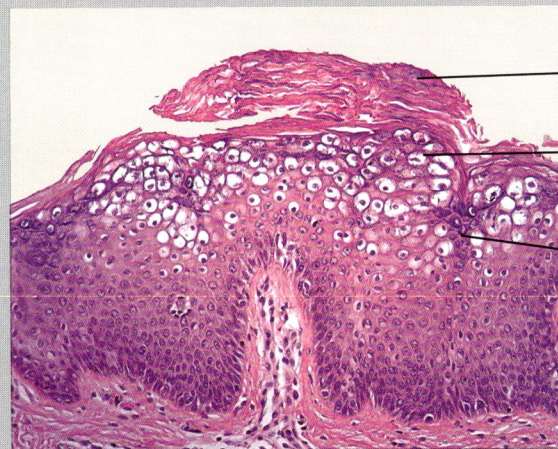

*ortho-
keratosis*

*hyper-
granulosis*

*spaces of
different
sizes*

*no distinct
cell
boundaries*

parakeratosis

*hyper-
granulosis*

*distinct large
nucleus*

*distinct halo
around
nucleus*

*halos of
nearly equal
size*

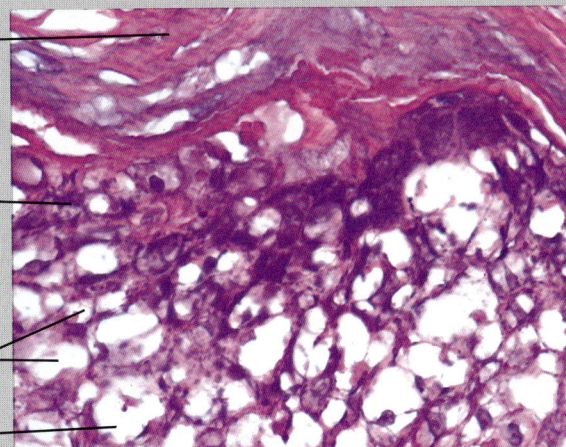

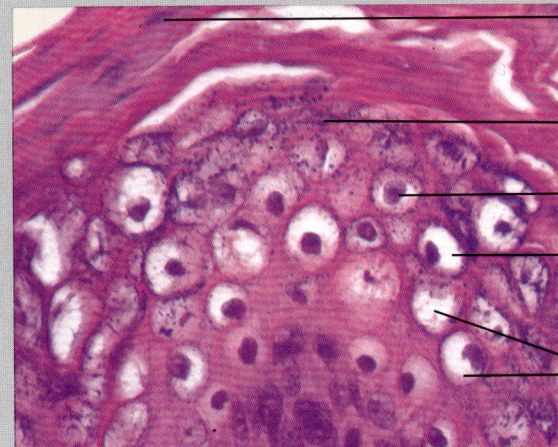

EPIDERMOLYTIC hyperkeratosis and plane warts share several histologic features, namely, papillated epidermal hyperplasia, hypergranulosis, and cells with pale cytoplasms within the epidermis.

Epidermolytic hyperkeratosis is a descriptive term for distinctive histologic changes that appear in several acquired and congenital lesions. Originally, epidermolytic hyperkeratosis was taken to be specific and diagnostic for and synonymous with bullous congenital ichthyosiform erythroderma. Subsequently, the histologic features of epidermolytic hyperkeratosis were found in cases of other nevoid conditions of the epidermis, particularly ichthyosis hystrix and some hereditary keratodermas of the palms and soles. In addition, the phenomenon of epidermolytic hyperkeratosis has been reported in widespread follicular eruptions, follicular cysts, benign solitary keratoses (epidermolytic acanthomas), solar keratoses, and in the form of tiny foci within the epidermis of various inflammatory diseases and benign and malignant neoplasms, especially malignant melanomas. As a pathologic phenomenon, epidermolytic hyperkeratosis has been compared to focal acantholytic dyskeratosis, and these conditions may occur in the epidermis of the same specimen, either in separate discrete foci or side by side. Other analogous pathologic phenomena in skin are cornoid lamellae and follicular mucinosis, both of which are found in a variety of circumstances and are not specific for any one disease.

Plane warts are slightly elevated, mostly flat-topped, relatively smooth-surfaced, discrete papules that vary in color from that of the normal skin of the patient to tan. They occur most commonly on the face and dorsal aspect of the distal parts of the upper extremities. The cause of verruca plana is *papova* virus.

Fully developed warts on the skin, muco-cutaneous surfaces, and mucous membranes have several different architectural patterns. For example, plane warts are characterized by slightly papillated epidermal hyperplasia, whereas condylomata acuminata show more markedly papillomatous epidermal hyperplasia, and verrucae vulgares exhibit digitated epidermal hyperplasia. In contrast, plantar warts are mostly endophytic, as a result of the pressure exerted upon them by walking.

The papova viruses responsible for warts also seem to be capable of causing squamous-cell carcinomas. Epidermodysplasia verruciformis, a condition consisting of numerous plane warts, is associated with the development of squamous-cell carcinomas at the sites of the plane warts. "Giant condyloma acuminatum of Buschke-Löwenstein" is a euphemism for verrucous squamous-cell carcinoma on the genitalia and, as the name suggests, is thought to arise in a pre-existing condyloma acuminatum.

Bowenoid papulosis consists of many small, innocuous-looking papules on the genitalia of young adults. The papules, when viewed by conventional microscopy, have the architectural features of condylomata acuminata, but the cytologic features of squamous-cell carcinomas in situ. It may be inferred that bowenoid papulosis represents condylomata acuminata eventuating in squamous-cell carcinomas in situ. It may also be that carcinoma cuniculatum originates from plantar warts and that the carcinomas of florid oral papillomatosis originate from oral warts. Rarely, we have seen carcinomas that seem to arise from verrucae vulgares.

24. Nevus Verrucosus
vs. Acanthosis Nigricans

Nevus Verrucosus	*Acanthosis Nigricans*
1. Compact orthokeratosis	1. Delicate orthokeratosis with basket-weave and laminated patterns
2. Hyperplastic epidermis, either papillated or digitated	2. Thin epidermis
3. Hypergranulosis usually	3. Granular zone normal or slightly diminished
4. Epidermis sometimes hyperpigmented	4. Epidermis consistently hyperpigmented
5. Papillomatosis (elongated projections of dermal papillae), but not prominent	5. Papillomatosis prominent

Nevus Verrucosus

Acanthosis Nigricans

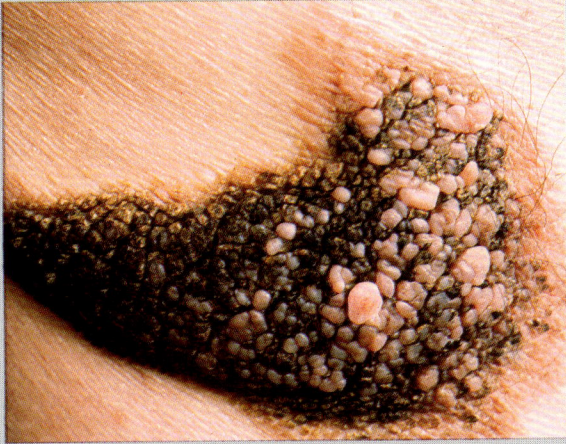

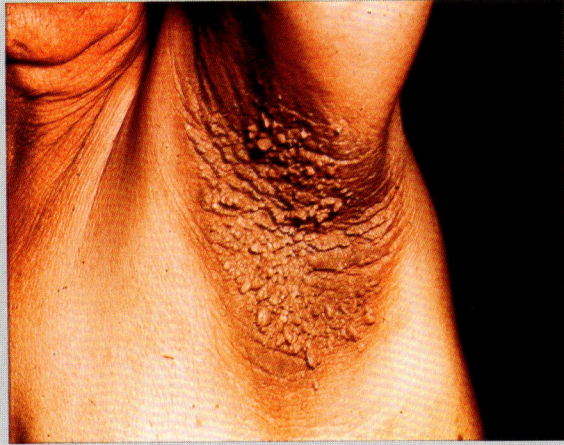

digitation of epidermis

compact ortho-keratosis

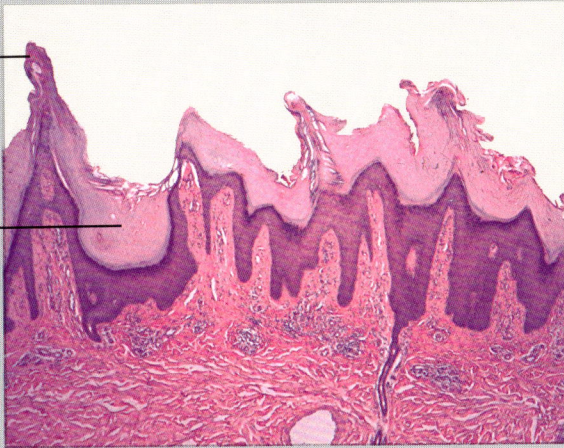

basket-weave pattern of cornified cells

thinned suprapapillary plate

papillo-matosis

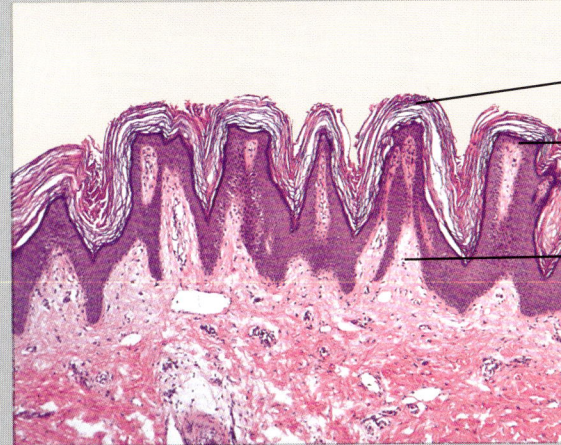

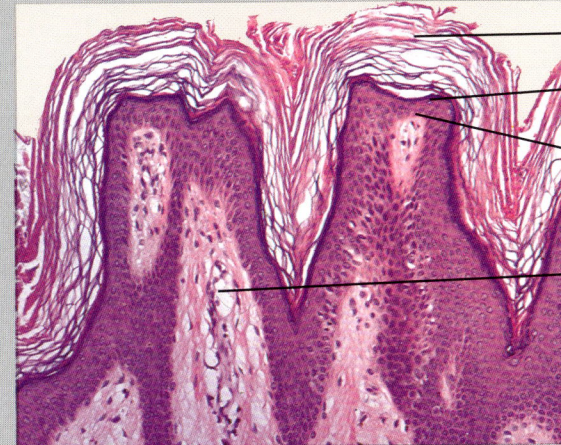

thin rete ridge

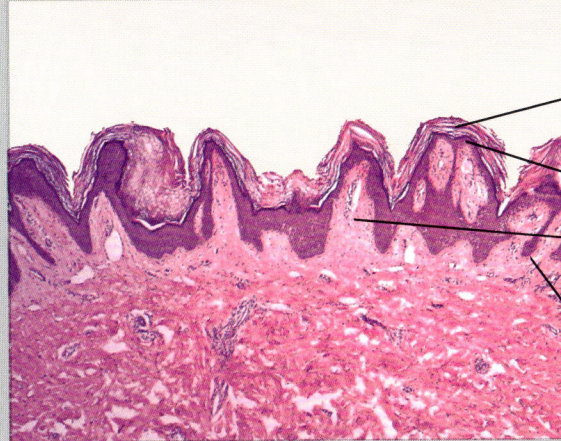

compact ortho-keratosis

hyper-granulosis

hyperplastic epidermis

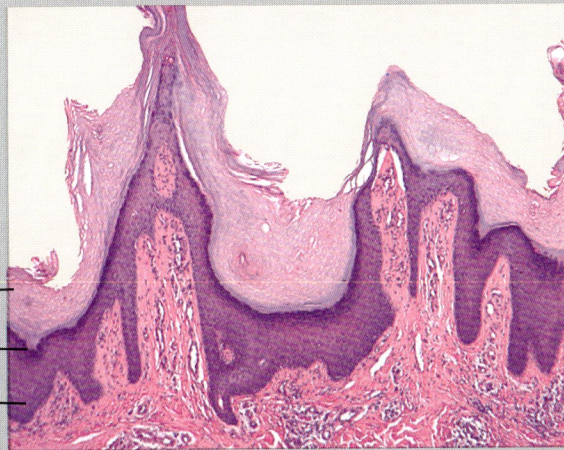

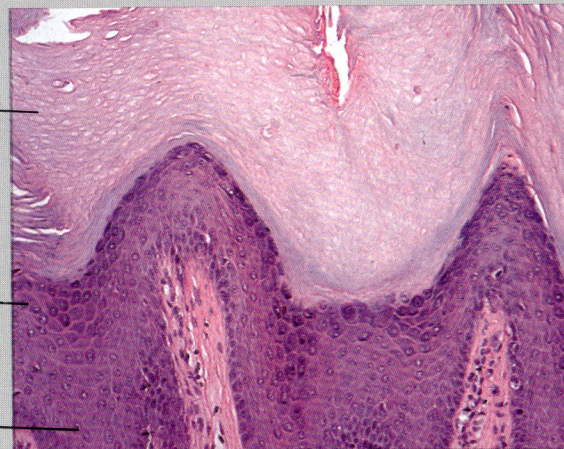

cornified cells in basket-weave array

thin suprapapillary plate

papillo-matosis

compact ortho-keratosis

hyper-granulosis

hyperplastic epidermis

basket-weave pattern

thin granular layer

thin suprapapillary plate

papillo-matosis

ACANTHOSIS nigricans and nevus verrucosus are processes that affect the papillary dermis and the epidermis. Both conditions may show hyperkeratosis, epidermal hyperpigmentation, papillomatosis, melanophages, and an increased number of fibroblasts in a thickened pale-staining papillary dermis.

Nevus verrucosus is an epidermal nevus, one among many. It usually starts to develop at birth or shortly thereafter in the form of tan to brown, rough-surfaced, warty lesions. Like most other epidermal nevi of this type, nevus verrucosus is usually distributed in a circumscribed or systematized fashion, i.e., unilaterally in linear or zosteriform pattern and occasionally widespread, e.g., to half the body. All epidermal nevi that are unilateral are also termed nevus unius lateris. Rarely, nevus verrucosus may be universal. These criteria for nevus verrucosus apply equally to other epidermal nevi such as those characterized histologically by epidermolytic hyperkeratosis (traditionally known as bullous congenital ichthyosiform erythroderma when widespread and as ichthyosis hystrix when limited), focal acantholytic dyskeratosis (which clinically resembles Darier's disease), cornoid lamellation (which clinically resembles porokeratosis), and seborrheic keratosis-like changes.

In contrast, acanthosis nigricans is of two types—one congenital, the other acquired. Clinically both are smooth rather than rough-surfaced and histologically they are papillomatoses rather than papillated epidermal hyperplasias. Histologically acanthosis nigricans is mostly an abnormality of the papillary dermis. The velvety, soft, tan to gray-brown excrescenses of acanthosis nigricans tend to develop especially in intertriginous regions such as the axillae and groins; the neck, umbilicus, and nipples are other favored areas. Acanthosis nigricans may develop as an autosomal dominantly transmitted congenital anomaly in childhood ("benign" acanthosis nigricans), as an aspect of underlying endocrinologic abnormality such as acromegaly, gigantism, diabetes insipidus, Cushing's disease; from obesity and ingestion of medications such as corticosteroids and nicotinic acid ("pseudo"-acanthosis nigricans); and finally as a portentous manifestation of an occult malignancy, usually an adenocarcinoma of the gastrointestinal or genital tracts, breast, or lung ("malignant" acanthosis nigricans). Each of these forms of acanthosis nigricans, irrespective of the underlying cause, has essentially the same clinical and histologic features.

There are other systematized congenital anomalies that have clinical and histologic features of acanthosis nigricans, some of such marked papillomatosis that they resemble confluent fibro-epithelial polyps or papillomas (skin "tags", acrochorda). Those that are marked by papillomatosis rather than by papillated epidermal hyperplasia should not be confused with epidermal nevi of the type in point, but rather malformations of the papillary dermis or perhaps mixed papillary dermal-epidermal nevi. The confluent and reticulated papillomatoses of Gougerot and Carteaud also resemble acanthosis nigricans histologically.

The rough surface of nevus verrucosus signifies that it is fundamentally a verrucous hyperkeratosis, whereas the smooth papillated surface of acanthosis nigricans indicates that it is primarily a papillomatosis rather than a hyperkeratosis.

25. Porokeratosis *vs.* Inflammatory Linear Verrucous Epidermal Nevus

<table>
<tr><th>Porokeratosis</th><th>Inflammatory Linear Verrucous Epidermal Nevus</th></tr>
<tr><td>1. Tall, thin, sharply circumscribed columns of parakeratosis (cornoid lamellae)</td><td>1. Moderately well circumscribed, short, broad columns of parakeratosis</td></tr>
<tr><td>2. Columns of parakeratosis are usually slightly off perpendicular to the skin surface</td><td>2. Columns of parakeratosis are perpendicular to the skin surface</td></tr>
<tr><td>3. Parakeratotic columns may arise from epidermis, acrosyringia, or infundibula</td><td>3. Parakeratotic columns arise from epidermis only</td></tr>
<tr><td>4. Columns of parakeratosis are usually situated in the valleys between papillations of hyperplastic epidermis</td><td>4. Columns of parakeratosis are usually at the summits of the epidermal papillations</td></tr>
<tr><td>5. Between areas of parakeratosis the stratum corneum is hyperkeratotic, alternating in basket-weave and compact pattern</td><td>5. Between areas of parakeratosis the stratum corneum is hyperkeratotic in compact pattern</td></tr>
<tr><td>6. Beneath the parakeratotic zones, no granular layer, but dyskeratotic and vacuolated cells</td><td>6. Beneath the parakeratotic zones, no granular layer and no dyskeratotic or vacuolated cells</td></tr>
<tr><td>7. Beneath areas of orthokeratosis, granular layer normal or thickened</td><td>7. Beneath areas of orthokeratosis, granular layer thickened</td></tr>
<tr><td>8. Epidermis papillated, psoriasiform, or atrophic depending upon the type of porokeratosis and the stage of the disease</td><td>8. Epidermis hyperplastic, usually papillated and psoriasiform</td></tr>
<tr><td>9. Lichenoid infiltrate of lymphocytes and histiocytes in early lesions of the disseminated superficial type</td><td>9. Superficial perivascular lympho-histiocytic infiltrate</td></tr>
</table>

Porokeratosis

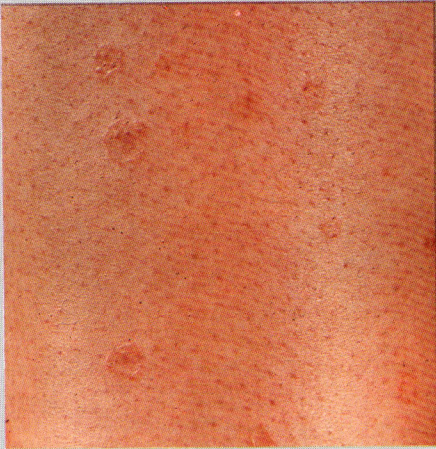

Inflammatory Linear Verrucous Epidermal Nevus

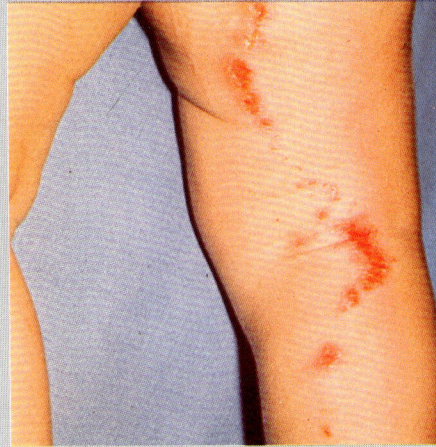

thin zone of para-keratosis

perivascular infiltrate of lymphocytes

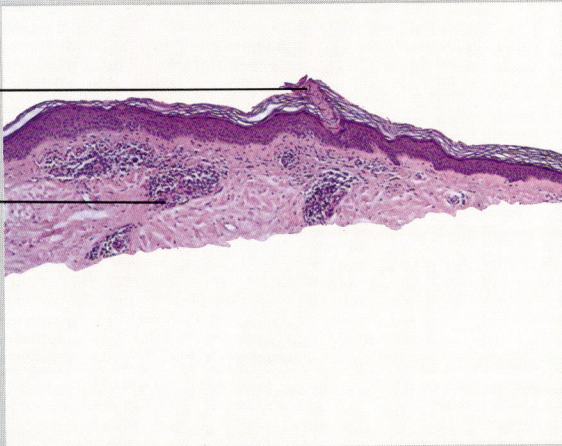

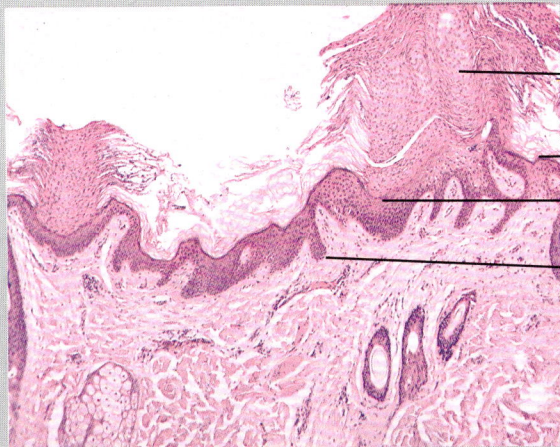

discrete broad zone of parakeratosis

orthokeratosis

focal hypo-granulosis

slight psoriasiform hyperplasia

cornoid lamella oriented at an angle

basket-weave cornified layer

lymphocytes

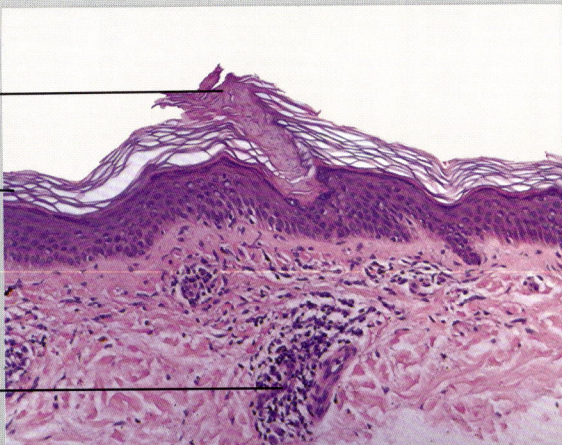

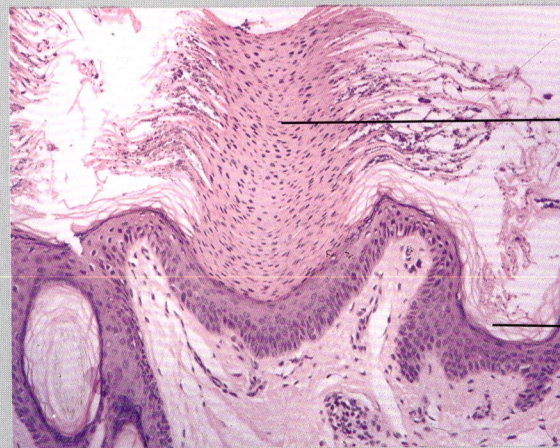

broad focus of parakeratosis in vertical orientation

basket-weave orthokeratosis

cornoid lamella

cornified cells in basket-weave pattern

hypo-granulosis

dyskeratotic cell

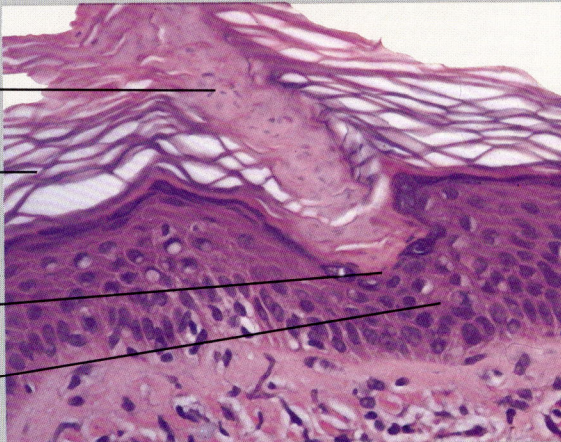

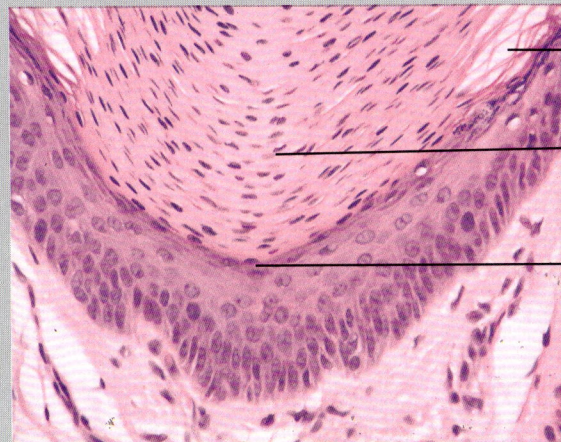

basket-weave orthokeratosis

parakeratosis

hypo-granulosis

HE various forms of porokeratosis and the inflammatory linear verrucous epidermal nevus have in common well circumscribed zones of parakeratosis beneath which the granular layer is absent and a lympho-histiocytic infiltrate around telangiectases in the upper part of the dermis. The porokeratoses and inflammatory linear verrucous epidermal nevi are diseases that involve the epidermis predominantly, but also the papillary dermis to some extent.

There are several varieties of porokeratosis, namely, porokeratosis of Mibelli, nevoid linear porokeratosis, punctate porokeratosis of the palms and soles, widespread punctate porokeratosis, and disseminated superficial porokeratosis (actinic and non-actinic). The first of these to be recognized was porokeratosis of Mibelli, a genodermatosis that is inherited as an autosomal dominant trait. It may appear at any age, usually early in childhood. The clinical lesions are papules and plaques that are sharply delimited from the surrounding normal skin by a keratotic ridge with a slight central depression in it. The centers of the lesions eventually become atrophic. Lesions of porokeratosis of Mibelli may appear on any part of the skin and may even involve mucous membranes. They are asymptomatic and tend to increase in number and size; some may resolve spontaneously.

A disseminated superficial type of porokeratosis, which is now the commonest form of porokeratosis, was described in recent years by Chernosky. It appears as a few or many round or oval lesions rimmed by a thread-like keratotic border. Early in their evolution the centers are erythematous but, in time, they become whitish and atrophic. Lesions of disseminated superficial porokeratosis have a predilection for sites that are ordinarily exposed to sunlight, but indistinguishable lesions may appear on other parts not sun-exposed, such as the palms, soles, and genitals. Prior to their recognition as distinctive, the lesions of disseminated superficial actinic porokeratosis were usually deemed to be nothing more than solar keratoses.

Thin cornoid lamellae make up the thread-like rims of lesions in all forms of porokeratosis and dense lichenoid lympho-histiocytic infiltrates around dilated blood-filled vessels are responsible for the erythematous centers of early lesions of the disseminated superficial type. Clinical atrophy results from both alteration of the papillary dermis by coarse collagen fibers and from effacement of the normal undulating pattern between rete ridges and dermal papillae. Rarely, a squamous-cell carcinoma may develop in the atrophic center of a lesion of porokeratosis.

The inflammatory linear verrucous epidermal nevus appears at birth or shortly thereafter as a linear or patchy aggregation of reddish, scaly papules, usually, for reasons hard to understand, on the left leg. An arm may also be involved. Clinically, the condition must be differentiated from other examples of nevus unius lateris and from linear psoriasis, linear lichen planus, and lichen striatus.

26. Amputation Neuroma Secondary to Supernumerary Digit *vs.* Acquired Digital Fibrokeratoma

Amputation Neuroma Secondary to Supernumerary Digit	*Acquired Digital Fibrokeratoma*
1. Increased number of large nerve trunks (axons) throughout the specimen	1. Normal number and size of nerve structures within the specimen
2. Nerve trunks and collagen bundles perpendicular to the skin surface (i.e., parallel to the original elongated anomaly)	2. Collagen fibers arranged haphazardly
3. Fibroblasts increased in number occasionally, but in the main of normal morphology	3. Fibroblasts markedly increased in number and large, stellate, or multinucleated usually
4. Collagen bundles thick and coarse	4. Collagen mostly fibrillar, but coarse

Amputation Neuroma Secondary to Supernumerary Digit

Acquired Digital Fibrokeratoma

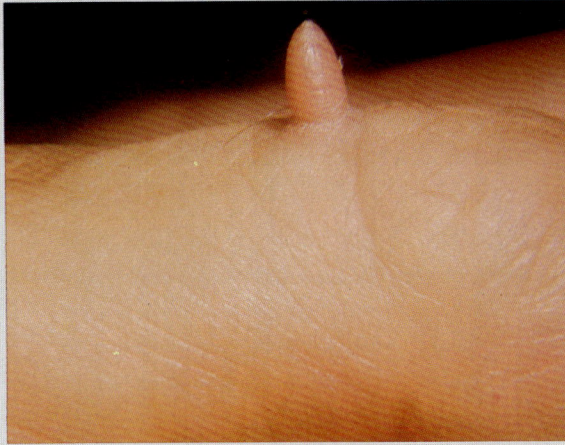

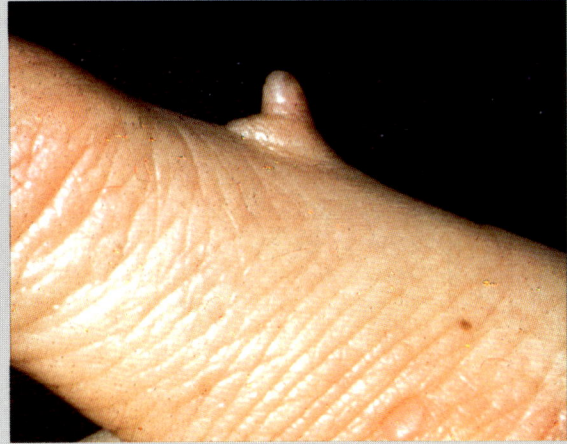

cornified layer of volar skin

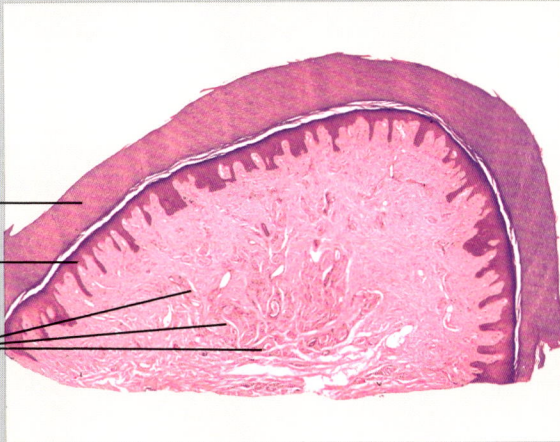

nearly normal epidermis

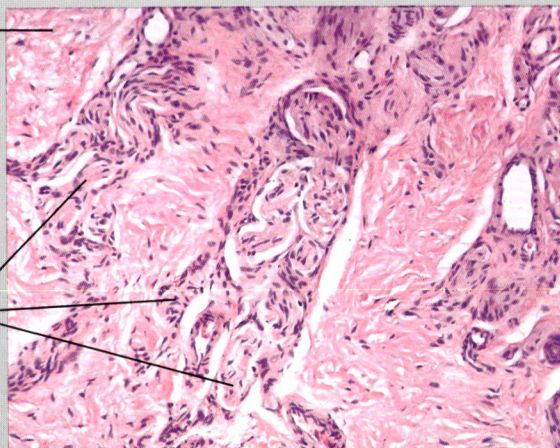

nerve fascicles

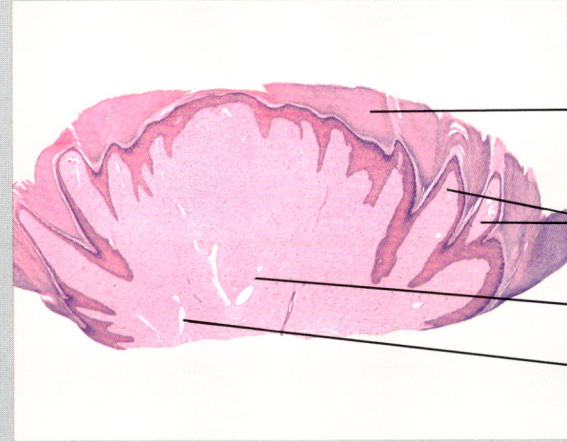

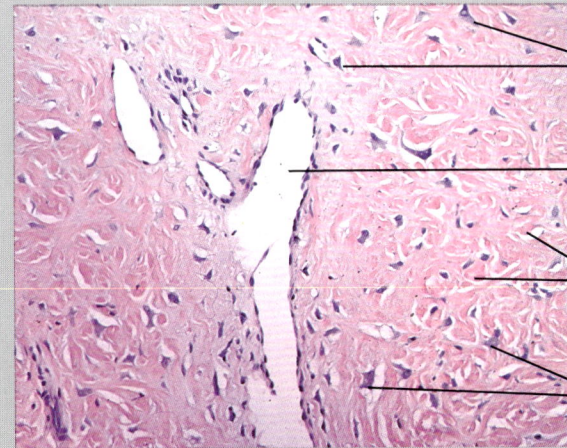

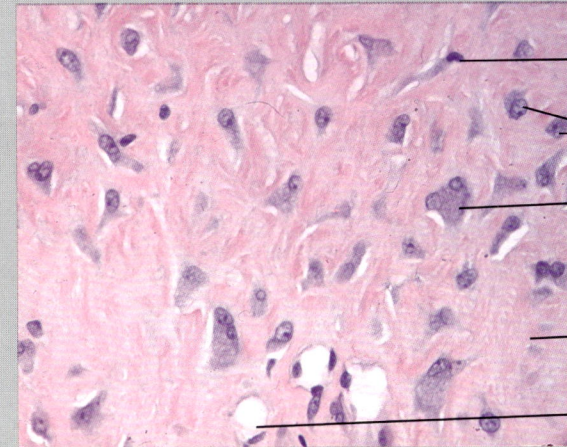

cornified layer of volar skin

papillomatosis beneath thinned epidermis

fibromatous dermis

dilated blood vessel

normal dermis

nerve fascicles

stellate fibroblasts

widely dilated blood vessel

short collagen bundles in haphazard array

multinucleated stellate fibroblasts

normal bundle of collagen

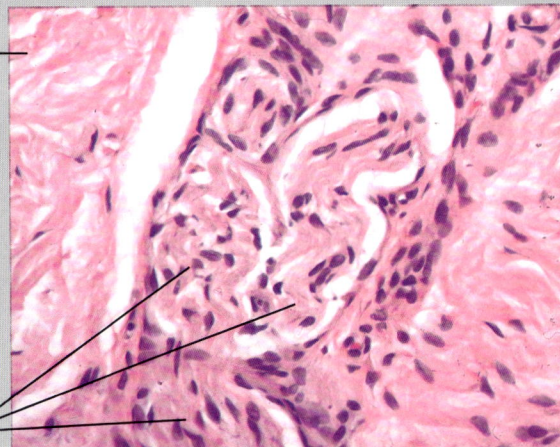

nerve fascicles

elongated fibroblast

plump fibroblasts

multinucleated stellate fibroblast

coarse collagen

dilated blood vessel

THE clinical features common to amputation neuroma secondary to rudimentary supernumerary digit and acquired digital fibrokeratoma are location and shape. Both occur on or near fingers and both are polypoid projections. In addition, both lesions are firm and keratotic because they are abnormalities of connective tissue covered by hyperkeratotic hyperplastic epidermis. The amputation neuromas are constituted mostly of neural tissues; acquired digital fibrokeratomas have fibrous tissue cores. In both conditions, widely dilated blood vessels are usually present in the uppermost portion of the dermis, as are extravasated erythrocytes, which often are found in the epidermis, too.

Amputation neuromas secondary to supernumerary digits are present at birth and are stubs that represent neural remnants in skin from supernumerary digits lost, presumably, in utero. Amputation neuromas usually occur in pairs at the lateral aspects of the fifth fingers of the hands. They are comparable to those neuromas that develop later in life at sites of surgical amputations, but are differentiated from them histologically by the polypoid shape and the cornified layer characteristic of volar skin.

A persistent supernumerary digit is not a neuroma, but a miniature digit composed of bone, cartilage, muscle, and other components of a normal finger such as nail plate.

In contrast, an acquired digital fibrokeratoma usually presents itself as a solitary excrescence that arises from the skin near interphalangeal joints of a finger of an adult. The projection is usually elongated (polypoid), sometimes domed (sessile), but always keratotic.

Histologically, acquired digital fibrokeratoma is a type of angiofibroma and is similar to the sub- and periungual fibromas that develop in children with tuberous sclerosis. Other angiofibromas that have histologic features in common with acquired digital fibrokeratomas are the papules of adenoma sebaceum, fibrous papules of the face, some perifollicular fibromas, pearly penile papules, and oral fibromas. The common denominators of these angiofibromas are marked vascularity and fibroplasia of mostly fibrillar collagen associated with an increased number of large, stellate, and often multinucleated fibroblasts. Such fibroblasts suggest active proliferation and manufacture of connective tissue. Darkly staining inclusions are sometimes present in the cytoplasms of these striking-looking fibroblasts.

There is an interesting parallel between fibrous papules of the face and acquired digital fibrokeratomas on the one hand, and the cutaneous angiofibromas of tuberous sclerosis on the other. Fibrous papules of the face are histologically indistinguishable from the lesions of adenoma sebaceum in tuberous sclerosis, and acquired digital fibrokeratomas are also microscopically indistinguishable from the subungual and periungual fibromas in tuberous sclerosis. It also may be worthy of notice that the strikingly apparent fibroblasts in the cutaneous angiofibromas of tuberous sclerosis resemble closely the glial cells in the intracranial tubers of that multisystemic disease.

27. Verruca Vulgaris
vs. Digitated Solar Keratosis

Verruca Vulgaris	Digitated Solar Keratosis
1. Compact orthokeratosis with focal parakeratosis mostly at the tips of the digitations	1. Parakeratosis in well-circumscribed broad columns alternating with thin columns of orthokeratosis
2. Hemorrhage in the parakeratotic foci at the tips of epidermal projections	2. No hemorrhage at tips of epidermal projections usually
3. Granular zone intact or thickened	3. Granular zone diminished or absent beneath areas of parakeratosis
4. Clear spaces of various sizes around nuclei ("owl eyes") in the spinous and granular zones	4. No cells with "owl eyes"
5. Few atypical keratinocytes, dyskeratotic cells, and mitotic figures, but those usually in the region of the basal layer	5. Many atypical keratinocytes, some dyskeratotic cells, and mitotic figures in the lower half of the epidermis
6. No buds of atypical keratinocytes	6. Buds of atypical keratinocytes extend into papillary dermis
7. No suprabasal clefts	7. Suprabasal clefts occasionally, often containing acantholytic dyskeratotic cells
8. Arborization (inward turning of outermost elongated epithelial adnexa)	8. No arborization
9. Intraepidermal epithelial structures of adnexa (acrosyringia and acrotrichia) affected by the pathological process	9. Intraepidermal epithelial structures of adnexa (acrosyringia and acrotrichia) spared by the pathological process
10. Marked tortuosity of blood vessels in elongated dermal papillae	10. Slight tortuosity of blood vessels in elongated dermal papillae
11. Slight to moderately dense lympho-histiocytic infiltrate in the upper part of the dermis	11. Moderately to markedly dense lympho-histiocytic infiltrate in the upper part of the dermis
12. Solar elastosis uncommon and incidental	12. Solar elastosis always and essential

Verruca Vulgaris

Digitated Solar Keratosis

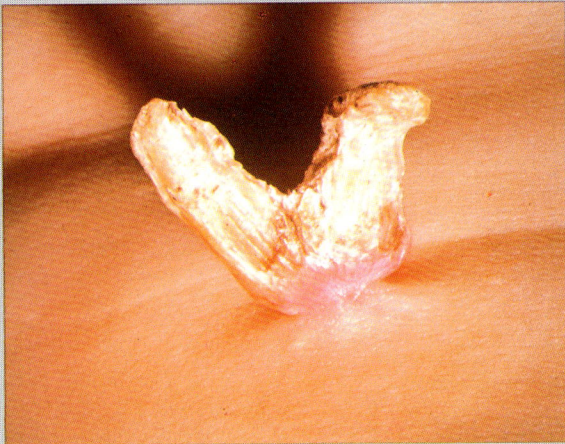

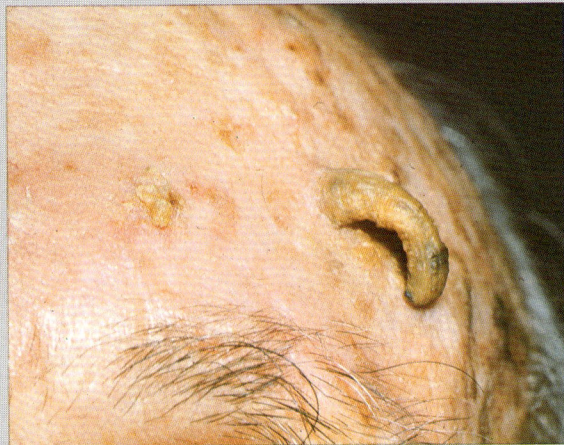

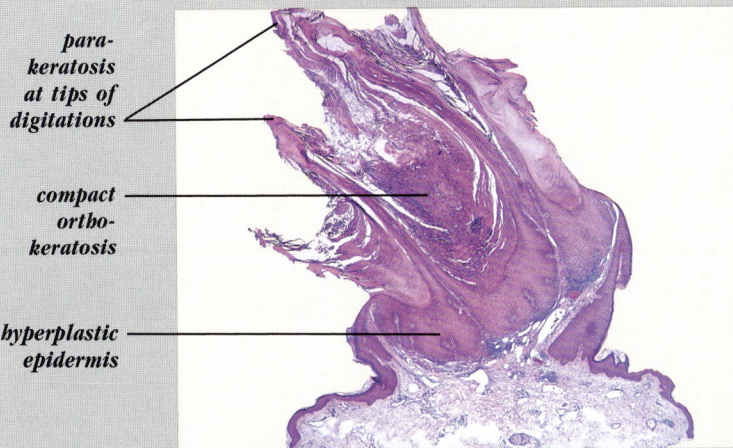

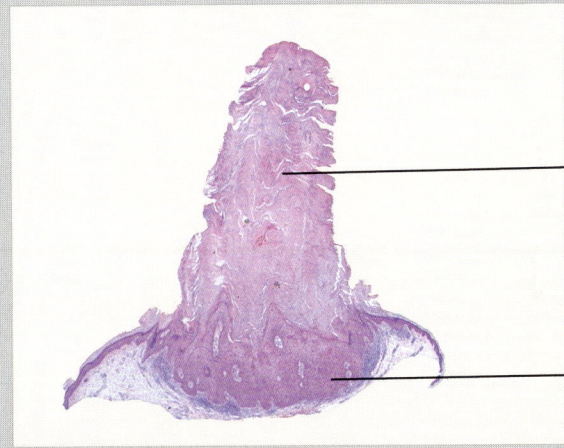

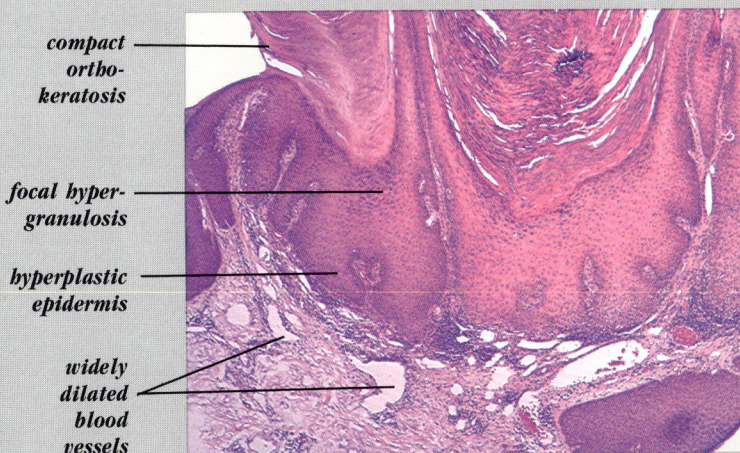

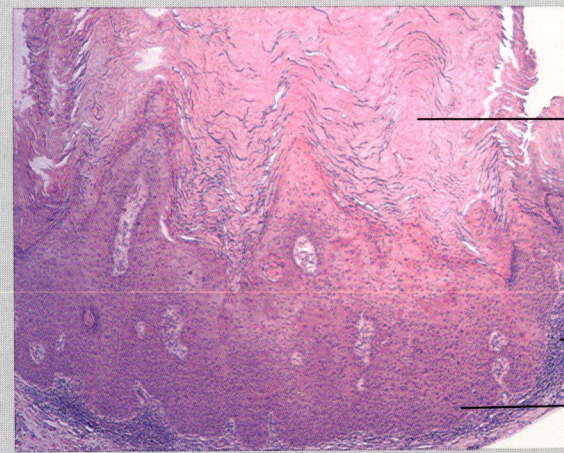

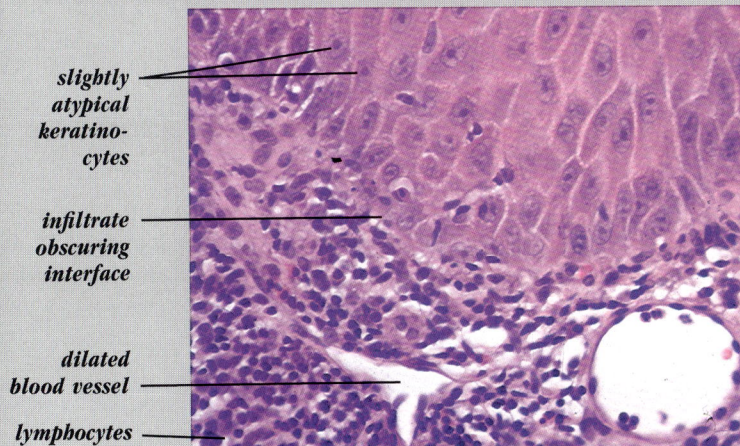

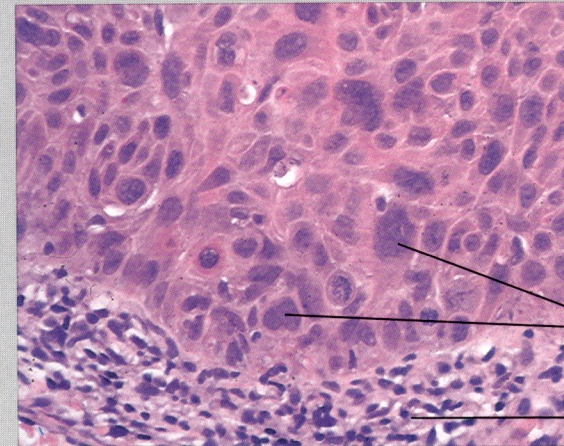

para-
keratosis
at tips of
digitations

mostly
parakeratosis

compact
ortho-
keratosis

atypical
keratinocytes
in thickened
epidermis

hyperplastic
epidermis

compact
ortho-
keratosis

parakeratosis

focal hyper-
granulosis

hyperplastic
epidermis

widely
dilated
blood
vessels

lymphocytes

atypical
keratinocytes

slightly
atypical
keratino-
cytes

infiltrate
obscuring
interface

dilated
blood vessel

atypical
nuclei of
keratinocytes

lymphocytes

lymphocytes

ALTHOUGH old verrucae vulgares and digitated solar keratoses are both examples of hyperkeratotic papillated epidermal hyperplasias, there are critical differences between them. Solar keratoses are atypical keratinocytic hyperplasias of epidermal keratinocytes, but not those of intraepidermal epithelial structures of adnexa, the eccrine sweat ducts (acrosyringia) and the hair follicles (acrotrichia). The cytologically atypical epidermal keratinocytes of solar keratoses produce parakeratosis. In contrast, the epidermal cells of old warts have only little cytologic atypicality and manufacture mostly orthokeratotic cells. The epithelial adnexa arborize in a wart, but not in a solar keratosis. Old warts differ from young warts by being less digitated and having no large nuclei in the cornified cells, less hypergranulosis, and less vacuolated cytoplasm in the upper portion of the epidermis.

The histologic differentiation of warts from solar keratoses is of more than academic interest because verrucae almost always behave in a wholly benign fashion, whereas solar keratoses tend to progress to squamous-cell carcinomas if untreated. In fact, however, squamous-cell carcinomas that develop in sun-damaged skin rarely metastasize.

Although the histologic differential between warts and solar keratoses may be difficult, their clinical differentiation often is even more so. Both may present themselves as cutaneous horns, i.e., hyperkeratotic projections above the skin surface. The term cutaneous horn is purely clinical. The clinician can but speculate about what lies beneath a cutaneous horn, a verruca, solar keratosis, squamous-cell carcinoma, and so on. Only histologic study of the lesion can resolve the uncertainty.

Verruca vulgaris may occur both in children and adults and on any area of the body, but they are more common on the fingers and hands. Warts are caused by a virus of the papova group.

Solar keratoses occur on areas of sun exposure, usually in older individuals with fair complexions. They are caused by the effects of sunlight on the epidermis and the dermis.

A subject of some debate among pathologists is the question of when a lesion marked by atypical keratinocytic hyperplasia (or neoplasia) should be diagnosed as "solar keratosis" and when it should be considered "squamous-cell carcinoma." The old shibboleth that the neoplasm is a squamous-cell carcinoma when it has "broken through the basement membrane" seems to have been abandoned by most pathologists. The concept of "invasion" is equally vague, because a wholly benign neoplasm like keratoacanthoma may be more "invasive" than many squamous-cell carcinomas.

What then is the boundary that enables a pathologist to separate solar keratosis (or any squamous-cell carcinoma in situ, for that matter) from squamous-cell carcinoma? There is no clear-cut boundary, like a goal line in football, because these two conditions often form a continuum. For purposes of communication, we diagnose as solar keratoses those lesions whose atypical keratinocytes are confined to the papillary dermis. If the same lesion at a later time had extended into the reticular dermis, we would have designated it a squamous-cell carcinoma.

Perhaps the thickness of neoplasms composed of atypical keratinocytes should be measured as they are for neoplasms composed of atypical melanocytes. Unlike the situation with malignant melanomas, a correlation between thickness of squamous-cell carcinomas and likelihood of metastasis has yet to be established.

28. Leukokeratosis

vs. Leukoplakia

Leukokeratosis

1. Orthokeratosis with few parakeratotic cells

2. Hypergranulosis

3. Slight to moderate regular epithelial hyperplasia.

4. No atypical keratinocytes

5. No dyskeratotic cells

6. Slight perivascular mononuclear-cell infiltrate

Leukoplakia

1. Parakeratosis with few orthokeratotic cells

2. No granular layer usually

3. Moderate to marked irregular epithelial hyperplasia

4. Atypical keratinocytes

5. Many dyskeratotic cells

6. Moderately dense perivascular mononuclear-cell infiltrate

Leukokeratosis

Leukoplakia

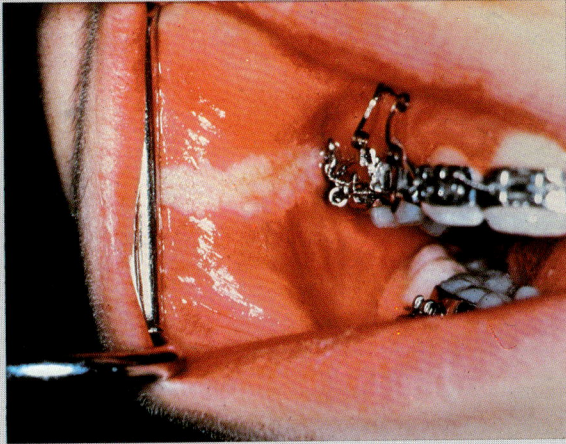

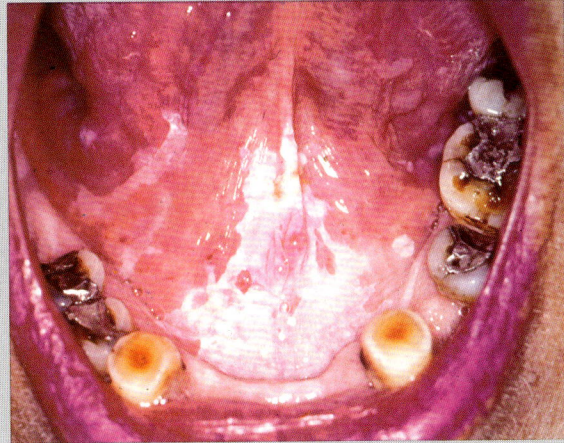

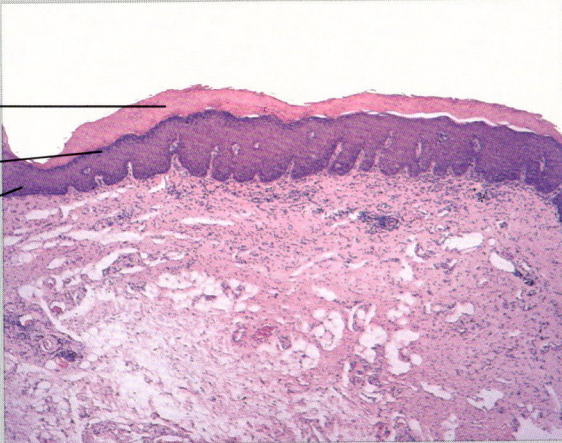

compact
ortho-
keratosis

hyper-
granulosis

epithelial
hyperplasia

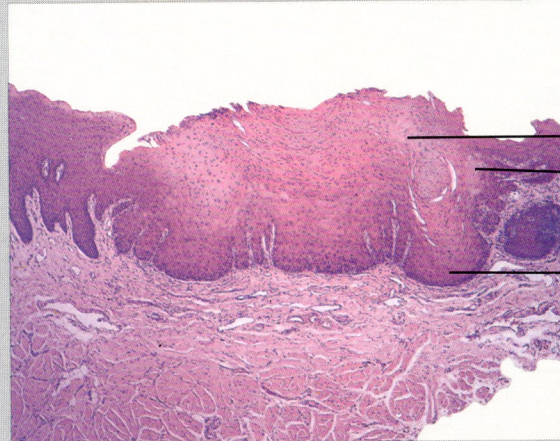

parakeratosis

no granular
layer

atypical
epithelial
neoplasia

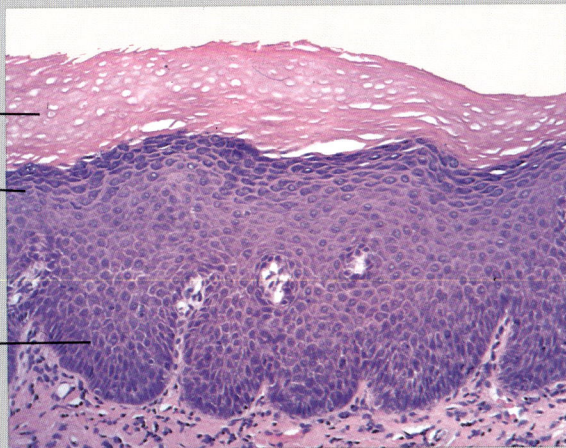

compact
ortho-
keratosis

hyper-
granulosis

no atypical
nuclei in
hyperplastic
epithelium

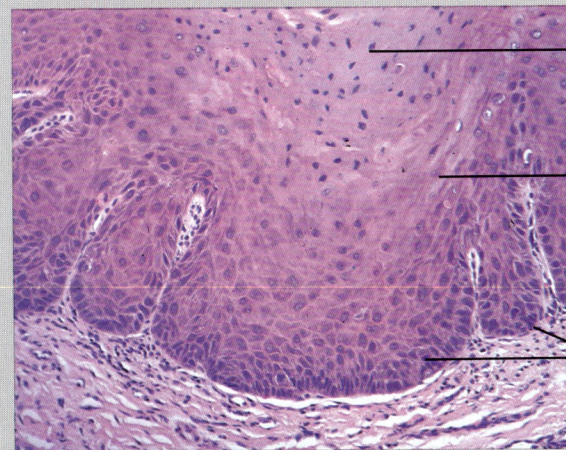

parakeratosis

no granular
layer

atypical
nuclei in
neoplastic
epithelium

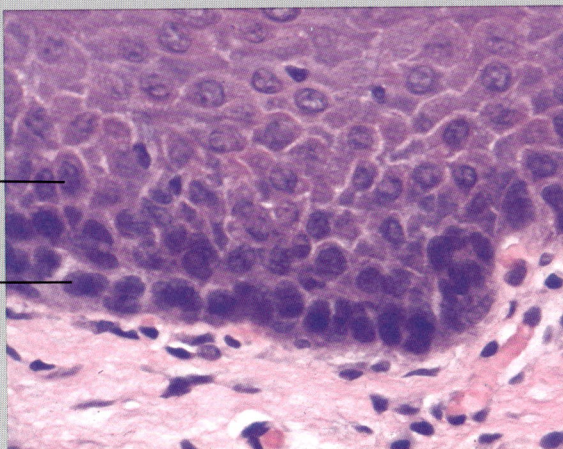

no nuclear
atypia

nuclei of
basal cells
aligned

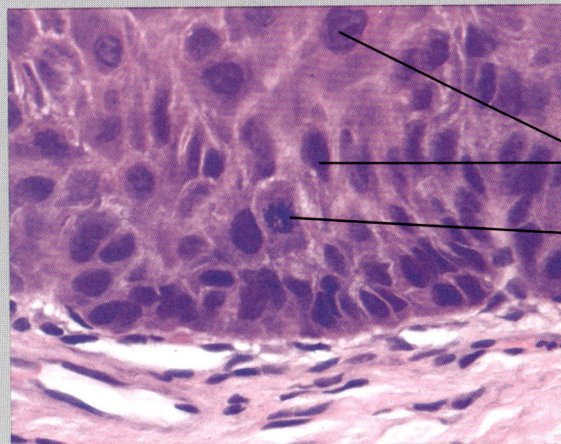

nuclear
atypia

mitotic
figure

nuclei of
basal cells in
disarray

L EUKOKERATOSIS and leukoplakia are white, relatively flat, nonindurated lesions of the mucosae (especially of the mouth, but also of the vagina, and so on) that have histologic features in common—hyperkeratosis, epithelial hyperplasia, and an inflammatory-cell infiltrate of mononuclear cells. The white color (leuko-) in both leukokeratosis and leukoplakia results from the abnormal production of cornified cells.

The main difference between them lies in the atypicality of the keratinocytes (large, hyperchromatic, and pleomorphic nuclei with mitotic figures) in leukoplakia. We advocate the use of the term leukoplakia for those white lesions characterized by the histologic changes enumerated above, and not as a clinical diagnosis for any white lesions on mucous membranes, such as those of lichen planus or lichen sclerosus et atrophicus.

Thus leukoplakia is the mucous membrane analogue of solar keratosis, namely, an atypical keratinocytic hyperplasia (or neoplasia) with characteristic clinical and histologic features. The cause of oral leukoplakia is elusive, but surely smoking is a factor in many instances. Another whitish lesion of mucous membranes that clinically may present a problem of differential diagnosis is candidiasis. The cornified layer of such a lesion teems with hyphae.

The importance of making a definite diagnosis of leukoplakia is that a neglected lesion may eventuate in a squamous-cell carcinoma, in the same manner in which solar keratosis may evolve into squamous-cell carcinoma. Unlike most cutaneous squamous-cell carcinomas of sun-damaged skin, however, mucosal squamous-cell carcinoma behaves biologically in a more aggressive fashion and may metastasize.

In contrast, leukokeratosis oris is a wholly benign condition that may revert to the normal condition once its cause is removed. The most common cause of leukokeratosis oris is persistent trauma or friction by dentures, maloccluded teeth, or habitual biting of the lips or buccal mucosa. In short, leukokeratosis is lichen simplex chronicus of the hyperkeratotic type on mucous membranes.

The atypical nuclei in leukoplakia, like those in solar keratosis, reside in the lower portion of the epithelium. In squamous-cell carcinoma in situ, atypical nuclei are present throughout the entire thickness of the epithelium. As long as the atypical keratinocytes are situated superficially in mucous membranes and in skin, as they are in leukoplakia, solar keratosis, and squamous-cell carcinoma in situ, the lesion is benign biologically, i.e., such lesions do not metastasize. Nevertheless, each of these atypical keratinocytic hyperplasias or neoplasias should be removed completely in order to prevent the development of true squamous-cell carcinomas that may metastasize.

Some clinical lesions of leukoplakia have reddish areas interspersed among the whitish zones, and still other lesions are mostly reddish. The name erythroplakia has been given to those mostly reddish lesions on mucous membranes that, like leukoplakia, are characterized histologically by atypical keratinocytes in the lower portion of the epithelium and that, if left untreated, may progress to indubitable squamous-cell carcinoma.

In summary, just as solar keratoses may be mostly whitish or reddish clinically depending on the amount of cornification, so too, their analogues on mucous membranes may be mostly whitish (i.e., leukoplakia) or reddish (i.e., erythroplakia) for the same reason.

29. Seborrheic Keratosis, Acanthotic Type *vs.* Eccrine Poroma

Seborrheic Keratosis, Acanthotic Type

1. Sharply circumscribed sessile exo-endophytic neoplasm

2. Delicate-basket-weave and laminated ortho-keratosis

3. Thick interlacing tracts of basaloid cells; tracts extend into the dermis to approximately the same level (usually only into the thickened papillary dermis)

4. Basaloid cells merge with spinous cells near the skin surface, around follicular epithelium, and around horn pseudocysts

5. Pale cells rarely present

6. Squamous eddies (whorls of squamous cells) common, especially secondary to irritation and consequent inflammation

7. No increased number of mitotic figures

8. Melanin in basaloid cells common

9. No necrotic cells as a rule

10. Horn pseudocysts usually

11. No ductal structures

12. No separation of the neoplasm from the surrounding stroma

13. Dilated blood vessels with numerous melanophages in the thickened papillary dermis occasionally

14. Lymphocytic infiltrate occasionally

15. In the same lesion other variants of seborrheic keratosis (e.g., verrucous, adenoid) occasionally

Eccrine Poroma

1. Sharply circumscribed polypoid or sessile predominantly endophytic neoplasm

2. Alternating ortho- and parakeratosis

3. Interconnected lobules of basaloid cells; lobules vary in sizes and shapes and extend from the epidermis into the dermis at different depths (often into the reticular dermis)

4. Basaloid cells at the periphery of the neoplasm are sharply demarcated from the contiguous spinous cells of the normal epidermis

5. Numerous foci of pale cells

6. Squamous eddies rare

7. Increased number of mitotic figures

8. Melanin in basaloid cells rare

9. Many necrotic cells, individual and in aggregate

10. No horn pseudocysts

11. Duct-like spaces lined by an eosinophilic cuticle frequent

12. Lobules of neoplasm separated from the surrounding stroma by clefts occasionally

13. Stroma composed of granulation tissue often; stroma sometimes mucinous

14. Lymphocytic infiltrate common

15. In the same lesion other hamartomas and neoplasms with eccrine sweat duct and gland differentiation occasionally

Seborrheic Keratosis, Acanthotic Type

Eccrine Poroma

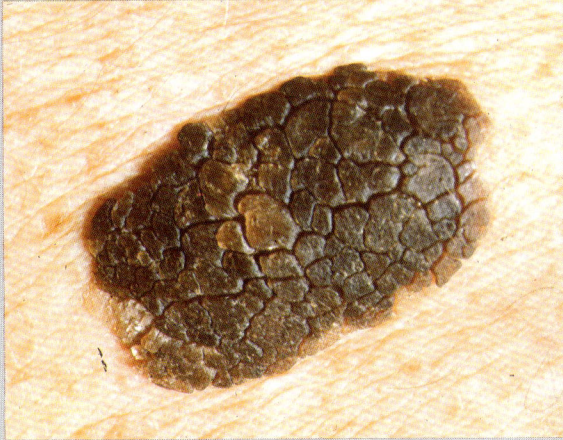

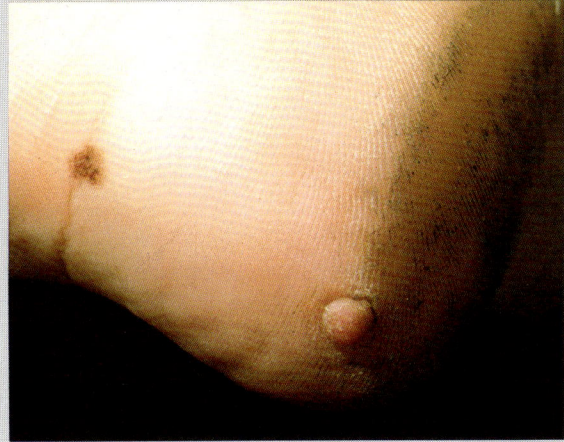

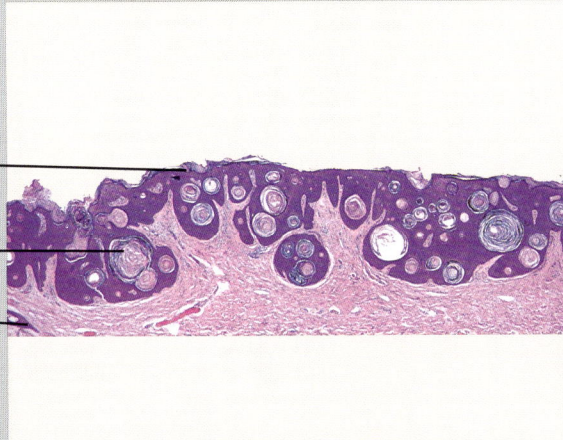

ortho-
keratosis

horn
pseudocyst

collarette of
epithelium

crust

focal
parakeratosis

prominent
stroma

basaloid cells

collarette of
epithelium

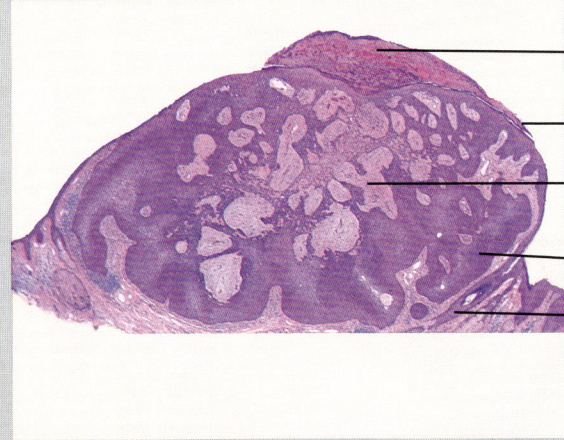

cornified
cells in
basket-
weave array

squamoid
cells

delicate
laminated
cornified
cells in
horn
pseudocysts

basaloid
cells

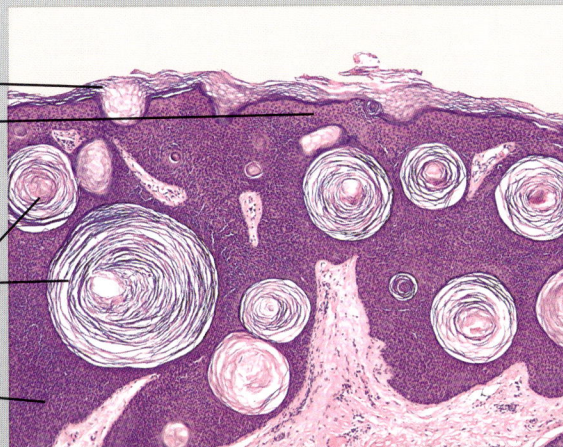

mucin in
stroma

basaloid cells

stroma highly
vascular

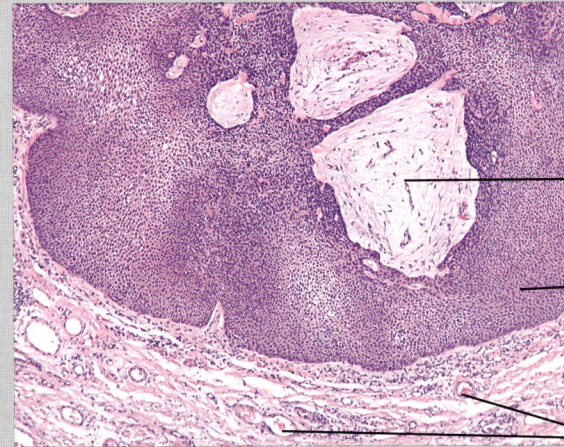

squamoid
cells

horn
pseudocyst

granular
cells around
pseudocyst

basaloid
cells

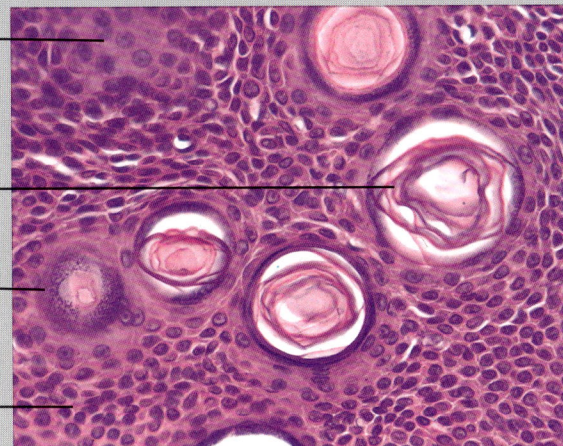

basaloid cells

structures
resembling
eccrine ducts

dilated blood
vessel

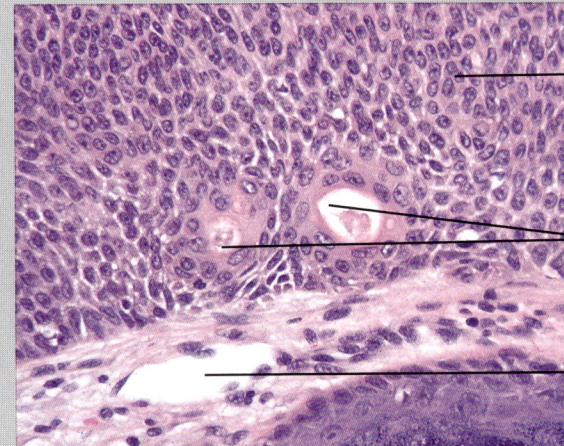

Seborrheic keratosis of the acanthotic type
and eccrine poroma are both benign epithelial growths, partially endophytic, composed of basaloid cells, and may be associated with amyloid in the dermis.

Seborrheic keratoses are common lesions that are often present in large numbers in older persons especially on the face, scalp, and trunk. They are relatively soft and have a surface that varies from flat to verrucous and a color that ranges from light tan to black. Because they are easily irritated, often artifactually by the patient, a variety of histologic changes develop in seborrheic keratoses. They range from squamous eddies to atypia that may simulate squamous-cell carcinoma. Of the three major patterns of seborrheic keratoses, namely acanthotic, adenoid (reticulated), and verrucous, only the acanthotic presents a problem in differential diagnosis from eccrine poroma.

Eccrine poroma is a relatively uncommon neoplasm that occurs predominantly on the palms and soles, but may also arise in any portion of the skin. Clinically, the eccrine poroma is usually a solitary firm lesion that may be a relatively flat-topped plaque, but more commonly is sessile or pedunculated. The abundant granulation tissue in some of these lesions gives them the clinical appearance of pyogenic granuloma. The neoplasm differentiates in the direction of the cells that line the eccrine duct and thus should really be termed eccrine periporoma. Some eccrine poromas extend from the epidermis into the dermis and even into the subcutis. Dermal lesions that are morphologically identical to eccrine poroma but that may or may not be connected to the epidermis are termed "dermal duct tumors."

If many sections are cut through specimens of dermal duct tumors, histologic features of eccrine poroma often emerge. In short, in our view, "eccrine poroma" (superficial lesion) and "dermal duct tumor" (deeper lesion) are different names for one pathologic process at different stages in its evolution.

Some pathologists tend to speak and write of adnexal neoplasms "arising from" particular structures such as the eccrine pore or the dermal duct. In truth, there is no compelling evidence that eccrine poroma arises from cells that line the intraepidermal eccrine pore, or that dermal duct tumor arises from cells of the dermal duct.

What can be asserted with some certainty is that eccrine poroma and dermal duct tumor *differentiate toward* eccrine ducts because structures that resemble eccrine ducts so commonly appear within these neoplasms. Theoretically, any epithelial germinative cell in the skin could give rise to any epithelial neoplasm, including eccrine poroma and dermal duct tumor. On morphologic grounds alone, one could conclude that superficial basal-cell carcinomas *arise from* basal cells of the epidermis because the neoplastic cells are continuous with the epidermal basal layer.

Prior to the original description of eccrine poroma by Pinkus in 1956, that neoplasm was generally misinterpreted histologically as an acanthotic type of seborrheic keratosis. From time to time, these two lesions continue to pose problems in histologic differential diagnosis, which usually may be resolved if the tabulated criteria are employed.

30. Sebaceous Gland Hyperplasia
vs. Nevus Sebaceus
of Jadassohn

Sebaceous Gland Hyperplasia	*Nevus Sebaceus of Jadassohn*
1. Dome-shaped papule with a small central depression	1. Relatively flat-topped plaque in early stages; papillated or digitated plaque in late stage
2. Basket-weave pattern to cornified layer	2. Laminated and compact orthokeratotic cornified layer
3. Thinned or normal epidermis	3. Slight papillated epidermal hyperplasia, early; marked papillated or digitated epidermal hyperplasia, late
4. No papillomatosis	4. Prominent papillomatosis
5. A solitary, circumscribed conglomerate of several large sebaceous lobules	5. Few scattered small sebaceous lobules in early lesions; many scattered large sebaceous lobules in late lesions
6. Each of several sebaceous lobules connects to its own sebaceous duct	6. Sebaceous lobules often open directly into the epidermis, but sometimes connect to a common sebaceous duct
7. Sebaceous ducts open into a widely dilated common follicular infundibulum	7. Sebaceous ducts enter directly and individually into the epidermis usually, and directly into the follicular infundibulum on occasion
8. Normal sebaceous follicles or vellus hair follicles usually present within the lesion	8. No normal hair follicles within the lesion usually
9. No apocrine glands within the lesion	9. Many apocrine glands and ducts, especially in late lesions, sometimes
10. Solar elastosis common	10. Solar elastosis rare and then only in late lesions
11. No basal-cell hyperplasia, basal-cell carcinoma, or neoplasms with adnexal differentiation within the lesion	11. Basal-cell hyperplasia, basal-cell carcinoma, and neoplasms with adnexal differentiation often within the dermis of late lesions

Sebaceous Gland Hyperplasia

Nevus Sebaceus of Jadassohn

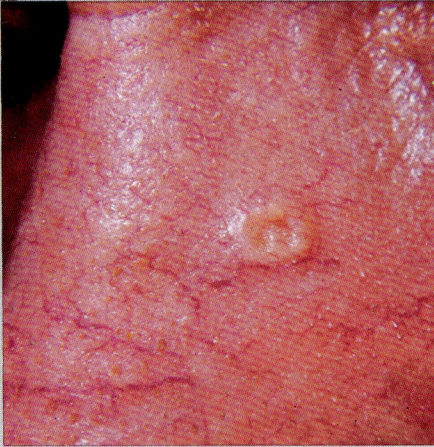

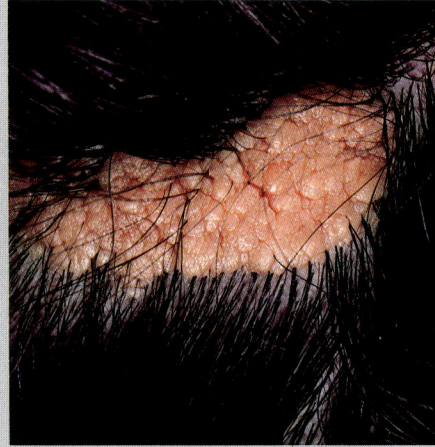

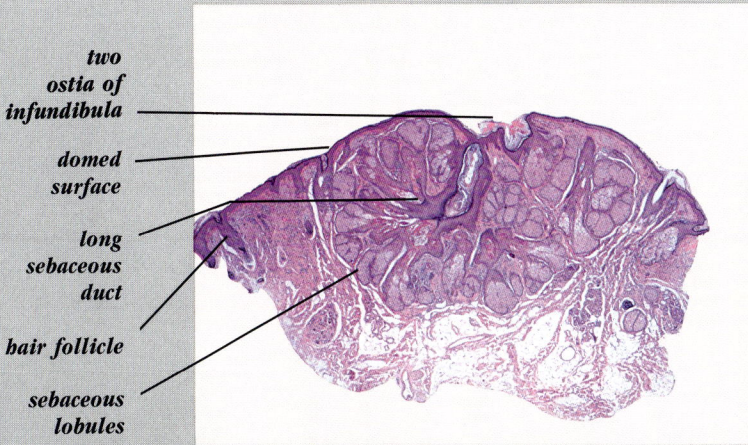

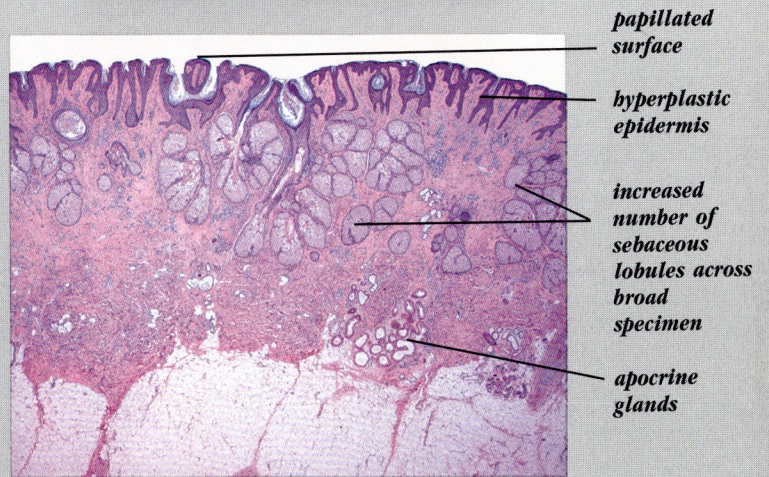

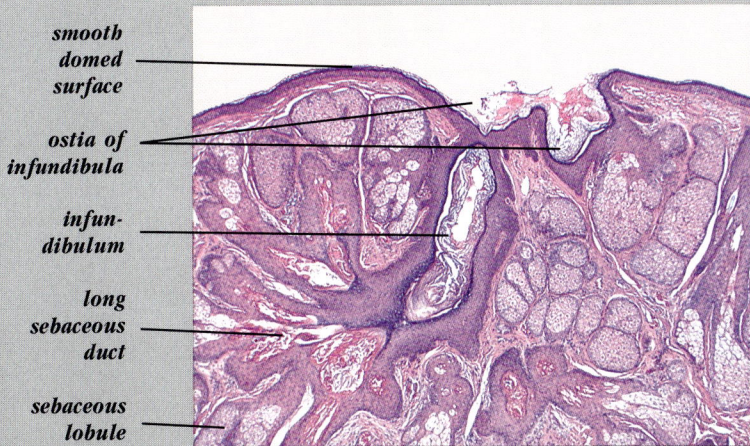

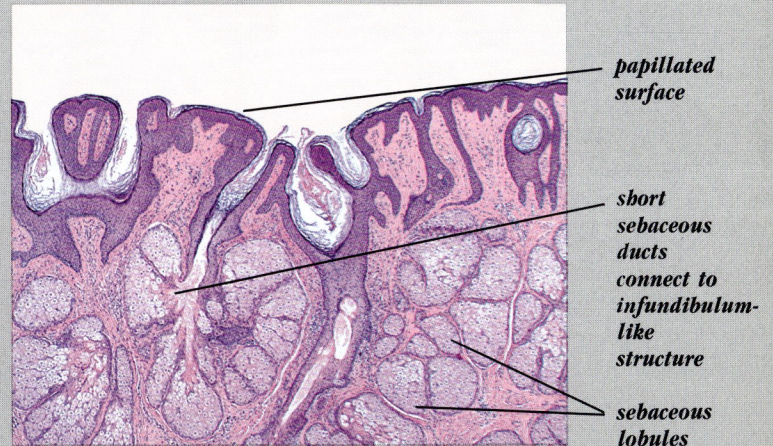

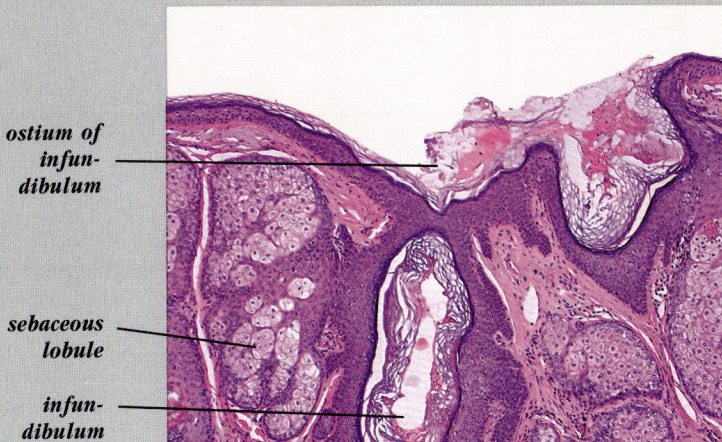

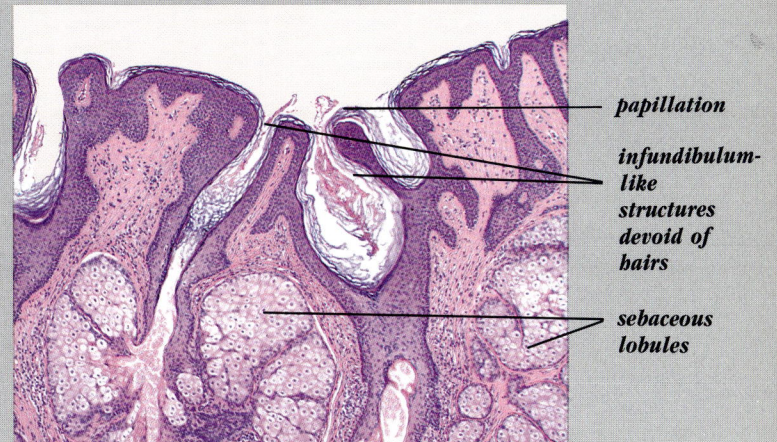

two ostia of infundibula

domed surface

long sebaceous duct

hair follicle

sebaceous lobules

papillated surface

hyperplastic epidermis

increased number of sebaceous lobules across broad specimen

apocrine glands

smooth domed surface

ostia of infundibula

infundibulum

long sebaceous duct

sebaceous lobule

papillated surface

short sebaceous ducts connect to infundibulum-like structure

sebaceous lobules

ostium of infundibulum

sebaceous lobule

infundibulum

papillation

infundibulum-like structures devoid of hairs

sebaceous lobules

BOTH sebaceous gland hyperplasia and nevus sebaceus of Jadassohn have abnormalities of sebaceous glands and both are also often associated with telangiectasias, a sparse to moderately dense lymphocytic infiltrate, and dilated sebaceous ducts. Sebaceous gland hyperplasia mostly affects sebaceous glands and follicular infundibula, whereas nevus sebaceus is a complex malformation that involves not only the sebaceous glands, but other adnexal epithelial structures, the epidermis, and the dermis.

The lesions of sebaceous gland hyperplasia are usually numerous, small, slightly yellowish papules with delicate rims and central depressions. They occur mostly in the elderly on the forehead, cheeks, and nose and a particular solitary lesion may be misinterpreted clinically as a basal-cell carcinoma because both conditions have slightly elevated borders and central dells. In basal-cell carcinoma the central depression often represents an erosion or ulceration, whereas in sebaceous gland hyperplasia it is the ostium of the dilated follicular infundibulum.

Sebaceous gland hyperplasia must also be differentiated histologically from sebaceous adenoma. Sebaceous hyperplasia is merely an exaggeration of a normal sebaceous follicle in which large lobules retain their original basic architecture and composition. The sebaceous adenoma also preserves the general architectural pattern of normal sebaceous follicles, but it is composed of many cell layers of peripheral germinative (undifferentiated basal) cells, rather than one germinative cell layer at the periphery, as is the case in the normal sebaceous lobule.

Nevus sebaceus of Jadassohn, usually a solitary lesion, tends to develop during prenatal life and is apparent at birth or early in neonatal life. Clinically and histologically, the lesions may be staged roughly in early (prepubertal) and late (post-pubertal) stages. Early lesions appear as smooth, relatively flat-surfaced, tan to brown, hairless plaques on the scalp, forehead, face, or neck. In time, they increase in size and in mass as patients bearing them grow. Their surfaces often develop cobblestone or warty appearances. As sebaceous glands enlarge at puberty, the anomalies take on a yellow-orange color. In late lesions many other abnormalities in association may become manifest, especially basal-cell carcinoma, syringocystadenoma papilliferum, various benign adnexal neoplasms of mixed sebaceous, eccrine, apocrine or follicular differentiation, and follicular and sweat duct cysts.

Despite the absence of any obvious abnormalities in the connective tissue of the dermis in nevus sebaceus of Jadassohn, it would seem that something must be faulty in the connective tissue there. Biochemical alterations in the connective tissue conceivably could induce the numerous and varied aberrations of epithelial structures that tend to occur within nevus sebaceus.

The presence of nevus sebaceus may presage congenital abnormalities of other systems, for example, the skeletal and cardiovascular systems. In this sense, nevus sebaceus is but one part of a multisystemic disease.

31. Keratoacanthoma
vs. Squamous-Cell Carcinoma

Keratoacanthoma	*Squamous-Cell Carcinoma*
1. Exo-endophytic neoplasm with a central horn-filled crater	1. Predominantly endophytic neoplasm (except for the verrucous form) with no horn-filled crater
2. Rarely ulcerated	2. Commonly ulcerated
3. Surface of horn-filled crater surrounded by overhanging "lips" of epithelium	3. No surrounding epithelial "lips"
4. Abundant pale-staining cytoplasms of keratinocytes	4. Little tendency to pale-staining cytoplasms of keratinocytes
5. Tongues of atypical epithelial cells interposed between collagen bundles approximately parallel to the skin surface	5. No tongues of atypical epithelial cells parallel to the skin surface
6. Intraepithelial abscesses within the neoplasm common	6. Intraepithelial abscesses within the neoplasm rare
7. Acantholytic cells within the intraepithelial abscesses often	7. Acantholytic cells form without associated neutrophils
8. Gland-like formations within the neoplasm rare	8. Pseudoglandular formations often
9. Many necrotic keratinocytes in aggregation when lesion is resolving	9. Individually necrotic keratinocytes (dyskeratotic cells) when lesion is growing
10. Lymphocytes and plasma cells early; neutrophils, eosinophils, histiocytes, and histiocytic giant cells later	10. Lymphocytes and plasma cells dominate
11. Granulation tissue appears prior to resolution	11. No prominent granulation tissue unless ulcerated
12. Granulomatous inflammation around extruded cornified cells of resolving lesions	12. No granulomatous reaction
13. Fibrosis present in a broad zone beneath spontaneously resolving lesions	13. Fibrosis, when present, is desmoplastic and around aggregates of neoplastic cells; this lesion does not resolve spontaneously

Keratoacanthoma

Squamous-Cell Carcinoma

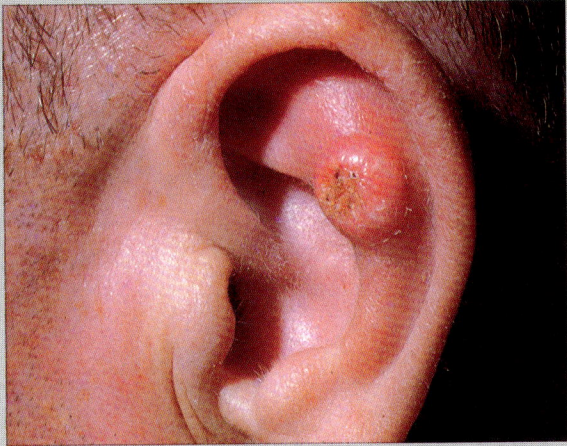
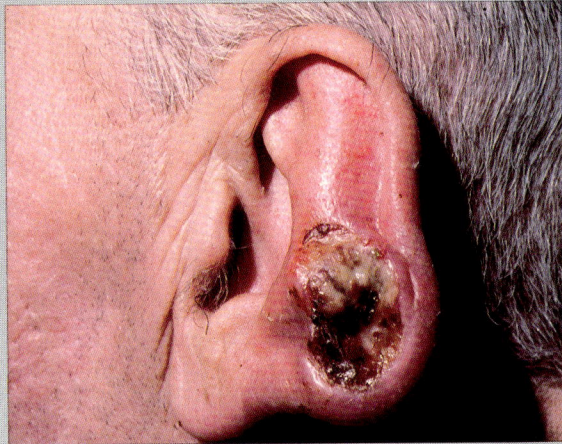

cornified cells atop central crater

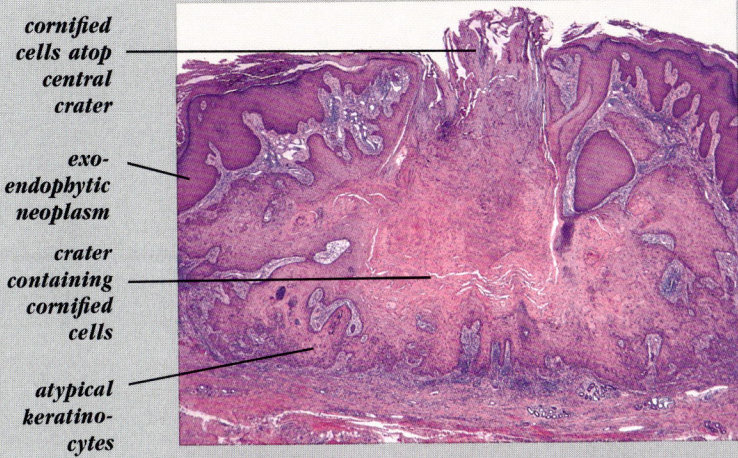

exo-endophytic neoplasm

crater containing cornified cells

atypical keratino-cytes

ulcer

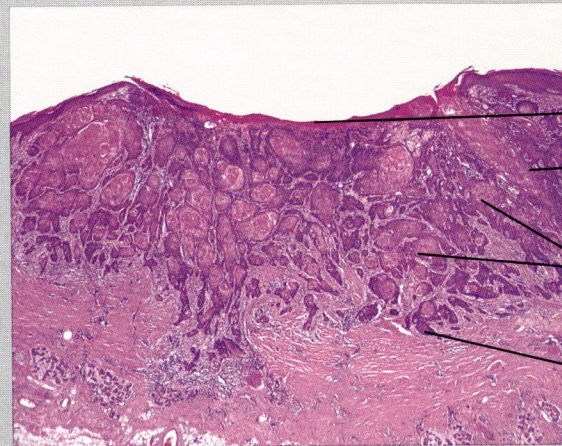

mostly endophytic neoplasm

whorls of cornified cells

atypical keratinocytes

atypical nucleus of keratinocyte

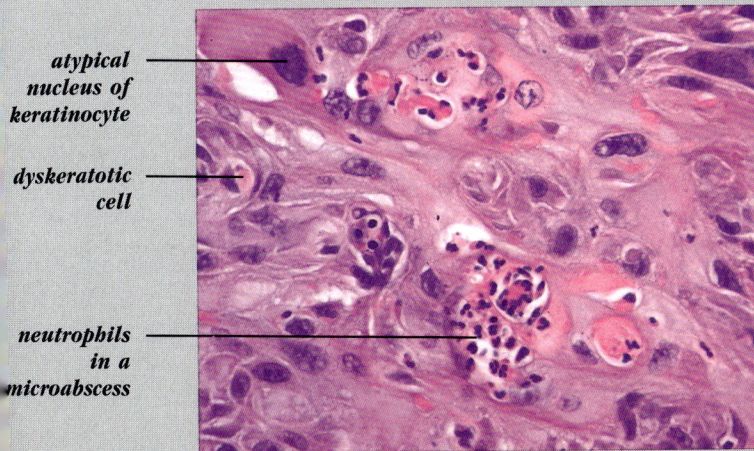

dyskeratotic cell

neutrophils in a microabscess

atypical nuclei of keratinocytes

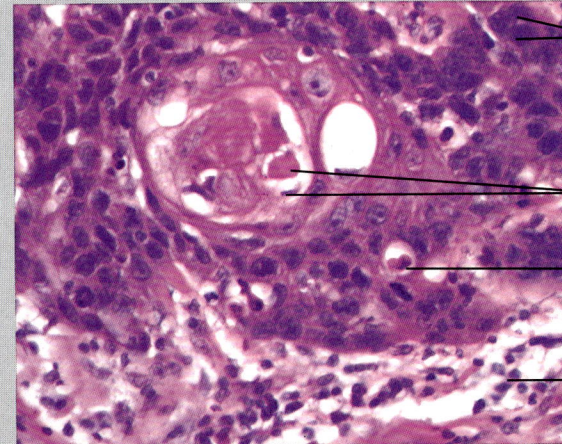

ortho- and parakeratotic cells

dyskeratotic cell

infiltrate of inflammatory cells

atypical nuclei

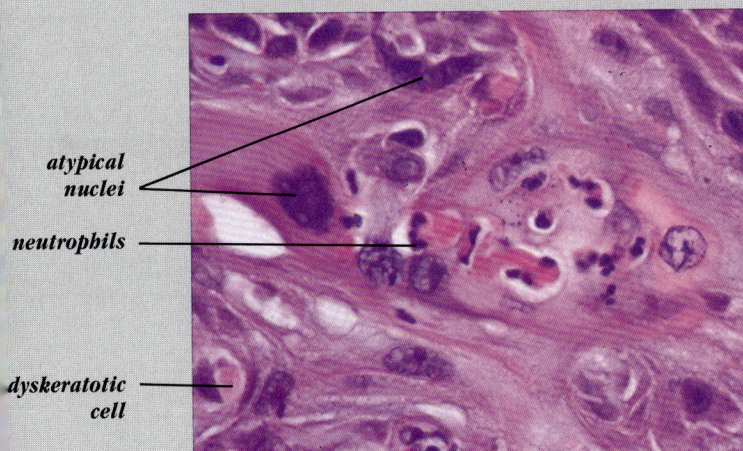

neutrophils

dyskeratotic cell

ortho- and parakeratotic cells

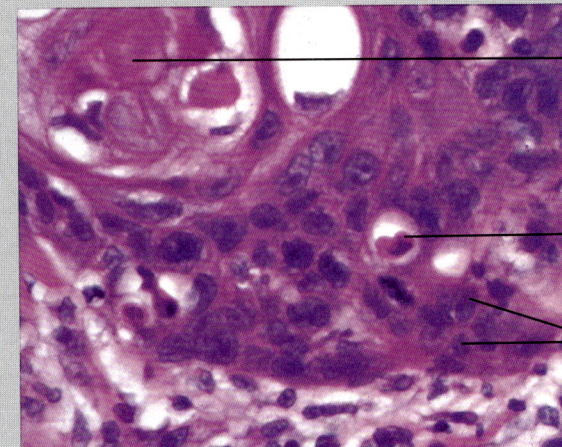

dyskeratotic cell

atypical nuclei

BOTH keratoacanthoma and squamous-cell carcinoma are neoplasms of keratinocytes that have many histologic features in common:

1. Atypical keratinocytes with large, hyperchromatic, pleomorphic nuclei and increased numbers of mitotic figures
2. Dyskeratotic cells
3. Inflammatory-cell infiltrates
4. Solar elastosis
5. Solar keratoses, basal-cell carcinomas, and even malignant melanomas in adjacent skin

The major histologic feature that distinguishes keratoacanthoma from squamous-cell carcinoma is their different and distinctive architectural patterns. The best biopsy specimen for revealing the characteristic diagnostic pattern of keratoacanthoma is one that extends from normal skin to normal skin through the center of the crater of the neoplasm. A biopsy of a squamous-cell carcinoma should also include sufficient adjacent or surrounding tissue to enable the pathologist to differentiate its pattern from that of keratoacanthoma. A punch biopsy specimen of either neoplasm is often insufficient for this important differentiation. Cytologic features, such as nuclear atypia, are not helpful in differentiating keratoacanthoma from squamous-cell carcinoma. In fact, some keratoacanthomas show a greater degree of nuclear atypia than do some squamous-cell carcinomas. If a proper biopsy is submitted, an accurate differentiation of a keratoacanthoma from a squamous-cell carcinoma may be made in almost every case.

Clinically, a keratoacanthoma usually presents itself as a solitary lesion, most commonly on sun-exposed areas of older individuals. More than one lesion may develop in the same individual. The typical solitary keratoacanthoma goes through two stages. First, there is rapid evolution for one to two months of a firm, dome-shaped nodule in which a horn-filled crater forms. Then, in another month or two, the nodule resolves, leaving an irregularly-shaped depressed scar. Rarely, a keratoacanthoma may grow for many months and even years to gigantic proportions and be markedly destructive. Still more rarely, this neoplasm takes the form of multiple, eruptive, widespread nodules. In the skin, keratoacanthoma seems to emanate from contiguous follicular infundibula. However, keratoacanthomas may also occur rarely in sites that are devoid of hair follicles, such as the subungual region and on mucous membranes.

Squamous-cell carcinoma may arise anywhere on the skin or mucous membranes de novo, but most commonly develops on sun-damaged skin as a continuous progression of atypical keratinocytes, i.e., from solar keratosis to hyperplastic solar keratosis to squamous-cell carcinoma. Squamous-cell carcinomas appearing in skin not exposed to sun, such as those arising in radiodermatitis or burn scars, have a greater tendency to behave in a biologically malignant fashion and to metastasize than do those that arise in solar-damaged skin, which nearly never metastasize. Clinically, squamous-cell carcinoma of the skin usually appears as an ulcer surrounded by a firm border, but its surface may occasionally be verrucous, smooth, or adorned by a cutaneous horn.

The history of rapid growth of a crateriform nodular lesion characterized histologically by atypical keratinocytic neoplasia should alert the pathologist to the probability of keratoacanthoma rather than squamous-cell carcinoma. It is imperative that clinicians not only provide adequate biopsy specimens of such lesions, but also ample historical information to the pathologist.

32. Pagetoid Bowen's Disease *vs.* Extramammary Paget's Disease

Pagetoid Bowen's Disease	*Extramammary Paget's Disease*
1. Parakeratotic hyperkeratosis usual	1. Orthokeratotic hyperkeratosis usual
2. No atypical pale cells within the stratum corneum usually	2. Atypical pale cells within the stratum corneum often
3. Cells with atypical nuclei and pale cytoplasms, singly but more usually in nests, at all levels of the epidermis equally	3. Cells with atypical nuclei and pale cytoplasm, singly and in nests, predominantly at lower levels of the epidermis
4. Nests of atypical cells merge with the surrounding epidermis at some points usually	4. Nests of atypical cells sharply demarcated from the keratinocytes in the surrounding epidermis
5. Intercellular bridges visible between pale cells in nests usually	5. Intercellular bridges not visible between pale cells in nests
6. Epidermal cells between the nests of pale cells have atypical nuclei usually	6. Epidermal cells between the nests of pale cells have normal nuclei
7. Atypical epidermal cells multinucleated sometimes	7. No multinucleated epidermal cells
8. Dyskeratotic cells in epidermis	8. No dyskeratotic cells in epidermis
9. No acinar structures within the epidermis	9. Acinar structures within the epidermis occasionally
10. Cells of basal layer not flattened by nests of atypical cells	10. Cells of basal layer often flattened by nests of atypical cells
11. Atypical cells spare the epithelial structures of adnexa usually	11. Atypical cells extend far down follicular infundibula and eccrine ducts

Pagetoid Bowen's Disease

Extramammary Paget's Disease

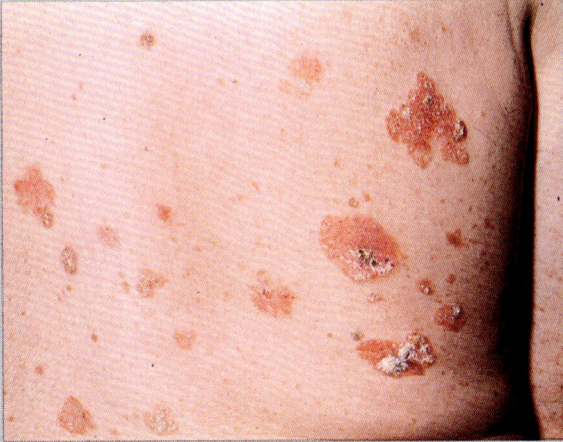

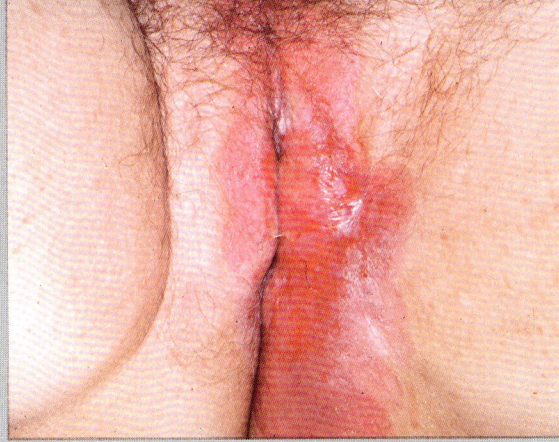

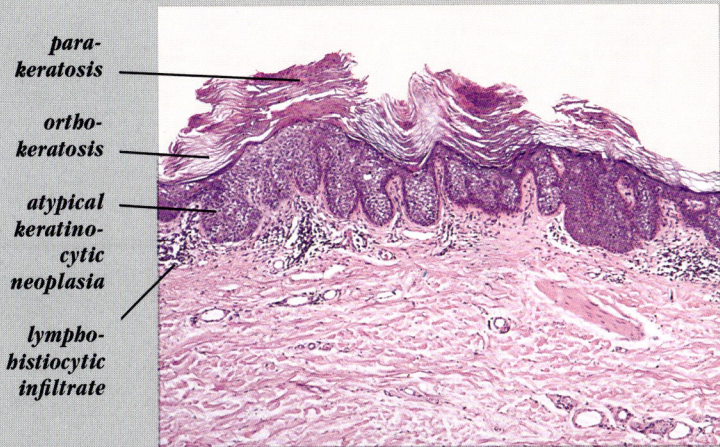

para-keratosis

ortho-keratosis

atypical keratino-cytic neoplasia

lympho-histiocytic infiltrate

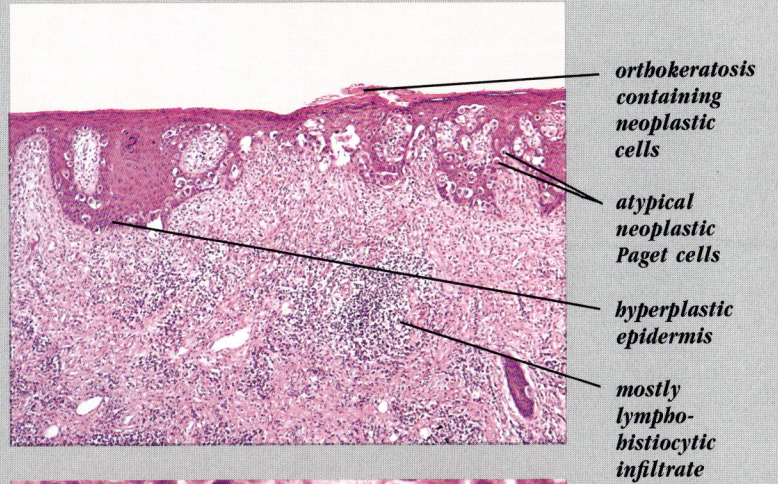

orthokeratosis containing neoplastic cells

atypical neoplastic Paget cells

hyperplastic epidermis

mostly lympho-histiocytic infiltrate

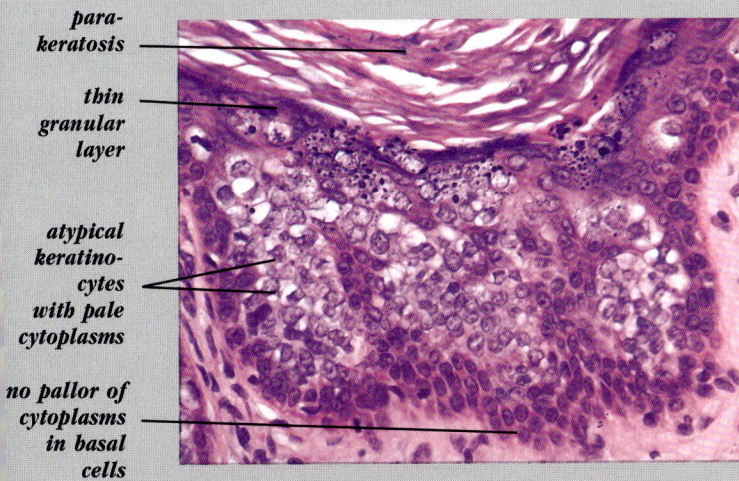

para-keratosis

thin granular layer

atypical keratino-cytes with pale cytoplasms

no pallor of cytoplasms in basal cells

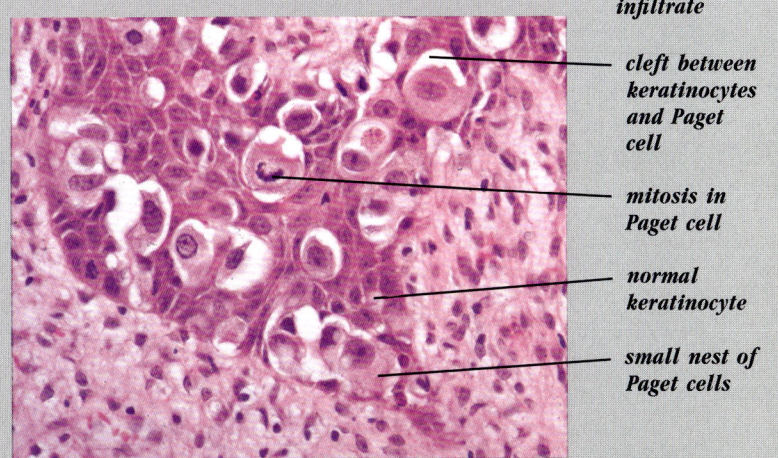

cleft between keratinocytes and Paget cell

mitosis in Paget cell

normal keratinocyte

small nest of Paget cells

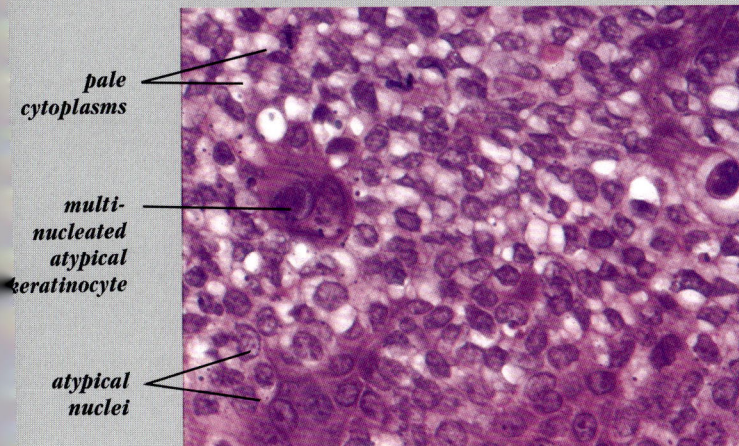

pale cytoplasms

multi-nucleated atypical keratinocyte

atypical nuclei

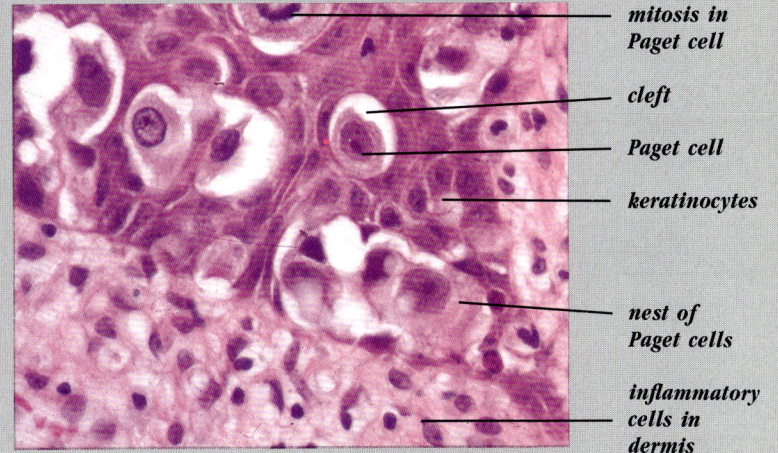

mitosis in Paget cell

cleft

Paget cell

keratinocytes

nest of Paget cells

inflammatory cells in dermis

BOTH pagetoid Bowen's disease and extramammary Paget's disease begin as intraepidermal carcinomas. Whereas Bowen's disease is a carcinoma in situ with squamous differentiation (it cornifies), extramammary Paget's disease is a carcinoma in situ with glandular differentiation (it goes to eccrine or apocrine differentiation). Despite the tabulated histologic differences between them, pagetoid Bowen's disease and extramammary Paget's disease have several histologic features in common:

1. Atypical cells with abundant pale-staining cytoplasms
2. An increased number of mitotic figures among the atypical cells
3. Atypical pale cells arranged singly and in nests within a hyperplastic epidermis
4. Carcinomas in situ, in time, may progress by extension downward into the dermis
5. An inflammatory-cell infiltrate is present in the upper part of the dermis

Ordinarily, Bowen's disease is not confused microscopically with extramammary Paget's disease; Bowen's disease usually is not nested, but confluently involves the entire thickness of the epidermis. However, in pagetoid Bowen's disease, intraepidermal aggregates of atypical pale cells mimic the nests of extramammary Paget's disease.

The histologic distinctions between pagetoid Bowen's disease and extramammary Paget's disease are made readily using the aforementioned criteria in sections stained merely by hematoxylin and eosin. Special stains serve only to confirm the diagnosis made with hematoxylin and eosin. In extramammary Paget's disease, the pale cytoplasms of atypical cells contain PAS positive neutral mucopolysaccharides that are not removed by diastase, whereas PAS positive material, when present in the cytoplasms of atypical cells in pagetoid Bowen's disease, is completely removed by diastase. Furthermore, the cytoplasms of cells in extramammary Paget's disease are positive with colloidal iron and mucicarmine stains, indicating the presence of acid mucopolysaccharides; those of pagetoid Bowen's disease are negative.

Bowen's disease is a form of intraepidermal squamous-cell carcinoma. It may occur anywhere on the skin and be a solitary lesion or multiple. The lesions are usually sharply marginated, brown-red plaques covered by scales and crusts. Bowen's disease on the genitalia is termed erythroplasia of Queyrat. In our experience, there is no increased incidence of internal malignant neoplasms in patients who have Bowen's disease. Bowenoid papulosis refers to numerous condylomata acuminata on the genitalia of young adults, which in time develop all of the histologic features of Bowen's disease, i.e., squamous-cell carcinoma in situ.

Extramammary Paget's disease is an intraepidermal adenocarcinoma with glandular differentiation that occurs in the axillary and anogenital regions. The disease generally consists of a solitary, irregularly shaped, often eroded plaque that varies in color from white to red and tends to progress centrifugally. There are two forms of the disease: a common form that originates in the epidermis as an adenocarcinoma and an uncommon form that extends into the epidermis from a contiguous adenocarcinoma of the genitourinary (e.g., the cervix) or the gastrointestinal (e.g., the rectum) tracts. The neoplastic cells in the common type of extramammary Paget's disease spread horizontally within the epidermis and vertically down the epithelial structures of adnexa for years (like atypical melanocytes in malignant melanoma) before entering the dermis from whence they may metastasize.

Extramammary Paget's disease is a wholly different pathological process from mammary Paget's disease in which neoplastic cells of an adenocarcinoma originate in the lactiferous ducts and ascend from there into the epidermis.

Pagetoid Bowen's disease and extramammary Paget's disease must also be differentiated histologically from pagetoid malignant melanoma in situ, because some examples of malignant melanoma in situ, especially those situated on the trunk and extremities, are characterized by atypical pagetoid melanocytes. This differentiation is especially difficult in those unusual instances in which the pagetoid cells of Bowen's disease and the pagetoid cells of extramammary Paget's disease contain melanin within their cytoplasms. However, some pagetoid cells of malignant melanoma in situ are always present at the dermo-epidermal junction, often in nests, whereas the nests of pagetoid cells of extramammary Paget's disease lie in or above the basal layer of the epidermis. The pagetoid cells of Bowen's disease may involve the basal layer, but not in nests at the dermo-epidermal interface. Furthermore, the atypical pale cells of pagetoid malignant melanoma are PAS negative and DOPA positive, another feature which differentiates them from both Bowen's and extramammary Paget's diseases.

33. Trichoepithelioma *vs.* Nodular Basal-Cell Carcinoma

Trichoepithelioma	*Nodular Basal-Cell Carcinoma*
1. Neoplasm symmetrical	1. Neoplasm asymmetrical
2. Ulceration infrequent	2. Ulceration frequent
3. Lesion well circumscribed with smooth margins	3. Lesion poorly circumscribed with irregular margins
4. Primitive hair structures common in the form of papillae and bulbs; uncommon as small hair follicles containing hairs	4. Primitive hair structures rare
5. Cribiform pattern of basaloid cells	5. No cribiform pattern of basaloid cells
6. Necrotic neoplastic cells rare	6. Necrotic neoplastic cells common and often in aggregates
7. No melanin in basaloid cells usually	7. Melanin in basaloid cells often
8. Acid mucopolysaccharides unusual in the epithelial aggregates or the stroma	8. Acid mucopolysaccharides usual in the epithelial aggregates and the stroma
9. No clefts between aggregates of neoplastic cells and stroma, but clefts between stroma of the neoplasm and the surrounding normal dermis	9. Artifactual clefts between aggregates of neoplastic cells and stroma common, but no clefts between stroma and surrounding dermis
10. Cornification of proliferating epithelial cells (i.e., cornified cysts) common	10. Cornified cysts uncommon
11. Foreign-body granulomas around cornified cells from ruptured cysts common	11. No granulomatous inflammation as a rule
12. Prominent fibrosis between and around aggregates of basaloid cells	12. Prominent fibrosis unusual
13. Inflammatory-cell infiltrates unusual	13. Inflammatory-cell infiltrates usual
14. No stromal edema	14. Stromal edema

Trichoepithelioma

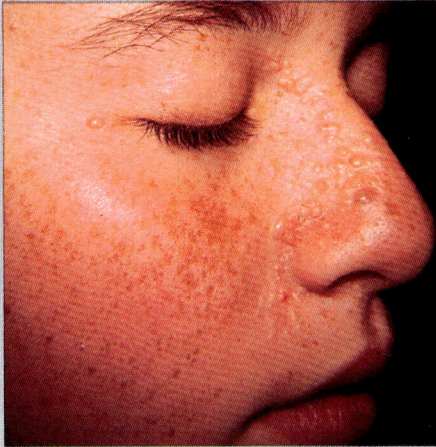

Nodular Basal-Cell Carcinoma

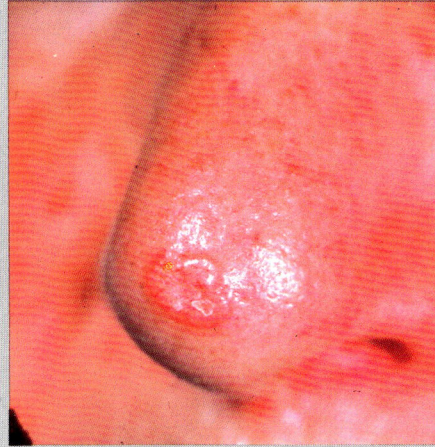

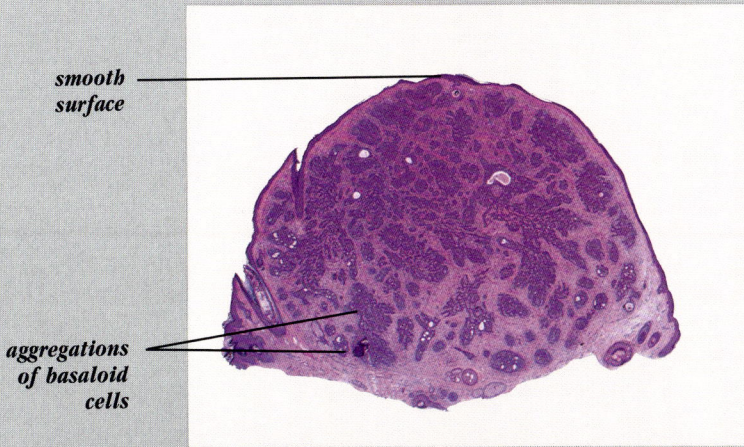

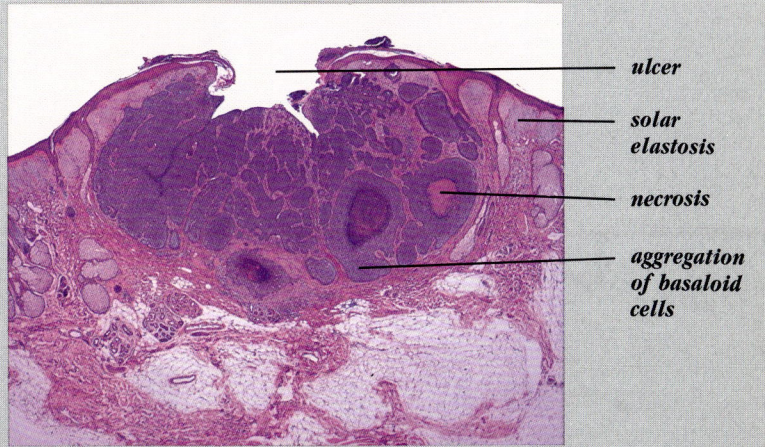

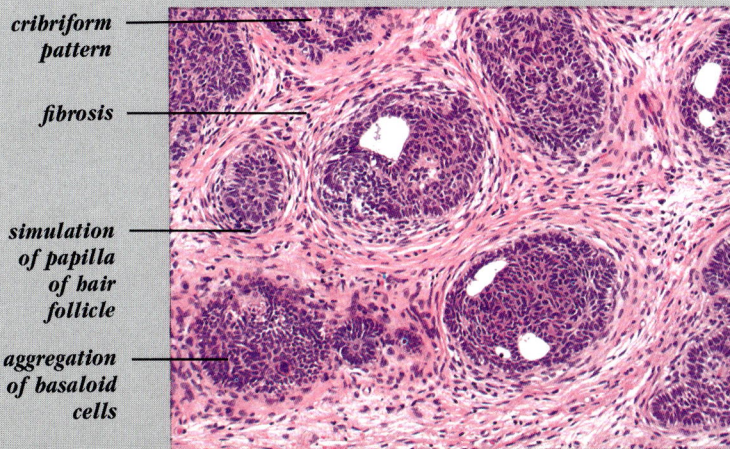

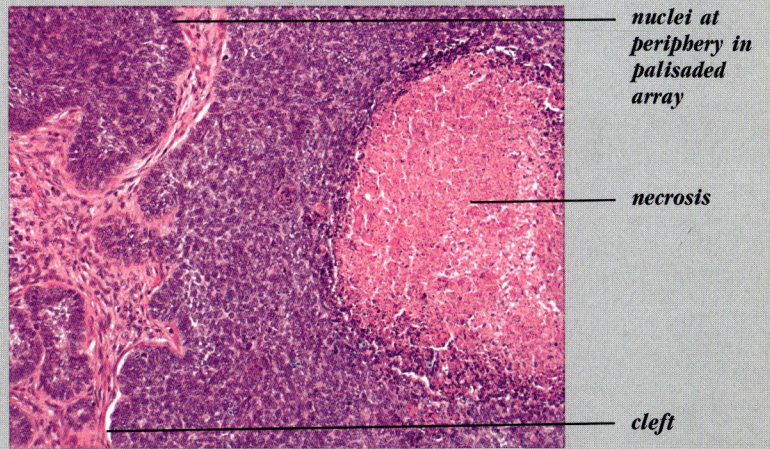

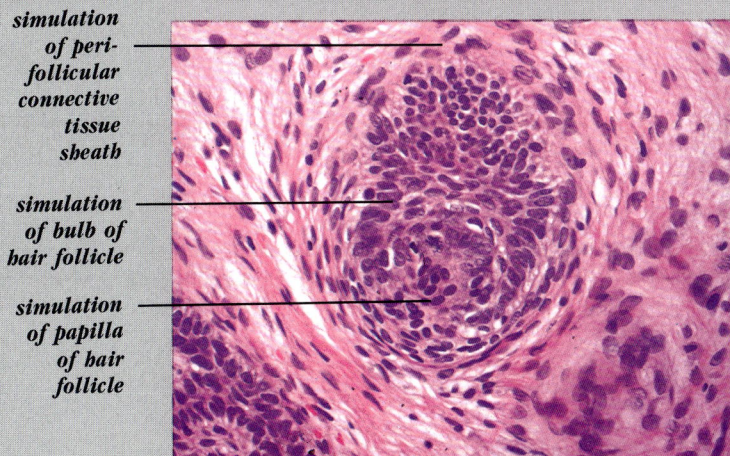

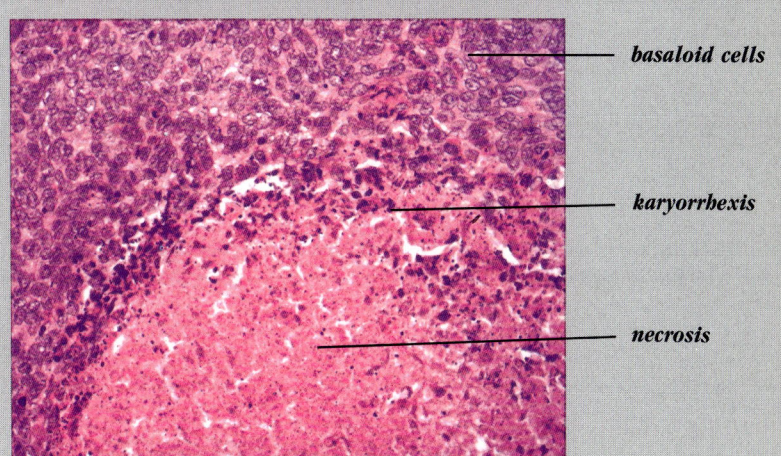

smooth
surface

aggregations
of basaloid
cells

ulcer

solar
elastosis

necrosis

aggregation
of basaloid
cells

cribriform
pattern

fibrosis

simulation
of papilla
of hair
follicle

aggregation
of basaloid
cells

nuclei at
periphery in
palisaded
array

necrosis

cleft

simulation
of peri-
follicular
connective
tissue
sheath

simulation
of bulb of
hair follicle

simulation
of papilla
of hair
follicle

basaloid cells

karyorrhexis

necrosis

TRICHOEPITHELIOMAS and nodular basal-cell carcinomas are epithelial neoplasms with the following histologic features in common:

1. Dome-shaped lesions
2. Aggregates of basaloid cells
3. Cells at the peripheries of the epithelial aggregates tend to be palisaded
4. Necrotic cells may be present within epithelial aggregates
5. Amyloid deposited in stroma commonly

Generally, these two neoplasms of basaloid cells may be differentiated from one another with confidence if the tabulated criteria are sought. This is especially true when biopsy of the entire lesion is submitted for microscopic examination. However, in some instances the differentiation between them may be nearly impossible and, in still others, there may be histologic features of both trichoepithelioma and of basal-cell carcinoma in the same specimen.

Clinically, trichoepitheliomas usually occur as multiple lesions on the face, but sometimes the process may appear as a solitary papule or nodule. Such lesions are skin-colored and often traversed by telangiectases. In cases of multiple trichoepitheliomas, inheritance is from an autosomal dominant trait, whereas the solitary trichoepithelioma is not inherited. Epithelioma adenoides cysticum is another older appellation for multiple trichoepitheliomas. An interesting association of benign neoplasms with adnexal differentiation is the concurrence of trichoepitheliomas and cylindromas in the same patient.

An uncommon variant of trichoepithelioma is the desmoplastic type in which cords and strands of basaloid cells, as well as cornifying duct-like structures, are present in an exuberant, fibrotic stroma. The desmoplastic trichoepithelioma must be differentiated histologically from the fibrosing (morphea) type of basal-cell carcinoma.

Nodular basal-cell carcinoma usually occurs as a single lesion on the sun-damaged skin of individuals with fair complexions; however, multiple basal-cell carcinomas sometimes are found in the same person. Basal-cell carcinoma is generally a neoplasm of middle-aged or older individuals, except in the systemic condition of nevoid basal-cell carcinoma syndrome where children may be affected. Basal-cell carcinomas develop in a variety of atrophic scars, such as those caused by radiotherapy, vaccinations, burns, lupus vulgaris, and discoid lupus erythematosus.

Besides the nodular type of basal-cell carcinoma, there are the nodulo-ulcerative, pigmented, morphea-like (fibrosing, syringomatous), superficial, cystic, adamantinoid, and the premalignant fibroepithelioma. This is but a partial list of the many histologic "faces" of basal-cell carcinoma.

34. Metastatic Carcinoma from the Breast *vs.* Morphea-like Basal-Cell Carcinoma

Metastatic Carcinoma from the Breast	*Morphea-like Basal-Cell Carcinoma*
1. Solitary neoplastic cells are found within the dermis in "Indian file" between collagen bundles often	1. Strands of several neoplastic cells are found within the dermis, but not in single file as a rule
2. Differentiation may be ductal	2. Differentiation is rarely ductal
3. The strands of neoplastic cells do not branch	3. The strands of neoplastic cells tend to branch
4. The neoplastic cells may be entirely within the deep dermis	4. The neoplastic cells are never entirely within the deep dermis
5. The neoplastic cells are often within lymphatics	5. The neoplastic cells are never within lymphatics
6. Nuclei of neoplastic cells pleomorphic	6. Nuclei of neoplastic cells monomorphic
7. Nucleoli prominent	7. Nucleoli not noticeable usually
8. The collagen surrounding the neoplastic cells is thickened, sclerotic, and eosinophilic and the number of fibroblasts is often decreased	8. The collagen surrounding the neoplastic cells is fibrillar and amphophilic, and the number of fibroblasts is increased

Metastatic Carcinoma from the Breast

Morphea-like Basal-Cell Carcinoma

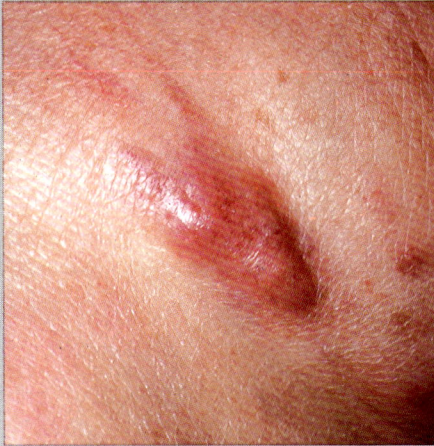

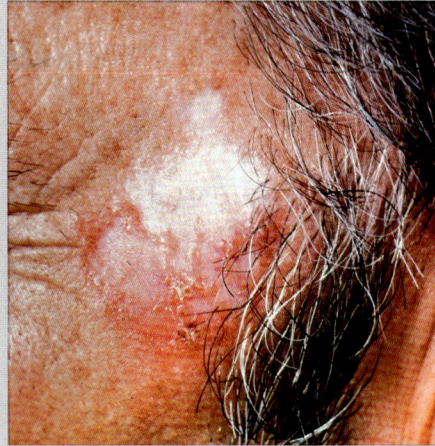

irregularly
shaped
aggregations
of atypical
epithelial
cells

solar
elastosis

cords of
basaloid cells

strands of
atypical
epithelial
cells

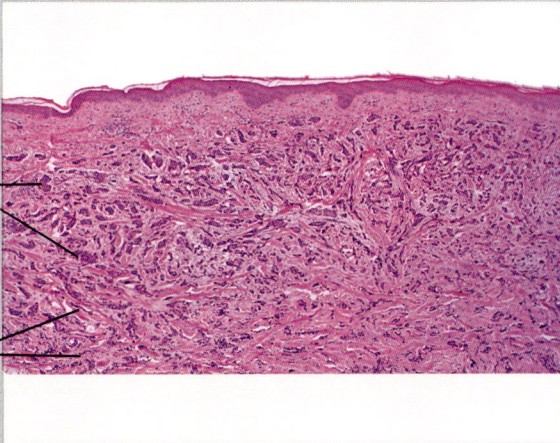

aggregates of
basaloid cells

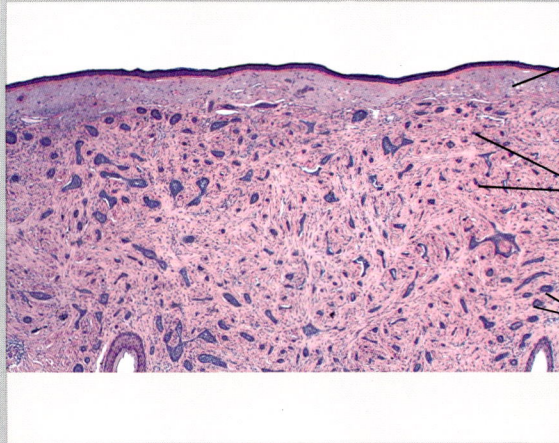

aggregations
of atypical
epithelial
cells

branching
from
aggregate
of basaloid
cells

strands of
atypical
epithelial
cells

cords of
basaloid cells

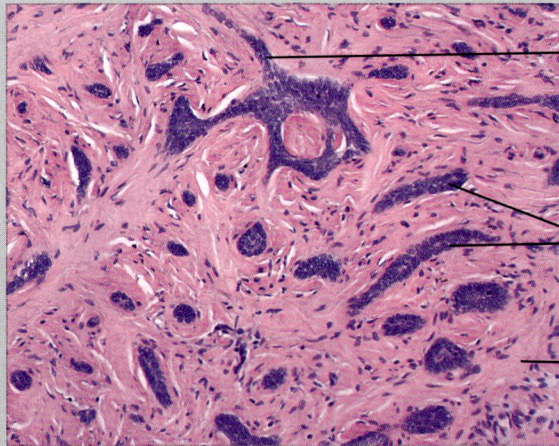

thickened
collagen
bundle

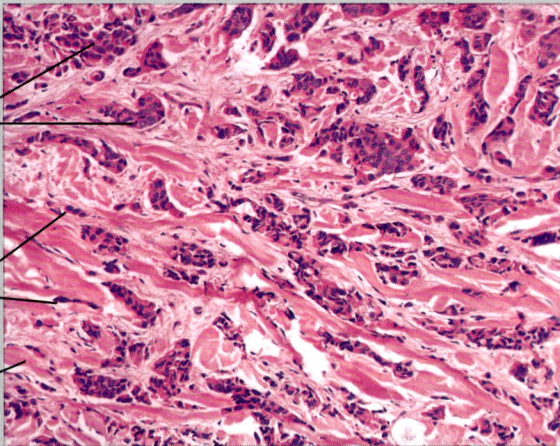

sclerosis

thickened
collagen
bundle

sclerosis

nuclei at
periphery in
palisaded
array

strand of
atypical
epithelial
cells

cleft

pleomorphic
nuclei

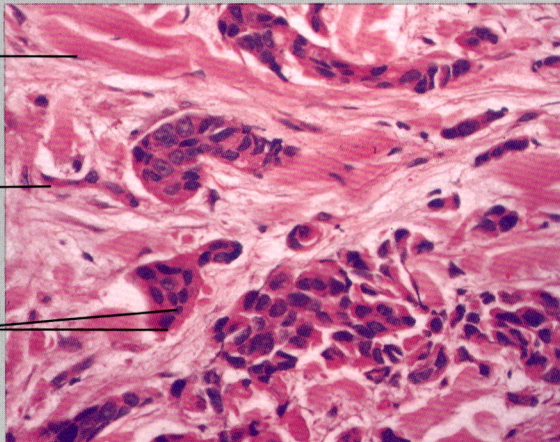

nuclei
relatively
uniform in
size and
shape

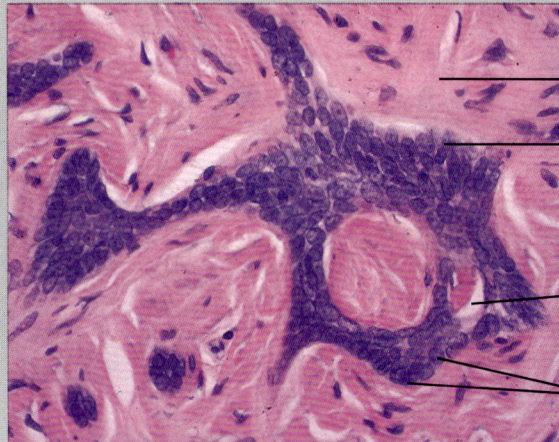

I N general, neoplasms metastatic to the skin from other organs present no great difficulty in differential diagnosis from neoplasms primary in the skin. Carcinoma of the breast is the one that most often presents difficulty in differential diagnosis. Metastatic carcinoma from the breast may be confused with a wholly inflammatory skin condition if the lesion consists of but few neoplastic cells and numerous inflammatory cells scattered diffusely among collagen bundles. In general, when diagnostic difficulties arise in differentiating metastatic carcinoma to the skin from carcinoma primary in the skin, fibrosing (morphea-like) basal-cell carcinoma is the one at issue. Other synonyms for fibrosing basal-cell carcinoma are sclerosing basal-cell carcinoma and syringomatosus basal-cell carcinoma.

Metastatic carcinoma from the breast and fibrosing (morphea-like) basal cell carcinoma have the following histologic features in common:

1. Epithelial cells arranged in linear fashion between collagen bundles
2. Epithelial cells embedded in a fibrotic stroma
3. Hyperchromatic nuclei within the epithelial cells

Metastatic carcinoma to the skin from the breast may present itself in four different clinical forms:

1. Inflammatory: the involved skin shows erythema, edema, and induration similar to erysipelas because of lymphatic involvement by the neoplastic cells
2. Telangiectatic: the affected skin has purple papules, nodules, and areas of hemorrhagic, spongy lesions that resemble vascular neoplasms
3. Nodular: the skin is characterized by deep-seated nodules, especially recurrences in mastectomy scars
4. Cancer en cuirasse: the malignancy takes the form of a diffuse, firm, brawny, tan plaque

Most commonly, metastasis occurs by way of the lymphatics, but occasionally by hematogenous routes. The scalp is the most common site of hematogenous spread, but any site on the skin may be affected.

Fibrosing basal-cell carcinoma presents itself clinically as an indurated yellow-tan patch or plaque coursed by telangiectases. The surface of the skin is usually intact, but rarely may be ulcerated.

Syringoma may be confused histologically with both metastatic carcinoma from the breast and with fibrosing basal-cell carcinoma. Syringomas are also composed of strands of epithelial cells and epithelial-lined small ducts may form within a fibrotic stroma. However, the ducts of syringoma, unlike ductal forms of metastatic carcinoma, often show comma-like extensions similar in appearance to tadpoles. Cornifying cysts and calcification may be seen in some lesions of syringoma, but not in breast carcinoma as a rule. Clinically, syringomas are small, yellowish-tan papules on the lower eyelids, but the lesions may occur in other areas of the skin (cheek, axillae, abdomen, chest, and so on). They tend to affect women more commonly than men.

Desmoplastic trichoepithelioma must also be differentiated from metastatic carcinoma in the skin and from morphea-type basal-cell carcinoma. The crucial feature in this differentiation is the tendency of the cords of cells in desmoplastic trichoepithelioma to be associated with cysts containing cornified cells that calcify.

35. Simple Lentigo

vs. Solar Lentigo

Simple Lentigo	*Solar Lentigo*
1. Laminated orthokeratotic cornified layer often contains abundant melanin	1. Compact orthokeratotic cornified layer contains relatively little melanin
2. Epidermal hyperplasia with thin elongated rete ridges	2. Epidermal hyperplasia with slightly bulbous rete ridges
3. Markedly hyperpigmented epidermis with abundant melanin throughout the entire thickness of the epidermis including the cornified layer	3. Moderately hyperpigmented epidermis, most discernible in the basal layer
4. Melanocytic hyperplasia, initially arranged individually at the dermo-epidermal junction	4. Little melanocytic hyperplasia as a rule
5. Melanocytes may form small nests at the bases of the rete ridges in time (junctional nevus)	5. No nests of melanocytes within the epidermis
6. Large globules of melanin (giant melanosomes) within some melanocytes usually	6. No large globules of melanin within melanocytes
7. Solar elastosis (elastotic material) uncommon and incidental	7. Solar elastosis always and significant pathogenetically
8. Lamellar collagen present around rete ridges often	8. No lamellar collagen
9. Melanophages numerous usually	9. Few melanophages usually

Simple Lentigo

Solar Lentigo

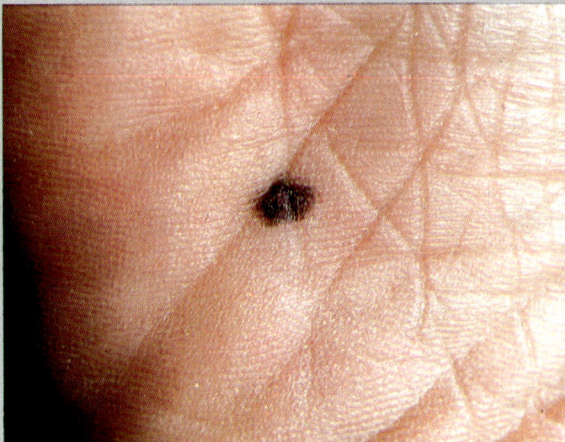

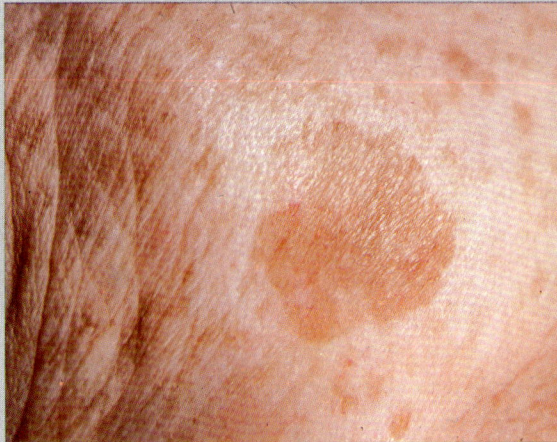

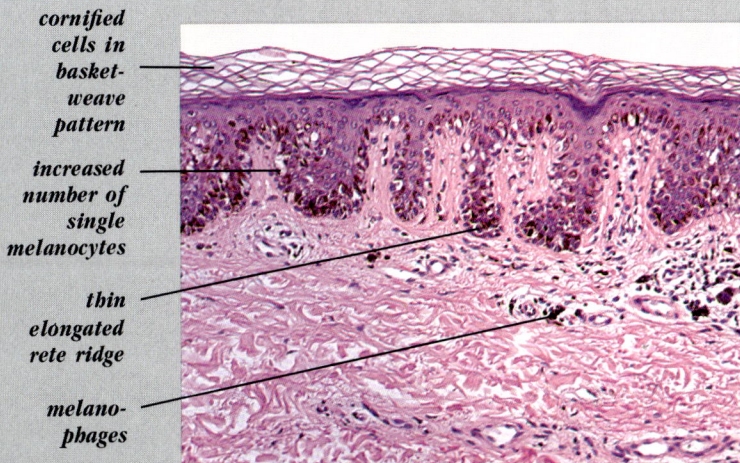

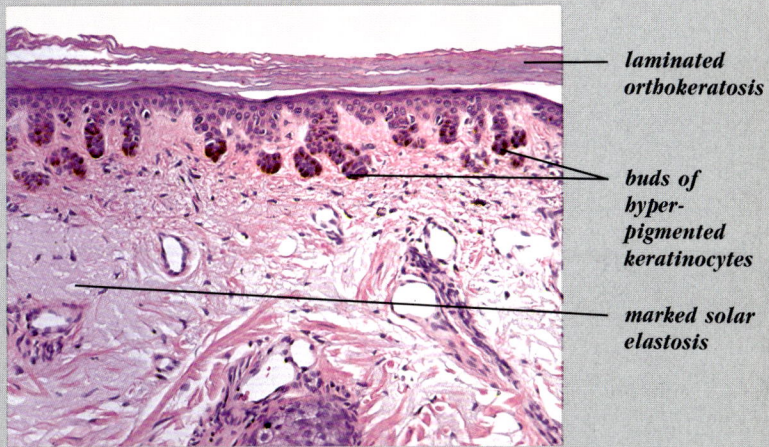

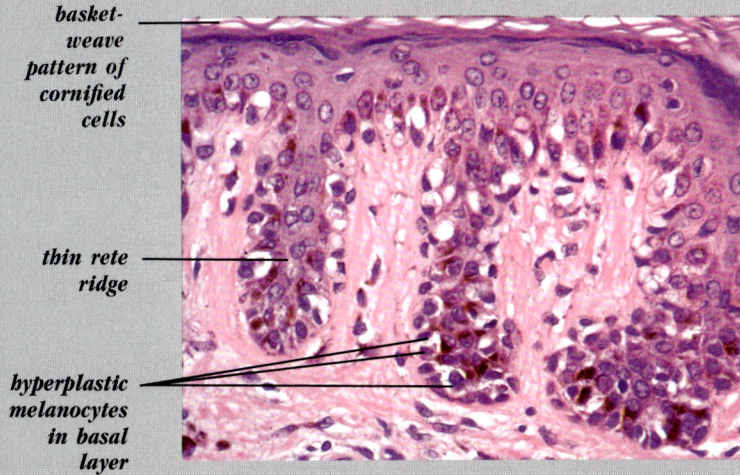

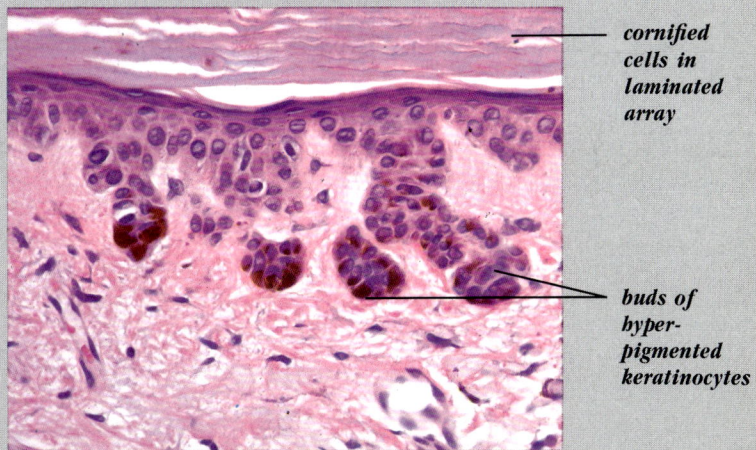

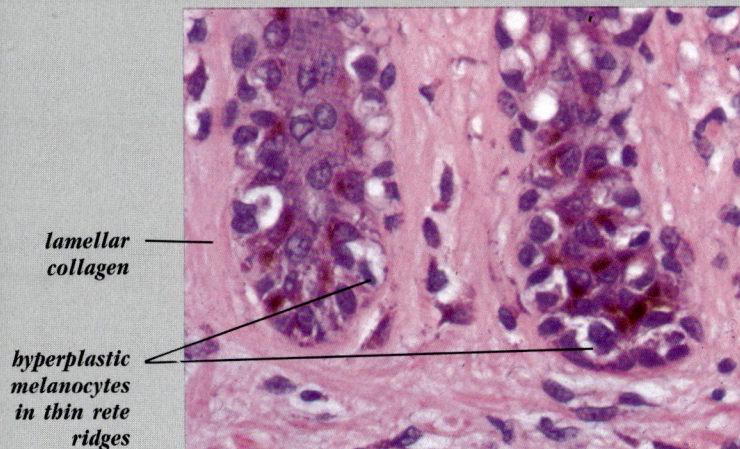

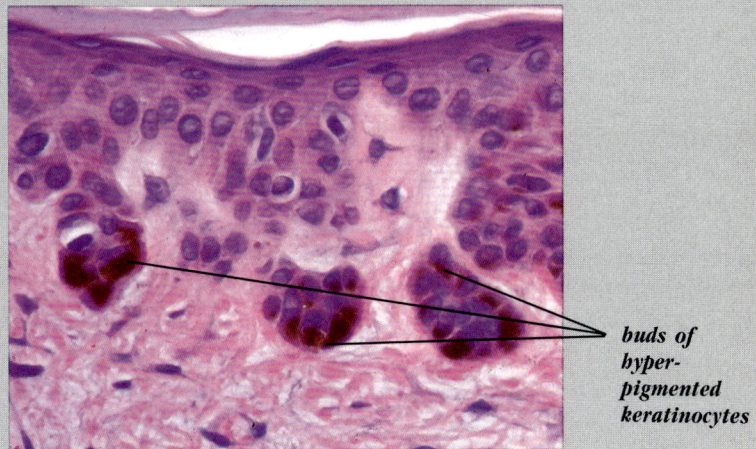

cornified cells in basket-weave pattern

increased number of single melanocytes

thin elongated rete ridge

melano-phages

laminated orthokeratosis

buds of hyper-pigmented keratinocytes

marked solar elastosis

basket-weave pattern of cornified cells

thin rete ridge

hyperplastic melanocytes in basal layer

cornified cells in laminated array

buds of hyper-pigmented keratinocytes

lamellar collagen

hyperplastic melanocytes in thin rete ridges

buds of hyper-pigmented keratinocytes

S IMPLE lentigo (also known as juvenile lentigo) and solar lentigo (also called senile lentigo) are common, wholly benign, pigmented lesions which share histologic features. Both are usually characterized by epidermal hyperplasia, hyperpigmentation, and melanophages in the upper part of the dermis. They differ principally in the shape of the rete ridges (thin and elongated in simple lentigo and relatively broad in solar lentigo) and in the number of melanocytes (increased more in simple lentigo than in solar lentigo).

Clinically, simple lentigines are small, round to oval, dark brown to black macules that occur anywhere on the skin surface of young individuals. They usually appear after the age of 3 and begin to regress after the age of 30. They are not related causally to sun exposure.

Solar lentigines, in contrast, are relatively large, irregularly shaped, mottled, tan to brown, macular and subtly papular, slightly keratotic lesions that develop only in sun-exposed areas of the skin of older individuals, especially on the face and the dorsa of the hands and forearms. They generally begin to appear after the age of 40 and increase in number with age. Solar lentigines, as their name implies, are induced by sunlight and are always associated with solar elastosis in the dermis. In common parlance, solar lentigines are known as "liver spots."

Simple lentigines are related to junctional nevi as is evidenced by the not infrequent association of nests of melanocytes within the thin rete ridges of otherwise typical simple lentigines. These junctional nevi simply represent later stages of simple lentigines, the results of confluence and nesting of the increased numbers of melanocytes. In still other lesions with typical histologic features of simple lentigines, there are not only nests of melanocytes within the epidermis, but a few nests of nevus cells in the papillary dermis. For telegraphic communication, we term a lesion that combines features of simple lentigo and junctional nevus a "jentigo" and one that has features of simple lentigo and compound nevus a "compendigo."

If simple lentigines in some instances blend imperceptibly into junctional and compound nevi, so some solar lentigines merge with adenoid (reticulated) types of seborrheic keratosis.

Simple and solar lentigines are easily differentiated histologically from ephelids (freckles) in which there are normal rete ridges with normal complements of melanocytes and only slight epidermal hyperpigmentation, just barely noticeable in the basal layer. Clinically, freckles, like solar lentigines, result from sun exposure, but they are smaller and less keratotic.

Lentigo maligna (Hutchinson's freckle) is completely unrelated to simple lentigo, solar lentigo, and freckle. It is a form of malignant melanoma in situ that occurs in chronically sun-damaged skin of the head and neck of light-complexioned persons. Histologically, it may sometimes be confused with junctional nevi. The distinguishing features of these two melanocytic conditions are contrasted in Chapter 36.

36. Junctional Nevus *vs.* Malignant Melanoma in Situ on Sun-Damaged Skin of the Face

Junctional Nevus	*Malignant Melanoma in Situ on Sun-Damaged Skin of the Face (Lentigo Maligna)*
1. Epidermis normal or slightly hyperplastic	1. Epidermis thinned usually
2. Preservation of the normal pattern between rete ridges and dermal papillae	2. Loss of the normal pattern between rete ridges and dermal papillae
3. Sharp circumscription of the intraepidermal melanocytic component; individual melanocytes do not extend horizontally beyond the most peripheral nests	3. Poor lateral circumscription of individual melanocytes which extend horizontally beyond the most peripheral nests
4. Increased number of normal melanocytes within the epidermis, mainly in nests	4. Increased number of atypical melanocytes within the epidermis, initially as individual cells and later in nests
5. Individual melanocytes have round or oval nuclei and their nests are also round or oval	5. Atypical melanocytes tend to be oval, dendritic, or spindle-shaped and their elongated nests tend to be parallel to the skin surface
6. Nests of normal melanocytes do not vary much in size and shape	6. Nests of atypical melanocytes vary in size and shape
7. Nests of normal melanocytes well circumscribed and discrete	7. Nests of atypical melanocytes usually poorly circumscribed and often confluent
8. In older lesions, normal melanocytes present individually in basal layer of epidermis only	8. In older lesions, atypical melanocytes often present individually at all levels of epidermis
9. Few melanocytes in nests within epithelial structures of adnexa (except for congenital and Spitz's nevi)	9. Atypical melanocytes singly and in nests extend down epithelial structures of adnexa
10. Little or no inflammatory-cell infiltrate usually	10. Moderately dense lympho-histiocytic infiltrate around superficial dilated blood vessels usually
11. Few melanophages usually	11. Many melanophages usually
12. Extensive solar elastosis in the dermis rare and incidental	12. Extensive solar elastosis in the dermis always and probably important pathogenetically

Junctional Nevus

Malignant Melanoma in Situ on Sun-Damaged Skin of the Face (Lentigo Maligna)

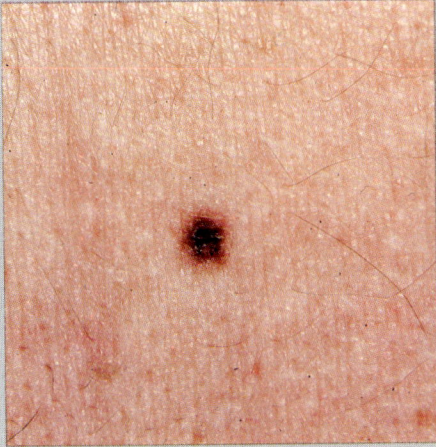

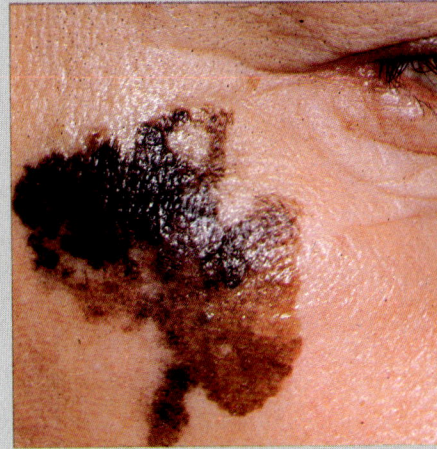

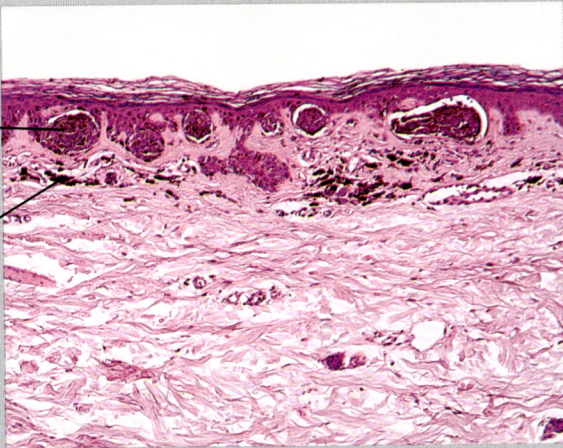

smooth-bordered nest of melanocytes

melanophages superficial in dermis

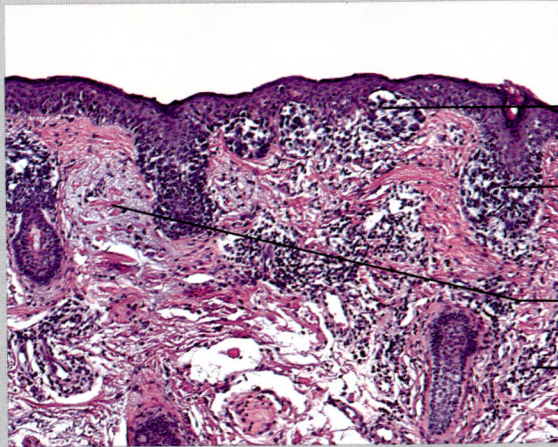

irregularly shaped nest of melanocytes

melanocytes in hair follicle

solar elastosis

inflammatory cells deep in dermis

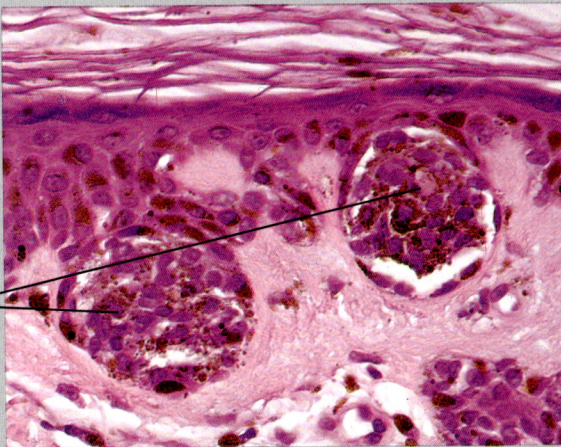

melanocytes in discrete nests of relatively uniform sizes and shapes

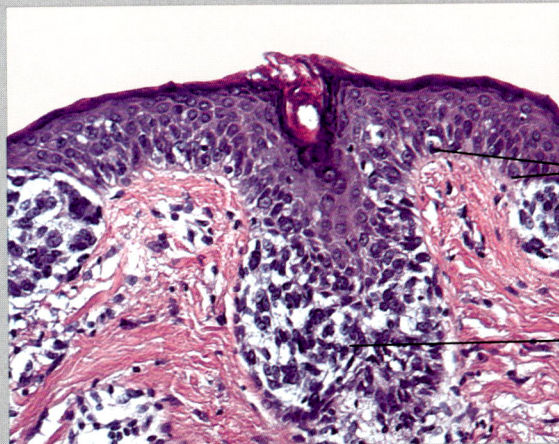

increased number of solitary melanocytes

nest of melanocytes within infundibulum

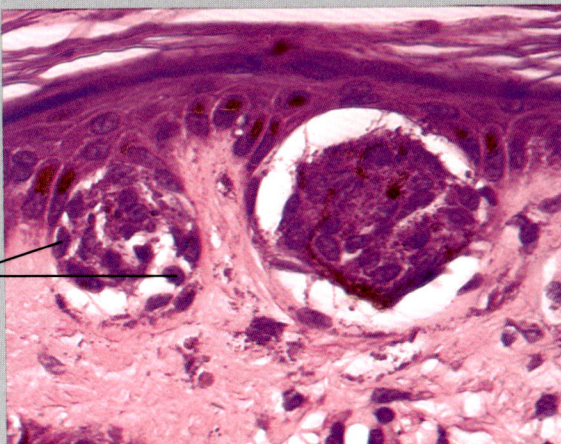

nuclei of melanocytes relatively uniform in sizes and shapes

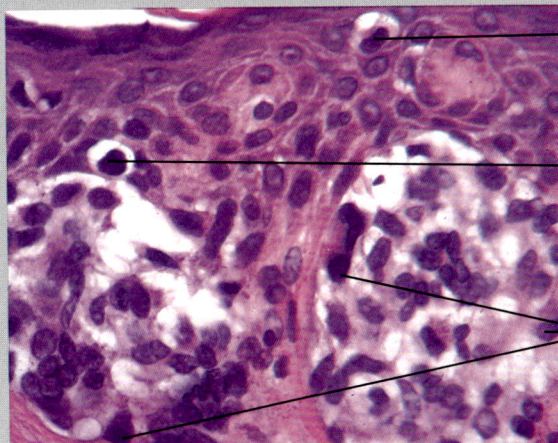

atypical melanocyte near granular layer

atypical melanocyte in spinous layer

pleomorphic nuclei in melanocytes

JUNCTIONAL nevus and malignant melanoma in situ on sun-damaged skin of the face (lentigo maligna) are both melanocytic processes in which nests of melanocytes tend to form within the hyperpigmented epidermis.

Acquired junctional nevi present themselves clinically as macules that are sharply circumscribed, ordinarily uniform in pigmentation, and smooth-surfaced. They vary in color from tan to brown and range in size from a few millimeters to about a centimeter. Junctional nevi usually appear during the first decade of life, but sometimes arise later. It is judicious in patients over 40 years of age to study carefully lesions that, at first glance under the microscope, appear to be junctional types of melanocytic nevi. More careful study may reveal some of them to be examples of malignant melanoma in situ, especially if they measure more than 6 mm in breadth.

Melanocytic nevi of junctional type may evolve from simple lentigines or arise de novo. They may remain junctional, regress, become compound, or come to be entirely intradermal. In former times it was widely believed that junctional nevi, especially those that were said to be "active" or those on palms, soles, and sites of irritation, were precursors of malignant melanomas. In fact, they are all benign. It is very exceptional for malignant melanoma to develop upon a pre-existing junctional nevus. Furthermore, the concept of "junctional activity" is an evasive judgment of benign or malignant nature and should be abandoned.

The cells that form nests in a junctional nevus are melanocytes, i.e., they make melanin and have all of the ultrastructural and biochemical characteristics of melanocytes. To refer to them exclusively as "nevus cells" beclouds their identity. By convention, melanocytes within the dermis of melanocytic nevi are termed "nevus cells" or "nevocytes."

Lentigo maligna (Hutchinson's freckle, melanosis circumscripta precancerose of Dubreuilh) begins clinically as an unevenly pigmented, light-brown macule that gradually extends centrifugally. Over a period of years it may attain several square centimeters or inches in an irregular outline. Well-developed lentigo maligna usually has gradations of color from brown to black within the lesion. The condition tends to develop on skin that has been chronically damaged by sunlight, almost always that of the face.

The histologic sequence of changes in lentigo maligna begins with hyperplasia of individual melanocytic cells, proceeds to hyperplasia of atypical melanocytes, and eventually to formation of nests of atypical melanocytes both within the epidermis and within adnexal epithelium. "Lentigo maligna" is simply a euphemism for a type of malignant melanoma in situ on sun-damaged skin of the face, comparable to squamous-cell carcinoma in situ. After several years, usually between 10 and 20, the atypical melanocytes from the epidermis descend into the dermis, at which time the lesion is a true malignant melanoma with the potential for metastasis. Clinically, the first evidence of descent into the dermis is a small papule which may eventually become nodular.

Malignant melanoma in situ on sun-damaged skin of the face, like the patch stages of Kaposi's sarcoma and mycosis fungoides (parapsoriasis en plaques) is not immediately life-threatening. It is only when papulation or nodularity supervenes (dermal involvement by atypical melanocytes) that the process has potential to metastasize and cause death.

Morphologically, if only the melanoma itself is studied, there is no single clinical or histologic feature or constellation of features that enables one to differentiate a malignant melanoma on sun-damaged skin of the face from a malignant melanoma on any other cutaneous site. The clues to the diagnosis of malignant melanoma on sun-damaged skin of the face are not to be found in the melanoma itself, but in the rest of the biopsy specimen, namely, numerous large sebaceous glands associated with vellus hair follicles and abundant solar elastosis.

37. Spitz's Nevus, Compound Type *vs.* Malignant Melanoma on the Trunk or Proximal Extremities

Spitz's Nevus, Compound Type (Nevus of Large Spindle and/or Epithelioid Cells)

1. Lesion symmetric
2. Lesion usually less than 6 mm in breadth
3. Sharp lateral demarcation of the intraepidermal melanocytic component (no horizontal spread of individual atypical melanocytes beyond the most peripheral nests)
4. Hyperkeratosis prominent usually
5. Hypergranulosis usually
6. Marked epidermal hyperplasia usual
7. Nests of melanocytes relatively uniform in size and shape
8. Nests of melanocytes within the epidermis are elongated and oriented perpendicular to the skin surface.
9. Homogeneous eosinophilic bodies singly and in nests within epidermis
10. Sharp circumscription of intraepidermal nests of melanocytes from keratinocytes
11. Clefts between nests of melanocytes and keratinocytes are the rule
12. Nests of dermal nevus cells tend to be discrete
13. Maturation of melanocytes (decrease in nuclear size) with descent into the dermis
14. Nevus cells at base of lesion commonly arranged as single cells
15. No pagetoid melanocytes
16. Mitotic figures near base of lesion rare
17. Inflammatory-cell infiltrate patchy around blood vessels throughout the lesion
18. No evidences of spontaneous regression

Malignant Melanoma on the Trunk or Proximal Extremities

1. Lesion asymmetric
2. Lesion usually greater than 6 mm in breadth
3. Poor circumscription of the intraepidermal component with horizontal extension of individual atypical melanocytes beyond the bulk of intradermal component of neoplasm
4. Hyperkeratosis not usually prominent
5. No hypergranulosis usually
6. Little epidermal hyperplasia usual
7. Marked variation in size and shape of nests of melanocytes
8. Nests of melanocytes within the epidermis neither elongated nor oriented perpendicular to the skin surface
9. No homogeneous eosinophilic bodies in nests within epidermis
10. Confluence of nests of melanocytes within the epidermis
11. Few, if any, clefts between melanocytes and keratinocytes as a rule
12. Nests of dermal melanocytes tend to become confluent and form sheets of cells
13. No maturation of melanocytes with descent into the dermis usually
14. Melanocytes at base of lesion not usually arranged as single cells
15. Pagetoid melanocytes often
16. Mitotic figures near base of lesion common
17. Inflammatory-cell infiltrate, when present, often band-like beneath the melanocytic component
18. Foci of spontaneous regression (fibrosis, telangiectases, melanophages) in the thickened papillary dermis common

Spitz's Nevus, Compound Type (Nevus of Large Spindle and/or Epithelioid Cells)

Malignant Melanoma on the Trunk or Proximal Extremities

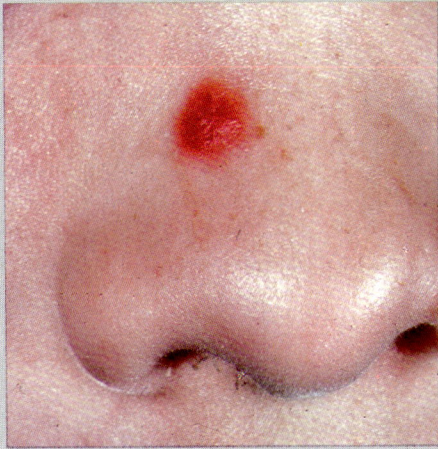

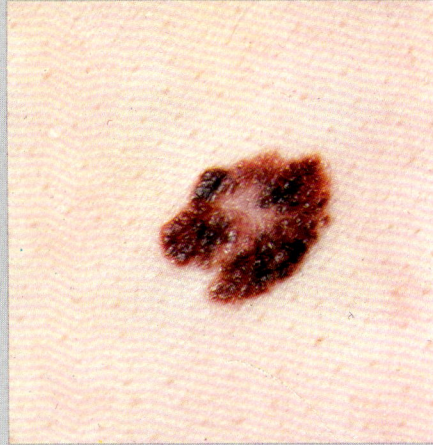

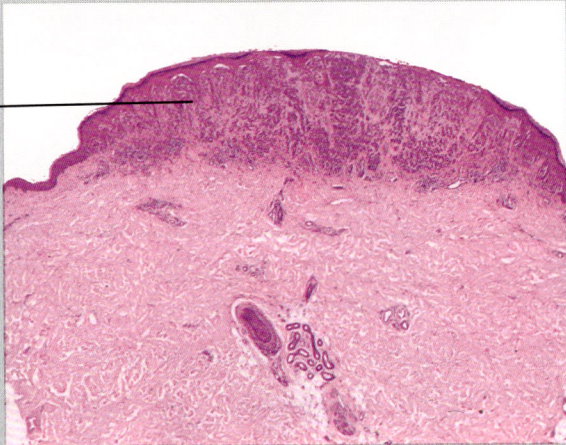

neoplasm symmetrical

neoplasm asymmetrical

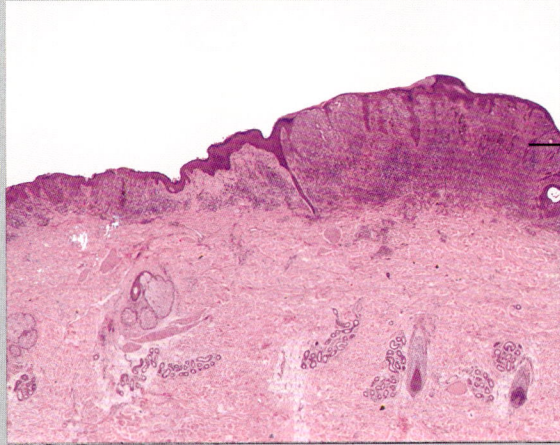

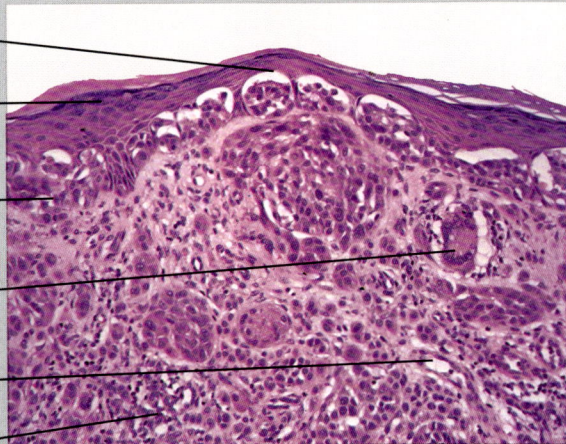

cleft

hyper-granulosis

epithelioid melanocytes at dermo-epidermal junction

multi-nucleated nevus cell

dilated blood vessel

lymphocytes

atypical melanocytes at all levels of epidermis

atypical pagetoid melanocyte

atypical melanocytes in infundibulum

melanophages

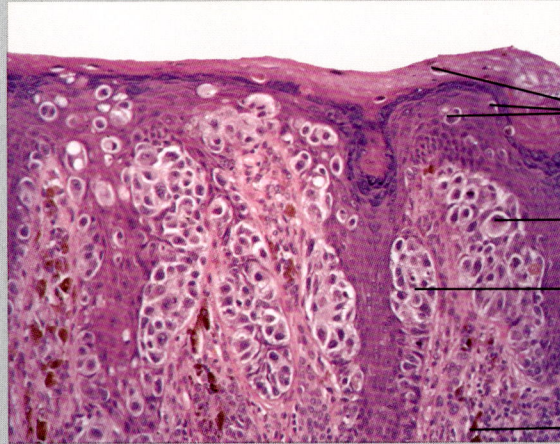

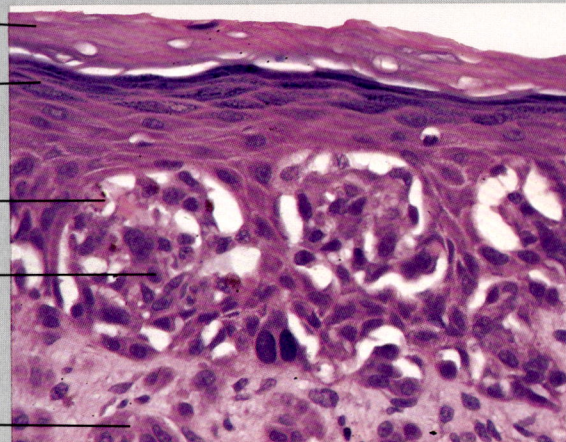

hyper-keratosis

hyper-granulosis

dull pink globule

nest of epithelioid melanocytes

nest of epithelioid nevus cells

atypical melanocytes in cornified layer

nests of atypical melanocytes differ in sizes and shapes

confluence of nests of atypical pagetoid melanocytes

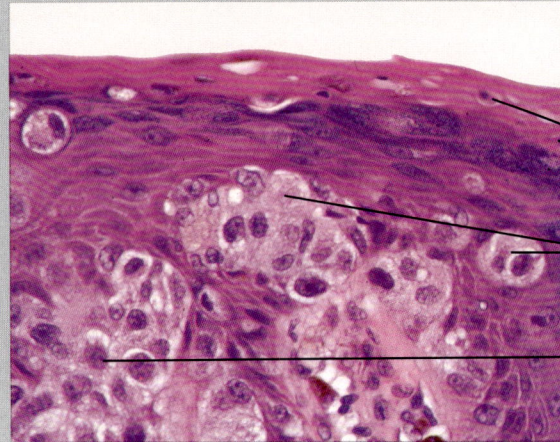

S PITZ'S nevus, compound type (the nevus of large spindle and/or epithelioid cells, benign juvenile melanoma) and malignant melanoma have in common nests of atypical melanocytes within the epidermis (often scattered at all levels of the epidermis) and the dermis, as well as an inflammatory-cell infiltrate in the dermis. In fact, nuclear atypia in some Spitz's nevi may be more striking than in many malignant melanomas.

The nevus of large spindle and/or epithelioid cells occurs in both children and adults and may or may not be pigmented. The nonpigmented type is often an orange-red, smooth-surfaced or papillomatous papule or nodule. The lesion in most instances is situated on the head or extremities (very commonly on the legs of women), but it sometimes occurs on the trunk. A desmoplastic variant of the nevus in point occurs in adults and because of the prominent fibrosis may be misinterpreted clinically and histologically as a dermatofibroma. The large size of some of the melanocytes is the common denominator of all forms of the nevus. Another important feature is the spindle and/or epithelioid morphology of the melanocytes and nevus cells. Spitz's nevus is merely one type of melanocytic nevus and like all of the others it behaves in a benign fashion biologically.

Malignant melanoma may develop anywhere on the body, but most often it appears on the legs of women and on the trunks of men. Clinically, malignant melanoma is characterized by variegation in its color (nuances of pink, brown, gray, black, blue), irregularity of its borders, and unevenness of its surface. Sometimes a nodule is present within such a lesion. Prognosis in malignant melanoma depends, in part, upon the extension in depth of the neoplastic melanocytes.

Virtually all malignant melanomas primary in the skin arise within the epidermis and extend horizontally there for varying periods before extending vertically into the dermis. In short, all primary malignant melanomas in skin are at first superficially spreading. There are differences in the cytologic features of atypical melanocytes in the epidermis of malignant melanomas on different anatomic sites; for example, those on the head and neck usually are oval or round, those on the trunk and extremities usually are pagetoid, and those on the palms and soles usually are dendritic. However, any of these cytologic variants of atypical melanocytes, as well as balloon and multinucleated ones, may be seen in malignant melanomas on any anatomic site. Furthermore, combinations of cytologic variants of atypical melanocytes may appear together in the same malignant melanoma. The criteria listed above for differentiating malignant melanomas from Spitz's nevi apply to malignant melanomas in general, irrespective of anatomic site.

In sum, the crucial features for histologic differentiation of these two lesions of atypical melanocytes are related to architectural pattern, especially symmetry, size, and circumscription. Too much concern for cytologic detail sometimes leads pathologists to "overdiagnose" Spitz's nevus as malignant melanoma. Such errors occur because melanocytes in some Spitz's nevi may show more striking nuclear atypia than do melanocytes in some malignant melanomas.

38. Pyogenic Granuloma *vs.* Kaposi's Sarcoma, Nodular Stage

Pyogenic Granuloma	*Kaposi's Sarcoma, Nodular Stage*
1. Exophytic growth predominantly	1. Endophytic growth predominantly
2. Epidermal collarette invariable	2. Epidermal collarette occasionally
3. Granulation tissue forms the entire early lesion	3. Granulation tissue superficial and then only in late ulcerated lesions
4. Endothelial cells and fibroblasts not arranged in any pattern	4. Spindle cells predominate and are arranged in interlacing fascicles
5. Erythrocytes within dilated endothelial-lined vascular spaces	5. Erythrocytes in slits formed by spindle cells
6. Focal extravasation of erythrocytes and hemosiderin in the stroma	6. Diffuse extravasation of erythrocytes and hemosiderin among spindle cells
7. Fibrous trabeculae separate vascular components into lobules often	7. No fibrous trabeculae
8. Moderately dense, mixed inflammatory-cell infiltrate throughout the stroma	8. Sparse mononuclear inflammatory-cell infiltrate in nonulcerated lesions

Pyogenic Granuloma

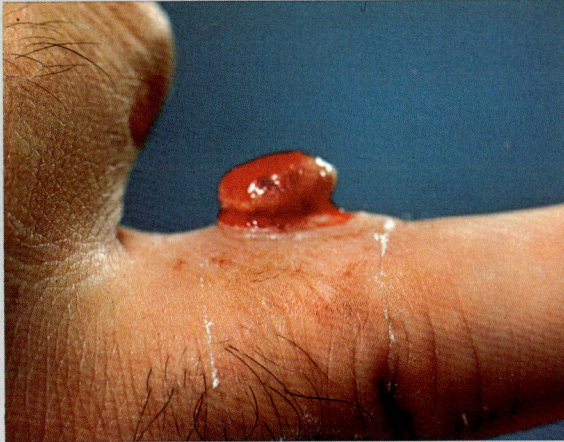

Kaposi's Sarcoma, Nodular Stage

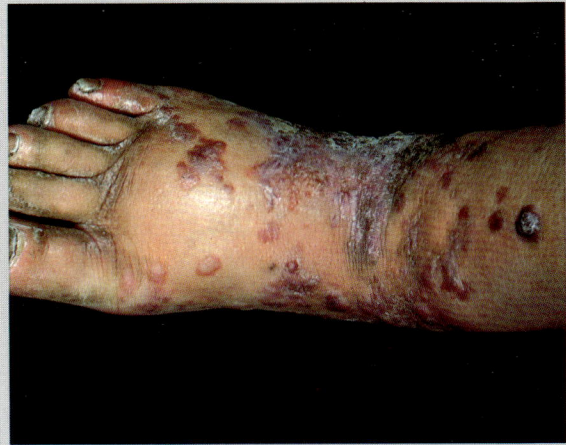

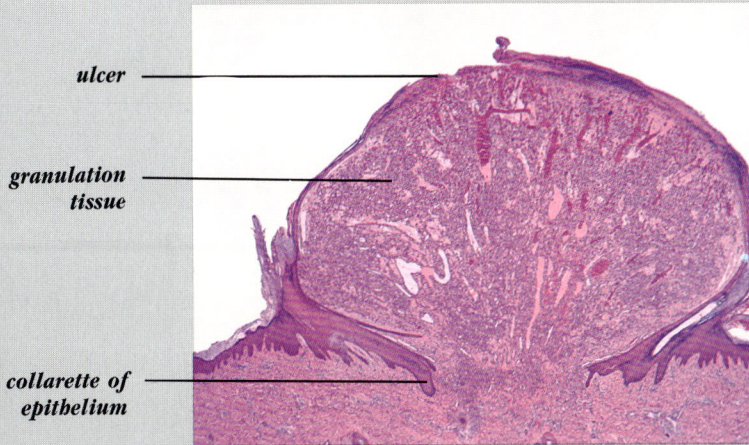

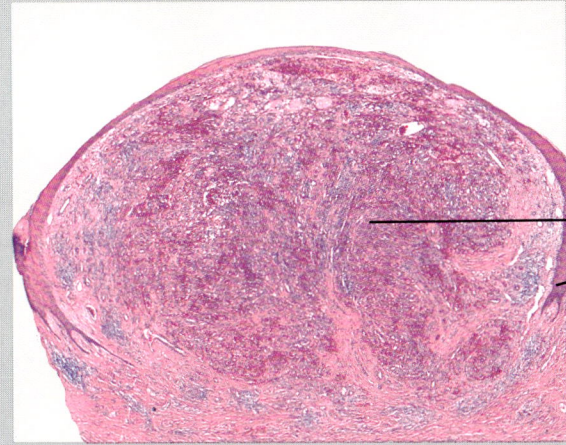

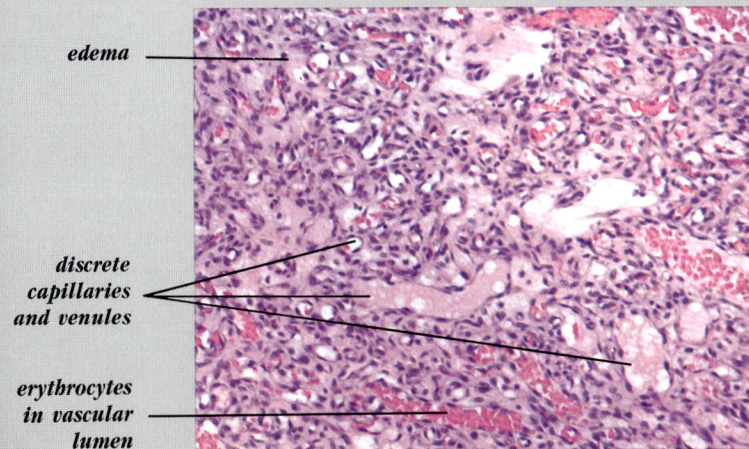

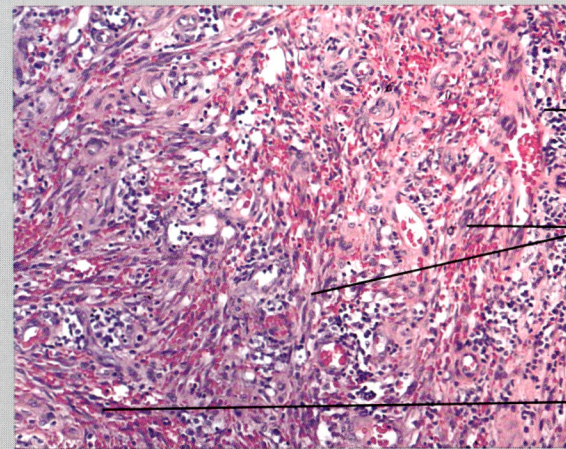

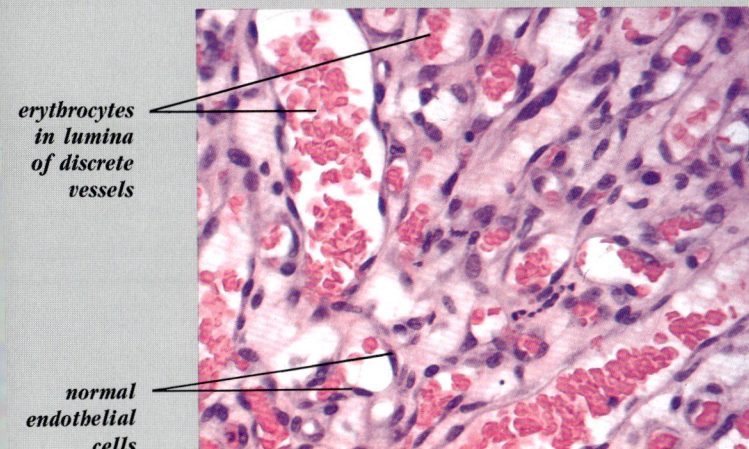

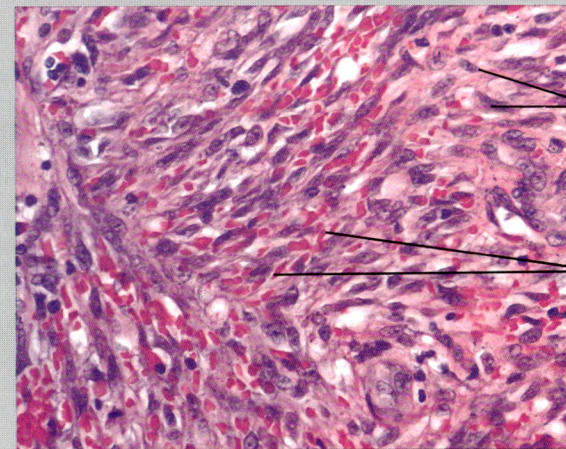

ulcer

granulation
tissue

spindle-cell
neoplasm

collarette of
epithelium

collarette of
epithelium

edema

lymphocytes
and plasma
cells

discrete
capillaries
and venules

fascicles of
spindle cells

erythrocytes
in vascular
lumen

erythrocytes
in slits
between
spindle cells

erythrocytes
in lumina
of discrete
vessels

atypical
spindle cells

erythrocytes
in slits
between
spindle cells

normal
endothelial
cells

Both pyogenic granuloma and Kaposi's sarcoma are vascular proliferations. In most instances, nodular lesions of Kaposi's sarcoma are easily differentiated histologically from those of pyogenic granuloma. Problems of differential diagnosis arise when lesions of Kaposi's sarcoma ulcerate and granulation tissue forms superficially, but exuberantly. In these more difficult cases, the preceding criteria are helpful in differentiating them. The histological features outlined for Kaposi's sarcoma apply only to nodules and not to earlier patches and plaques, which do not present a problem in differential diagnosis from pyogenic granuloma.

Clinically, both pyogenic granuloma and Kaposi's sarcoma are found predominantly on the skin of the extremities. The hands, fingers, and face (highly vascular regions) are more commonly affected by pyogenic granulomas, generally in the form of a solitary, reddish-orange to brown, translucent, ulcerated nodule, but rarely as multiple lesions. Nodular lesions of Kaposi's sarcoma also tend to affect the acral parts, but they are usually purple to dark brown and variably sized lesions. Occasionally, Kaposi's sarcoma may appear as a solitary lesion and remain that for a time.

Pyogenic granuloma and Kaposi's sarcoma may be said to evolve in three stages. A pyogenic granuloma begins as a result of trauma, often a penetrating injury; grows rapidly as "proud flesh" that histologically consists of ulcerated, exuberant granulation tissue; and, in time, comes to resemble a hemangioma, clinically and histologically. In resolution, a pyogenic granuloma re-epithelializes, develops thick, fibrous septa that intersect the angiomatous elements and, at long last, constricts by fibrosis.

Kaposi's sarcoma begins as a patch that is characterized histologically by an increased number of irregular, jagged-shaped endothelial-lined spaces in the upper part of the dermis that are surrounded by a sparse to moderately dense infiltrate of lymphocytes and plasma cells. Gradually, as plaques form, multiple foci of vascular proliferation and of spindle cells are seen throughout the dermis accompanied by extravasated erythrocytes, siderophages, and plasma cells. Finally, as nodules appear, Kaposi's sarcoma consists of a spindle-cell neoplasm throughout the dermis. The spindle cells are often arranged in large aggregates or fascicles and solitary erythrocytes are generally found in interstices (slits) between the closely packed spindle cells.

Whereas pyogenic granuloma occurs only in skin and mucous membranes, Kaposi's sarcoma, nearly always involving skin, may also involve internal organs, especially lymph nodes, lungs, and the gastrointestinal tract in as many as 10% of cases. Furthermore, patients with Kaposi's sarcoma have a greater incidence of other lymphoreticular disorders such as Hodgkin's disease and lymphocytic leukemia. Although not in itself lethal in most instances, many patients with Kaposi's sarcoma die of bleeding from gastro-intestinal or pulmonary lesions, from infections superimposed upon massively edematous ulcerated lower extremities, or from associated lympho-reticular diseases.

39. Angiolymphoid Hyperplasia with Eosinophilia *vs.* Angiosarcoma

Angiolymphoid Hyperplasia with Eosinophilia	Angiosarcoma
1. Dome-shaped lesion (clinically a nodule)	1. Flat-surfaced lesion (clinically a patch or plaque)
2. Ulceration rare	2. Ulceration common
3. Well circumscribed neoplasm of thick-walled vessels	3. Poorly circumscribed, diffusely infiltrating neoplasm of thin-walled vessels
4. Involves the dermis alone and/or the fat	4. Involves the dermis and the fat almost always
5. One pattern in each lesion, namely discrete, muscular, thick-walled blood vessels resembling veins of various sizes and shapes	5. Two patterns in the same lesion often: (a) ill-defined, bizarre-shaped, irregularly anastomosing, vascular channels, and (b) solid areas arranged as cords, fascicles, or sheets of cells with no or only slight suggestion of vascular differentiation
6. No projections into lumina	6. Bulbous, villous, or frond-like projections from vessel walls into the lumina often
7. Large, pleomorphic cells lining vascular channels; none in mitosis	7. Atypical cells lining vascular channels, i.e., with large, hyperchromatic, and pleomorphic nuclei; many in mitosis, some of them atypical
8. Endothelial cells protrude into lumina, but do not appear to lose contact with the vessel walls or with one another	8. Atypical endothelial cells that protrude into lumina often appear to lose contact with the vessel walls and with one another, giving the impression of cells floating free within a space
9. Erythrocytes wholly within vascular channels	9. Erythrocytes inside and outside vascular channels
10. Eosinophils (usually numerous), lymphocytes, and histiocytes within the stroma	10. Occasional eosinophils, lymphocytes, and histiocytes within the stroma
11. Lymphoid follicles common	11. Lymphoid follicles rare
12. Abundant acid mucopolysaccharides in the stroma	12. No acid mucopolysaccharides in the stroma

Angiolymphoid Hyperplasia with Eosinophilia

Angiosarcoma

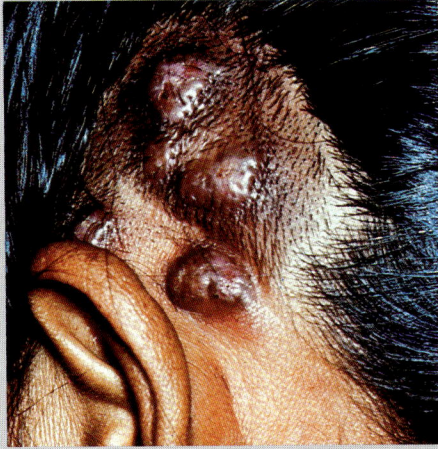

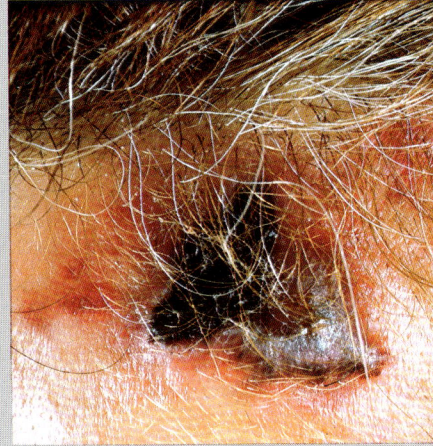

infiltrate of lymphocytes and eosinophils

discrete vascular spaces

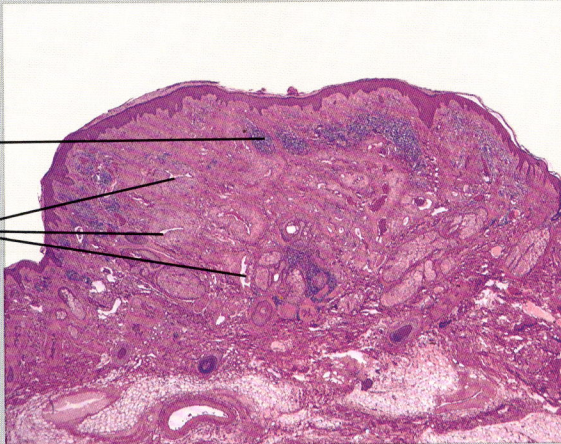

lymphocytes and eosinophils

discrete, large, irregularly shaped space lined by endothelial cells

mucin around blood vessel

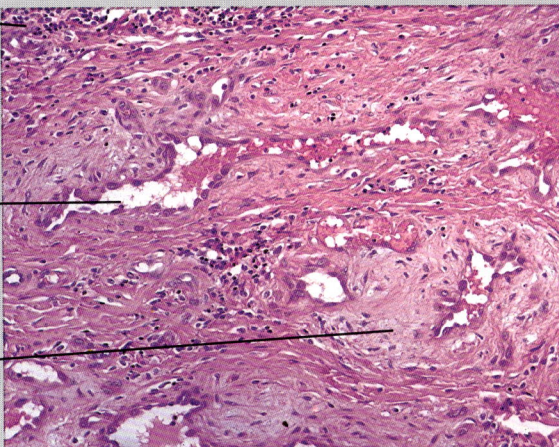

large endothelial cells protrude into lumen

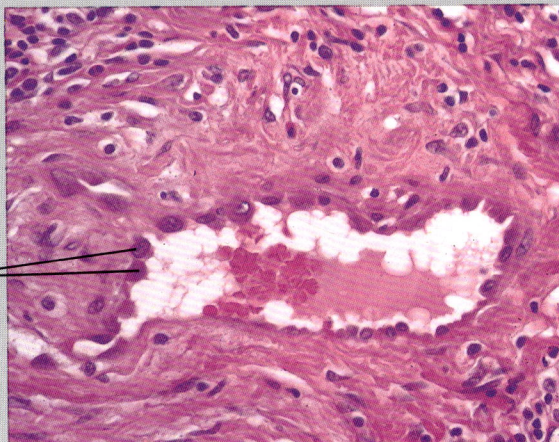

ulcer

neoplastic cells throughout dermis and subcutaneous fat

inflammatory and neoplastic cells in fascia

small irregularly shaped space

irregularly shaped spaces

space lined by atypical cells

zone of neoplastic cells devoid of spaces

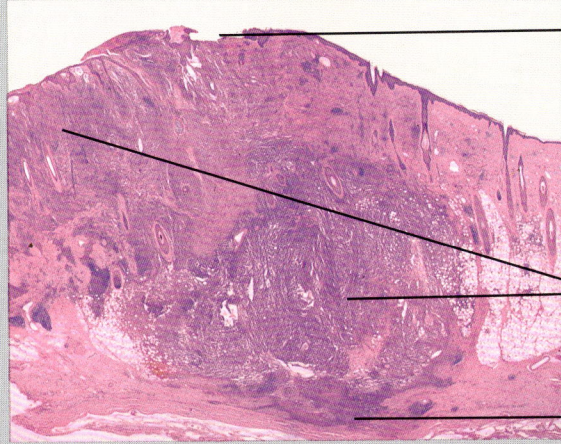

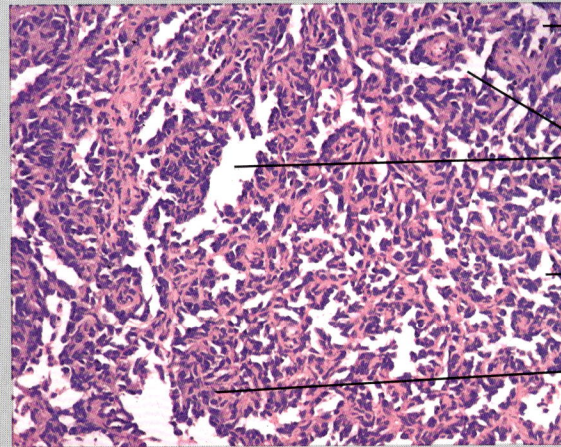

irregularly shaped spaces lined by numerous atypical cells

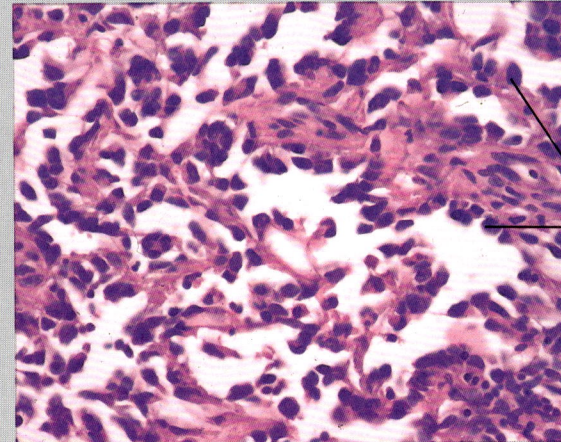

ANGIOSARCOMA, (also known as malignant hemangio- or lymphangio-endothelioma) and angiolymphoid hyperplasia with eosinophilia (known as Kimura's disease when there is systemic involvement) are pathological processes with vascular differentiation. Whereas angiolymphoid hyperplasia with eosinophilia is a benign vascular malformation that usually results from an arterio-venous shunt, angiosarcoma is a malignant neoplasm. Clinically and biologically they are very different from one another, but histologically they have features in common. Both may have vascular channels lined by large atypical cells that protrude into the lumina of the channels. For this reason, those not acquainted with angiolymphoid hyperplasia with eosinophilia may misinterpret the condition as angiosarcoma unless the many histologic differences enumerated above are taken into account. Clinically, angiolymphoid hyperplasia develops as nodules on the head, especially around the ears, of younger individuals. The nodules enlarge to sizes from 1 to 5 cm in diameter and then cease to grow. Some nodules even regress. Angiosarcomas, in contrast, tend to occur on the face, especially on the scalps of older individuals, as firm, bluish-purple patches and plaques which inexorably extend horizontally and deeply.

Angiolymphoid hyperplasia behaves in an utterly benign fashion. Angiosarcomas, on the other hand, even when ablated surgically and seemingly completely, almost always eventually metastasize and kill.

The Stewart-Treves syndrome is angiosarcoma (presumably lymphangiosarcoma) that develops in lymphedematous arms as a consequence of radical mastectomy (which includes lymphadenectomy) for carcinoma of the breast. The histologic features detailed for angiosarcomas in general apply equally to the lymphangiosarcomas described by Stewart and Treves. It is also possible to see histologic features focally in Kaposi's sarcoma that are indistinguishable from those in angiosarcomas.

It should be noted that several variants of angiolymphoid hyperplasia have been described, papular angioplasia as one example, pseudopyogenic granuloma as another. Histologically, angiolymphoid hyperplasia may involve the dermis only, the subcutaneous fat only, or the dermis and the subcutis together. The condition was termed angiolymphoid hyperplasia with eosinophilia because the individual lesions may consist of lymphoid follicles (germinal centers) and numerous eosinophils, as well as increased numbers of aberrant blood vessels.

As is so often the case in histologic differentiation between a malignant neoplasm like angiosarcoma and a pseudomalignant condition like angiolymphoid hyperplasia with eosinophilia, the pathologist is well advised to pay heed to their distinctively different architectural patterns, rather than to give too much attention to cytologic details. Not only are the endothelial cells in angiosarcoma and angiolymphoid hyperplasia marked by atypical nuclei, but their cytoplasm may contain characteristic, variably sized circular lacunae. In short, these two biologically different conditions of atypical endothelial cells are best differentiated when viewed by scanning rather than high power magnification.

40. Lymphomatoid Papulosis *vs.* Mycosis Fungoides, Plaque Stage

Lymphomatoid Papulosis	*Mycosis Fungoides, Plaque Stage*
1. Dome-shaped lesions	1. Flat-topped lesions
2. Erosion and/or ulceration common	2. No erosion or ulceration usually
3. Parakeratosis, often containing neutrophils	3. Ortho- and parakeratosis; no neutrophils
4. Wedge-shaped necrosis and individually necrotic keratinocytes in epidermis often	4. Only individually necrotic keratinocytes and uncommon at that
5. Intraepidermal vesicles or pustules often	5. No intraepidermal vesicles or pustules at all
6. Atypical mononuclear cells scattered singly in epidermis	6. Atypical mononuclear cells singly and in collections in epidermis
7. Atypical mononuclear cells in epidermis of about the same size as those in dermis	7. Atypical mononuclear cells in epidermis larger than those in dermis
8. Wedge-shaped infiltrate in the dermis	8. Infiltrate not wedge-shaped
9. Many extravasated erythrocytes in dermis and in epidermis	9. Few, if any, extravasated erythrocytes
10. Edema in papillary dermis usually; no sclerosis	10. No edema in papillary dermis; sclerosis common there
11. Increased mucin in reticular dermis often	11. Mucin in dermis not increased
12. Infiltrate perivascular and interstitial	12. Infiltrate perivascular in the reticular dermis
13. Neutrophils numerous in a mixed cellular infiltrate	13. Usually no neutrophils
14. Striking pleomorphism of atypical cells	14. Moderate pleomorphism of atypical cells
15. Plasmacytoid appearance of atypical cells often	15. No plasmacytoid atypical cells
16. Bi- and multinucleated atypical cells common	16. Bi- or multinucleated cells rare
17. Marked contrast in size between contiguous lymphoid cells	17. Lymphoid cells approximately the same size
18. Many mitotic figures in mononuclear cells, some atypical	18. Few mitotic figures in mononuclear cells
19. Nuclear dust and tingible bodies common	19. No nuclear dust or tingible bodies
20. Neutrophils in lumina of small blood vessels	20. No neutrophils in lumina of blood vessels
21. Blood vessels have thick walls and plump endothelial cells	21. No alterations in walls of blood vessels as a rule
22. Vasculitis of small and medium-sized blood vessels occasionally	22. No vasculitis
23. Degeneration of collagen and necrosis of adnexal epithelium secondary to vasculitis	23. No degeneration of collagen or necrosis of epithelium as a rule
24. No follicular mucinosis	24. Follicular mucinosis occasionally
25. Infiltrate in subcutaneous fat commonly	25. Infiltrate in subcutaneous fat rarely

Lymphomatoid Papulosis

Mycosis Fungoides, Plaque Stage

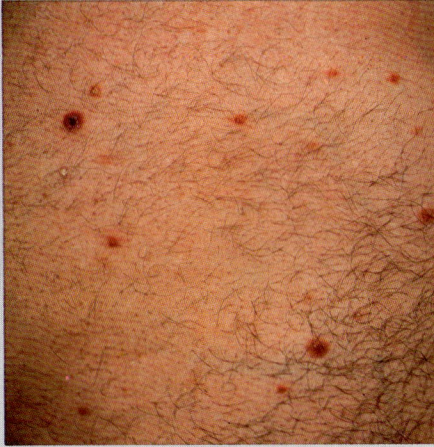

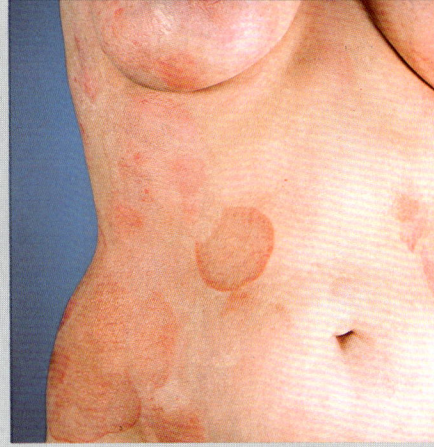

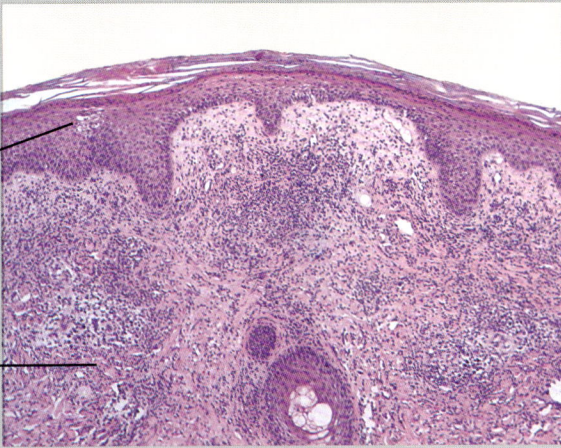

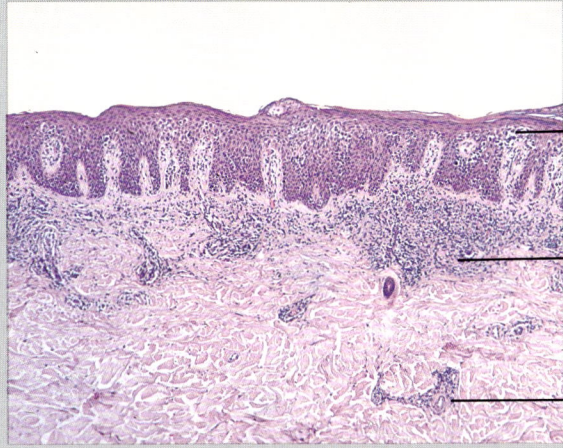

few inflammatory cells in epidermis

perivascular and interstitial mixed-cell infiltrate

nuclear "dust"

large atypical lymphoid cell

neutrophils

plasma-cytoid cells

plump endothelial cell

nuclear "dust"

neutrophil

large atypical lymphoid cells

many large atypical lymphoid cells in epidermis

lichenoid infiltrate of mononuclear cells

mononuclear cells around deep vascular plexus

small collection of atypical lymphoid cells

atypical lymphoid cells in epidermis

hyperplastic epidermis

mononuclear cells in dermis smaller than those in epidermis

large atypical lymphoid cells

small lymphocytes

L YMPHOMATOID papulosis and the plaque stage of mycosis fungoides have many histologic features in common. In both, the superficial and deep infiltrate may also be band-like in the papillary dermis and may contain eosinophils and atypical mononuclear cells. The atypical mononuclear cells are morphologically of two types—convoluted (cerebriform) with hyperchromatic nuclei and convoluted with pale-staining nuclei and prominent nucleoli. Typical and sometimes atypical mitotic figures may be seen. The histological differential diagnosis between the two conditions is sometimes difficult, but the listed differential features are helpful in correctly identifying them.

Clinically, lymphomatoid papulosis resembles pityriasis lichenoides et varioliformis acuta (Mucha-Habermann disease) by consisting of macules, papules, scaly papules, vesiculo-pustules, and small ulcers that heal leaving scars. Lymphomatoid papulosis usually starts in persons over 25 years of age, lasts for years, is much more common in women than in men, and is associated with nodular (and sometimes plaque) lesions, unlike Mucha-Habermann disease, which usually starts in persons under 25, is of relatively short duration (weeks or months), is more common in men, and is devoid of nodules.

Histologically, lymphomatoid papulosis and Mucha-Habermann disease both have superficial and deep wedge-shaped infiltrates which obscure the dermo-epidermal interface, necrosis and ulceration of the epidermis, and edema and hemorrhage in the papillary dermis. Despite these similarities, Mucha-Habermann disease may be differentiated from lymphomatoid papulosis because it contains lymphocytes and histiocytes only, no neutrophils within vascular lumina, mononuclear cells of relatively uniform size, no atypical mononuclear cells as a rule, no mitoses of the mononuclear cells, no binucleated or multinucleated cells, no tingible bodies, and no vasculitis. Because of the aforementioned many clinical similarities (and the few histological ones) between Mucha-Habermann disease and lymphomatoid papulosis, some of the cases reported as Mucha-Habermann disease in which biopsy revealed large mononuclear cells within the infiltrate were actually lymphomatoid papulosis.

The clinical spectrum of mycosis fungoides ranges from early macular lesions, through plaques (parapsoriasis en plaques) to nodules (tumors), and ulcers. Some plaques may resolve spontaneously and regress to atrophic patches (e.g., poikiloderma vasculare atrophicans). All of these stages may be present simultaneously in the same patient. During the patch stage of mycosis fungoides, the cellular infiltrate is lympho-histiocytic and no atypical mononuclear cells are usually discernible by conventional microscopy. However, even in patches of mycosis fungoides there are increased numbers of lymphocytes scattered singly within the epidermis in the absence of spongiotic microvesiculation. This finding enables accurate diagnosis and differentiation of mycosis fungoides from spongiotic dermatitides. As plaques develop there are still only lymphocytes and histiocytes in the lichenoid infiltrate, but in late plaques there are often eosinophils and plasma cells in addition to mononuclear cells, many of which are atypical. In fully developed plaques of mycosis fungoides, numerous atypical lymphoid cells are present within the epidermis singly and sometimes in collections of various sizes and shapes (Pautrier's microabscesses). Atypical mononuclear cells within the epidermis of mycosis fungoides are usually larger than those within the dermis. By the time nodules form, the dense, diffuse, monomorphous infiltrate of atypical mononuclear cells resembles what was formerly termed reticulum-cell sarcoma.

Mycosis fungoides usually begins in adulthood and tends to have a variable chronic course. The patch stage may persist for many years without apparent involvement of internal organs by the disease. As plaques develop, the prognosis worsens and the presence of nodules presages a grim end because by then there is frequently concomitant systemic disease.

What then is the relationship, if any, between lymphomatoid papulosis, mycosis fungoides, and other malignant lymphomas? The large atypical lymphoid cells of lymphomatoid papulosis, both the convoluted and hyperchromatic types, are virtually indistinguishable by conventional and electron microscopy from those in mycosis fungoides. Although most patients with lymphomatoid papulosis have an uneventful course, save for the coming and going of cutaneous lesions, some of them develop plaque lesions that are similar, clinically and histologically, to plaques of mycosis fungoides. A few patients with lymphomatoid papulosis, after years of evanescent skin lesions, have developed huge nodules in the skin that eventuated in large ulcers. These patients subsequently manifested evidences of systemic malignant lymphoma, to which some of them succumbed.

From what is currently known about lymphomatoid papulosis, it becomes apparent that this distinctive disease cannot be readily classified as inflammatory or neoplastic and benign or malignant. One hypothesis holds that immune factors of the host keep the atypical lymphoid cells of lymphomatoid papulosis in check. When these factors fail, the atypical cells proliferate unchecked and the result is malignant lymphoma in skin and internal organs. More about this enigmatic process must be learned before these issues will be resolved.

41. Pseudolymphoma *vs.* Malignant Lymphoma, B-Cell Type

Pseudolymphoma	*Malignant Lymphoma, B-Cell Type*
1. Epidermal hyperplasia occasionally; no ulceration usually	1. Epidermis thinned; ulceration occasionally
2. Involvement of the upper part of the dermis by cellular infiltrate markedly greater than that of the lower part	2. Involvement of the lower part of the dermis by cellular infiltrate approximately equal to or greater than that of the upper part
3. Germinal centers may be present	3. Germinal centers absent
4. Vasculature prominent with increased number of blood vessels which have plump endothelial cells	4. Vasculature not prominent
5. Mixed cellular infiltrate (lymphocytes and histiocytes at the least, but plasma cells and eosinophils often and neutrophils rarely)	5. Monomorphous cellular infiltrate
6. No inflammatory cells within the walls of blood vessels or epithelial structures of adnexa	6. Neoplastic mononuclear cells often within the walls of blood vessels and within epithelial structures of adnexa
7. Polychrome bodies (tingible bodies, nuclear dust) within macrophages common	7. Polychrome bodies rare
8. Histiocytic giant cells occasionally	8. No histiocytic giant cells
9. Mitotic figures not numerous usually, except in germinal centers	9. Mitotic figures may be numerous
10. No necrosis within cellular infiltrate	10. Necrosis within cellular infiltrate occasionally

Pseudolymphoma

Malignant Lymphoma, B-Cell Type

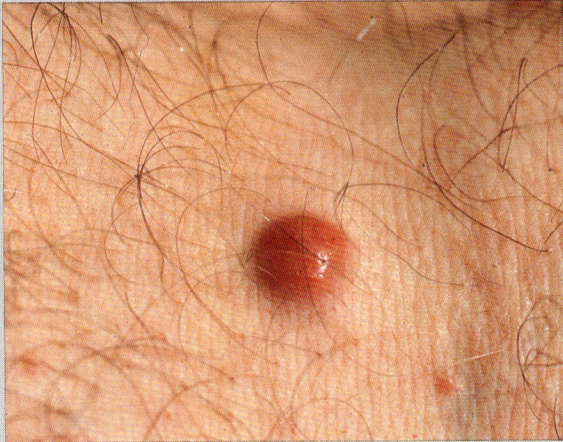

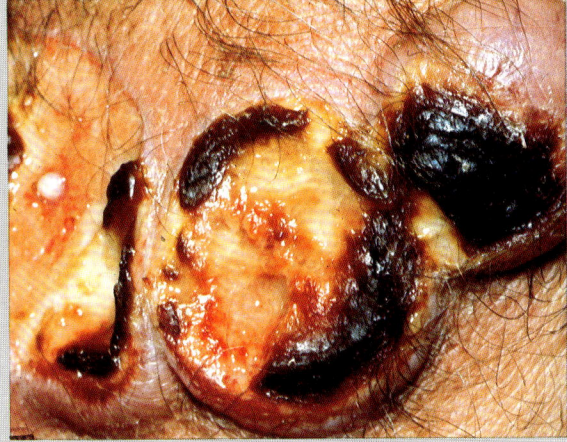

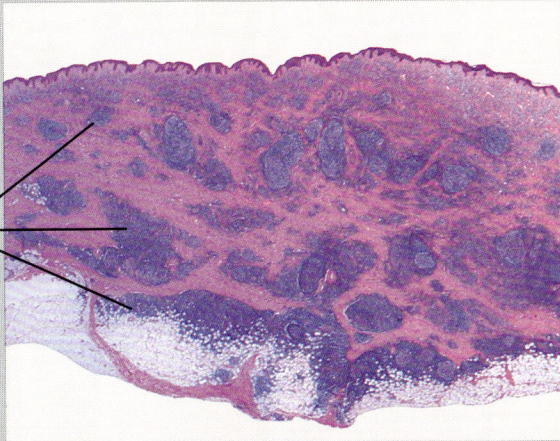

upper part of dermis spared

infiltrate equally dense throughout lesion

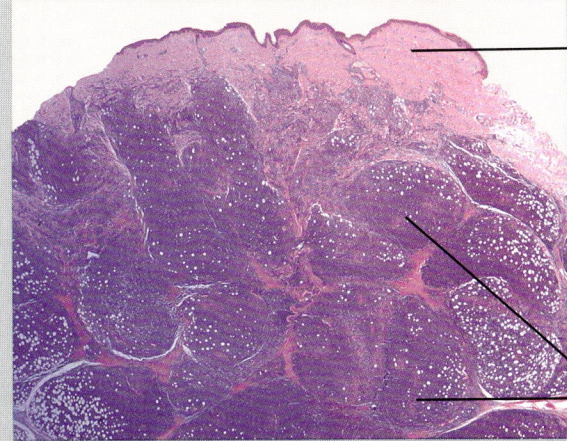

"bottom-heavy" infiltrate

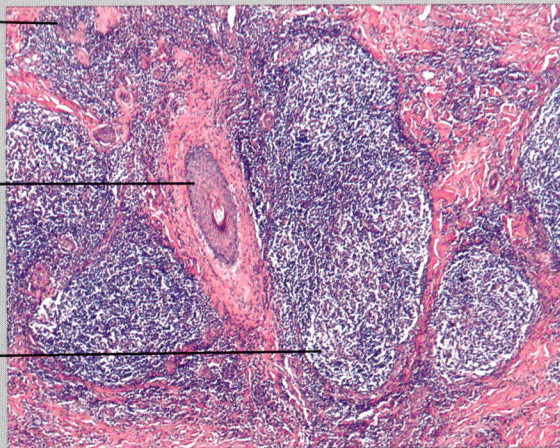

mixed-cell infiltrate

hair follicle uninvolved

lymphoid follicle in nodule of inflammatory cells

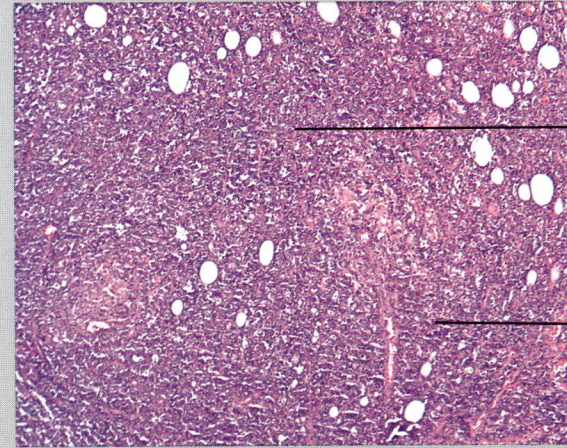

sheets of neoplastic cells

monomorphous infiltrate

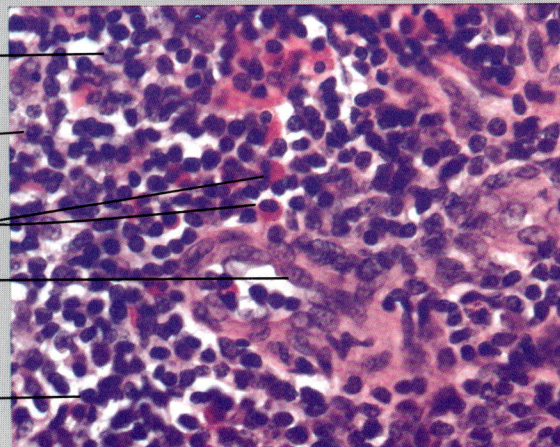

histiocyte

plasma cell

eosinophils

plump endothelial cell

lymphocyte

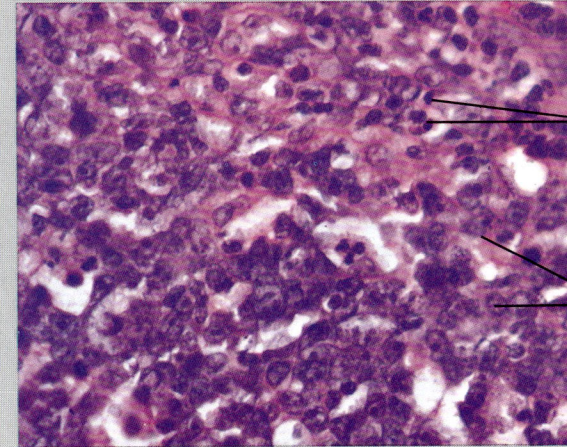

necrotic neoplastic cells

large atypical lymphoid cells in monomorphous infiltrate

Pseudolymphoma and malignant lymphoma are lymphoreticular processes that have histologic features in common, namely, dense nodular or diffuse infiltrates containing some atypical mononuclear cells, increased number of mitotic figures, and even atypical mitotic figures. These similar cytologic features make differentiation of pseudolymphomas from malignant lymphomas exceedingly difficult at times, especially when the biopsy is not wide and deep. The differences listed above are usually helpful, but the ultimate criterion is the biologic behavior of the process, i.e., the course of it over many years. Pseudolymphomas behave in an entirely benign fashion, whereas malignant lymphomas almost always end fatally. Occasionally, individual lesions of malignant lymphomas, like those of pseudolymphomas, undergo spontaneous resolution.

Malignant lymphomas are usually plum-colored nodules that often ulcerate. Although malignant lymphoma may, in rare instances, begin in the skin, the vast majority of them arise in internal organs and only secondarily involve the skin. There are two major categories of malignant lymphomas, the B-cell and the T-cell types. These can be subdivided by nuclear size into small, intermediate, and large. The T-cell types, of which mycosis fungoides is the prototype, tend to involve the epidermis, whereas the B-cell types do not. The criteria used here for the differentiation of pseudolymphoma from malignant lymphoma apply only to the B-cell types of malignant lymphoma. Of these criteria, the single most important one for diagnosis of B-cell malignant lymphomas is the monomorphous quality of the cellular infiltrate. Lymphocytic leukemias may be indistinguishable histologically from B-cell malignant lymphomas.

Pseudolymphomas may stimulate malignant lymphomas of both the B- and T-cell types. Pseudolymphoma, B-cell type, is a term we use to include lesions that have also been named Spiegler-Fendt sarcoid, lymphocytoma cutis, lymphadenosis benigna cutis, and cutaneous lymphoid hyperplasia. These have been reported following trauma, rupture of follicular cysts, insect bites, vaccinations and hyposensitization injections, although in most instances, the cause remains obscure. Clinically, pseudolymphoma of the B-cell type presents itself as a solitary pink-purple papule, nodule, or plaque on the face, but it may be multiple and may occur in other areas of the skin.

Pseudolymphoma, T-cell type, refers to inflammatory diseases in the skin that resemble mycosis fungoides because of the presence of atypical lymphoid cells within the epidermis. The two most common pseudolymphomas of the T-cell type are spongiotic simulators of mycosis fungoides and lymphomatoid papulosis. In some spongiotic dermatitides such as contact dermatitis, nummular dermatitis, and Gianotti-Crosti syndrome, lymphocytes within spongiotic foci may transform into blasts and thereby resemble Pautrier's microabscesses. In lymphomatoid papulosis, large atypical lymphoid cells, many with convoluted nuclei, tend to be scattered singly within the epidermis like the atypical convoluted lymphocytes in mycosis fungoides. The histologic features crucial to a differentiation between lymphomatoid papulosis and mycosis fungoides are listed on page 158.

An attempt should be made in the case of every pseudolymphoma to search for a cause and to give a precise etiologic diagnosis. Only when no cause is evident should the imprecise diagnosis of pseudolymphoma be rendered. Pseudolymphomas of the T-cell type such as spongiotic simulators of mycosis fungoides, e.g., nummular dermatitis, and lymphomatoid papulosis also may be diagnosed with more precision.

In conclusion, terms like pseudolymphoma, pseudosarcoma, pseudocarcinoma, and pseudomelanoma are helpful in alerting pathologists to pitfalls in the interpretation of benign and malignant conditions, but all of these pseudoterms are nonspecific and, wherever possible, should be avoided and replaced by specific diagnoses.

42. Xanthogranuloma *vs.* Reticulohistiocytic Granuloma

Xanthogranuloma	*Reticulohistiocytic Granuloma*
1. Very dense and diffuse infiltrate of mononucleated and multinucleated histiocytes	1. Moderately dense and diffuse infiltrate of large mononucleated and multinucleated histiocytes
2. Cytoplasm of histiocytes usually foamy	2. Cytoplasm of histiocytes usually eosinophilic and granular, resembling ground glass; sometimes foamy
3. Touton giant cells (also termed "wreath" cells because a wreath of nuclei often separates amphophilic-staining centers from foamy peripheries) usually numerous	3. No Touton giant cells as a rule
4. Mixed cellular infiltrate, often with lymphocytes, plasma cells, neutrophils, and eosinophils	4. Relatively monomorphous infiltrate of characteristic histiocytes; occasionally mixed-cell

Xanthogranuloma

Reticulohistiocytic Granuloma

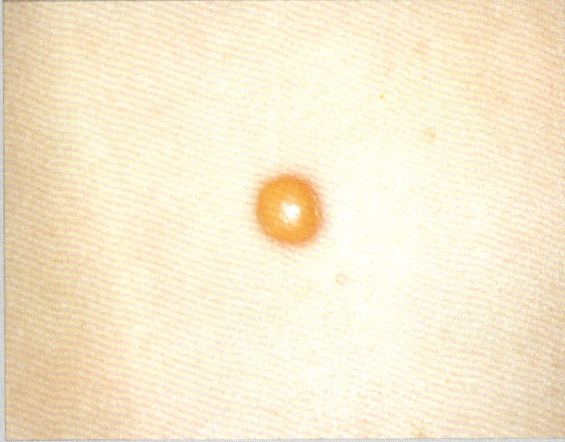
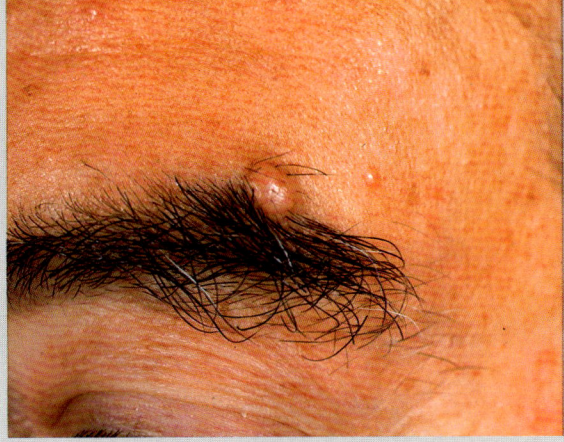

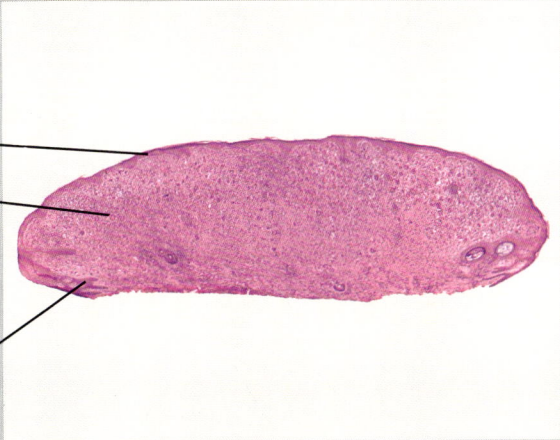

thinned epidermis

dense, diffuse, predominantly histiocytic infiltrate

epithelial collarette

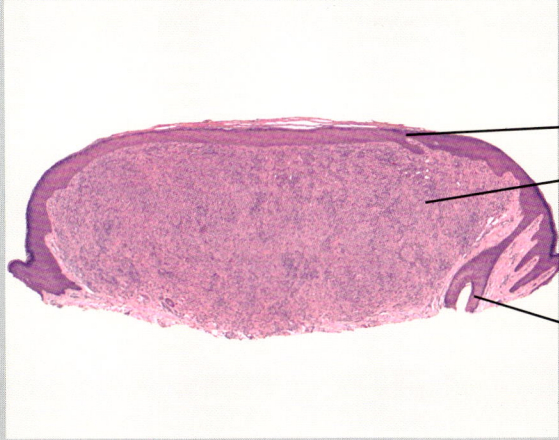

thinned epidermis

dense, diffuse, predominantly histiocytic infiltrate

epithelial collarette

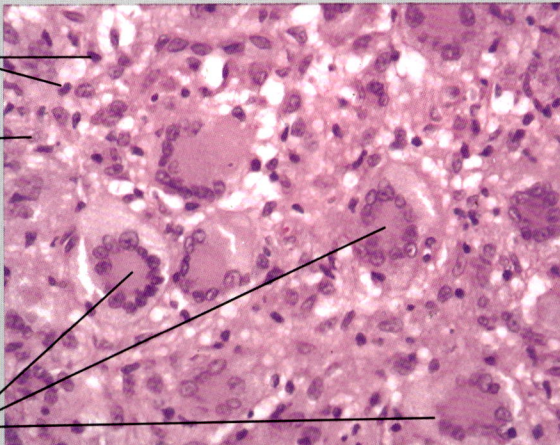

lymphocytes

histiocyte

Touton giant cells

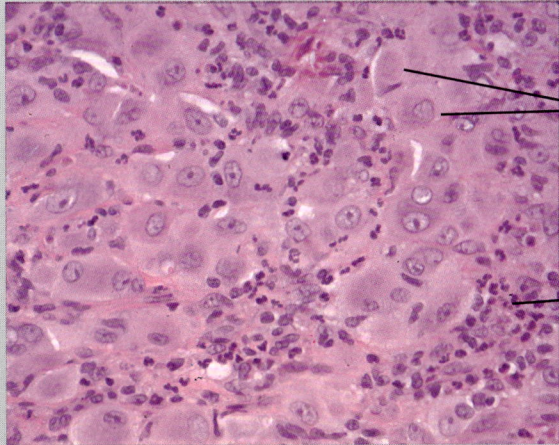

large histiocytes with "ground-glass" cytoplasms

neutrophils

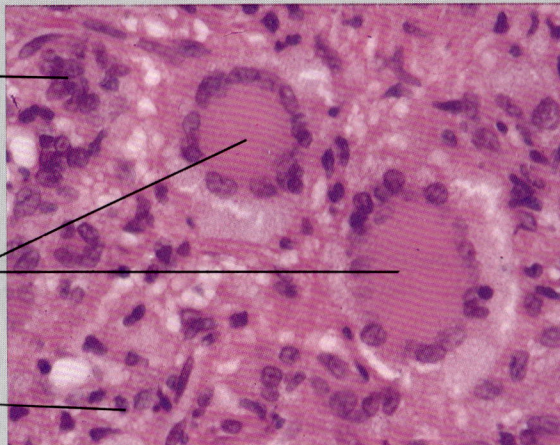

periphery of multinucleated histiocyte

Touton type of multinucleated histiocytes

lymphocytes and histiocytes

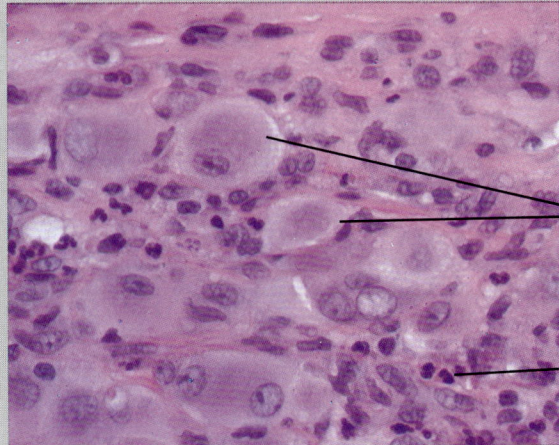

large histiocytes with "ground-glass" cytoplasms

neutrophil

XANTHOGRANULOMAS and reticulohistiocytic granulomas share histologic features in common, namely, relatively well-circumscribed, dense, diffuse, predominantly histiocytic infiltrates (granulomatous), multinucleated histiocytic giant cells, and resolution with fibrosis.

Clinically, xanthogranulomas are papules or nodules with a yellow, orange, or tan hue. The color results from abundant lipid within the histiocytes. The lesion is better termed xanthogranuloma than its former name, nevoxanthoendothelioma, which incorrectly implies that it is a nevoid condition related to blood vessels.

Although xanthogranulomas may occur at any age, they are more common in infants and young children. In youngsters, they are usually multiple, favor the face, and may involve organs besides the skin such as the eye and the gastrointestinal and genitourinary tracts. Hemorrhage into the anterior chamber from xanthogranuloma of the iris may lead to permanent blindness. The skin lesions of juvenile xanthogranuloma tend to resolve spontaneously in months. The clinical differential diagnosis of multiple lesions of juvenile xanthogranuloma is juvenile nodular urticaria pigmentosa. A solitary lesion of juvenile xanthogranuloma may be confused clinically with the nevus of large spindle and/or epithelioid cells (Spitz's nevus, benign juvenile melanoma). In contrast, xanthogranulomas in adults are usually solitary, do not involve organs other than the skin, and generally do not resolve without treatment. No abnormalities of serum lipids are found in either children or adults with xanthogranulomas.

Reticulohistiocytic granuloma may present itself as a single lesion or as widespread ones (multicentric reticulohistiocytosis). Both forms of reticulohistiocytic granuloma occur in adults rather than in children and have similar histologic findings. Persons with multicentric reticulohistiocytosis have an increased incidence of internal malignancies, especially carcinomas.

A solitary reticulohistiocytic granuloma is usually a dome-shaped nodule on the face or scalp. Multicentric reticulohistiocytosis also consists of dome-shaped nodules that tend to affect the face and hands. Polyarthritis of varying severity is often present in conjunction with the widespread form of the disease (lipoid dermatoarthritis). Biopsy specimens from the involved joints show the same kind of infiltrate as in the skin lesions.

The material resembling "ground glass" within the cytoplasm of reticulohistiocytic granuloma is PAS positive and diastase resistant, indicating that it is a neutral mucopolysaccharide, probably a glycolipid.

The lesions of histiocytosis-X are differentiated histologically from those of xanthogranuloma and reticulohistiocytic granuloma by having large atypical kidney-shaped nuclei but no Touton giant cells, and electro-microscopically by many Langerhans granules within the cytoplasms.

Touton giant cells are not specific for juvenile or adult xanthogranulomas. They may be seen in other xanthomas and, commonly, in the histiocytic stage of evolving dermatofibromas.

43. Dermatofibroma *vs.* Dermatofibrosarcoma Protuberans

Dermatofibroma

1. Well-circumscribed small lesion, usually less than 2 cm, often wholly contained within an excisional biopsy specimen

2. Epidermal hyperplasia and hyperpigmentation usually

3. Epidermal basal cells often hyperplastic to form buds with follicular differentiation; rarely authentic basal-cell carcinoma

4. Increased fibroblasts and coarse collagen fibers arranged in intersecting but haphazard pattern

5. Fibroblasts at the periphery of the lesion appear to wrap around thickened collagen bundles

6. Cellular infiltrate usually mixed (fibroblasts, histiocytes, lymphocytes, and plasma cells)

7. Histiocytic giant cells sometimes present

8. Hemorrhage, siderophages, and foam cells often

9. Cholesterol clefts occasionally

10. Sclerotic foci occasionally

11. Keloidal collagen bundles occasionally

12. Epithelial structures of adnexa destroyed by fibrosis

13. Acid mucopolysaccharides in connective tissue slightly increased

14. Increased number of prominent blood vessels with plump endothelial cells

15. Subcutaneous fat involved occasionally and focally

16. No melanocytes within lesion

Dermatofibrosarcoma Protuberans

1. Poorly circumscribed broad lesion, usually greater than 2 cm and practically never wholly contained within an excisional biopsy specimen

2. No epidermal hyperplasia or hyperpigmentation; epidermis often atrophic

3. No epidermal basal-cell hyperplasia or neoplasia

4. Increased spindle cells and fibrillar collagen often arranged in "cartwheel" pattern of short, interlacing fascicles

5. Fibroblasts at the periphery of the lesion diffusely infiltrate between normal collagen bundles

6. Cellular infiltrate usually monomorphous (spindle cells)

7. Multinucleated cells not present

8. Hemorrhage, rare; no siderophages or foam cells

9. No cholesterol clefts

10. No foci of sclerosis

11. No keloidal collagen

12. Epithelial structures of adnexa constricted by impingement

13. Acid mucopolysaccharides in connective tissue usually markedly increased

14. Blood vessels not prominent

15. Subcutaneous fat involved usually and diffusely, beginning in the fibrous septa

16. Melanocytes within lesion rarely

Dermatofibroma

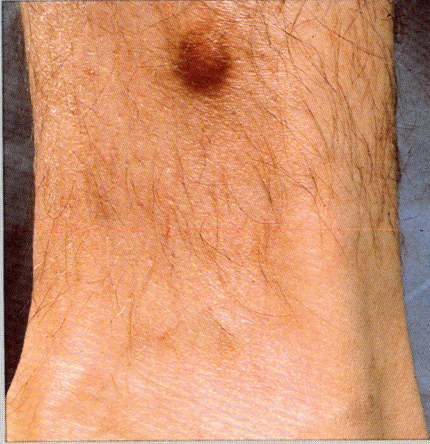

Dermatofibrosarcoma Protuberans

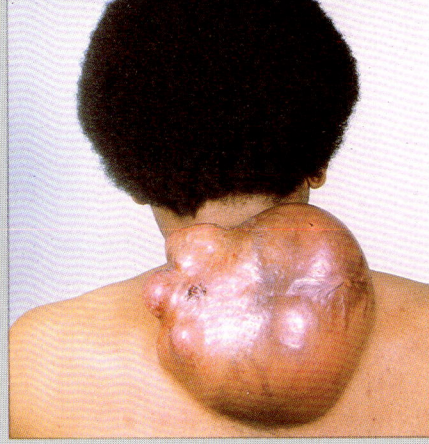

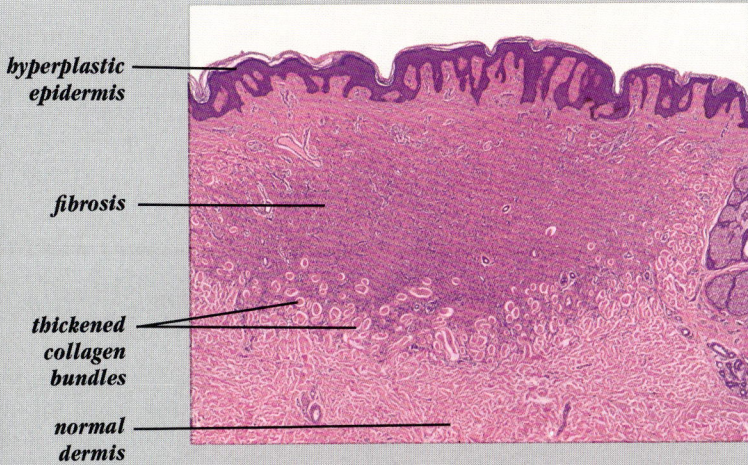

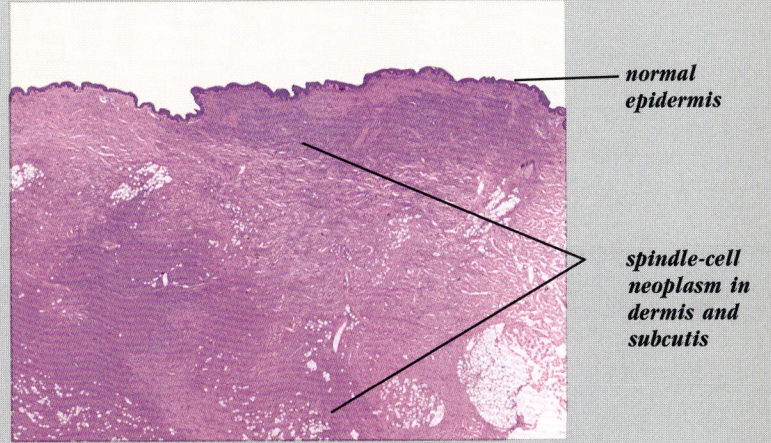

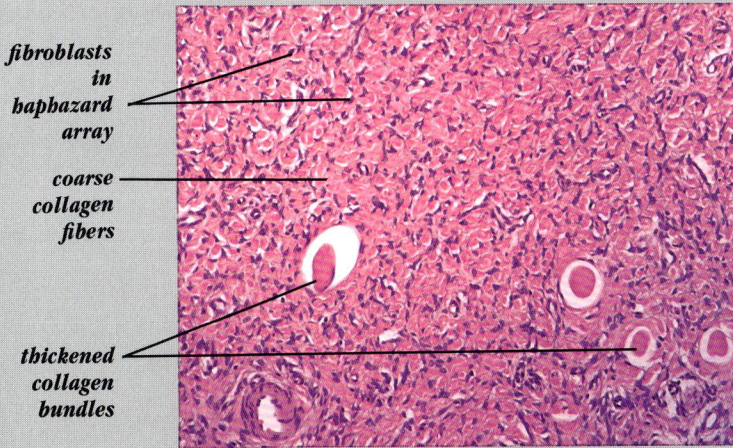

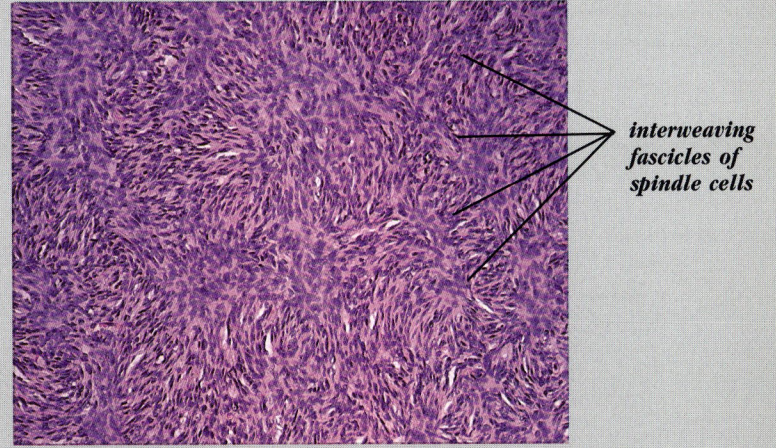

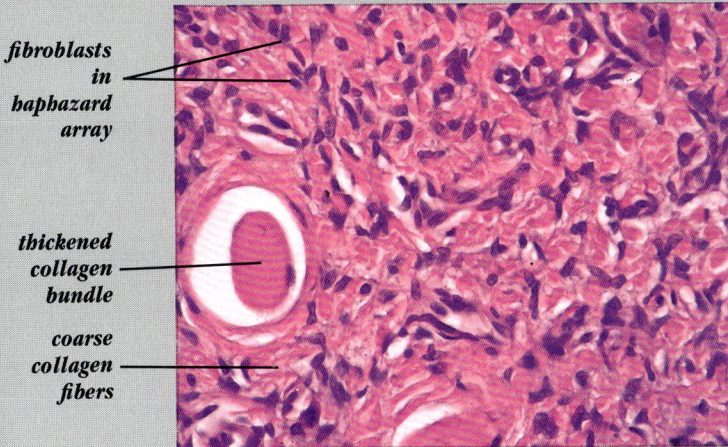

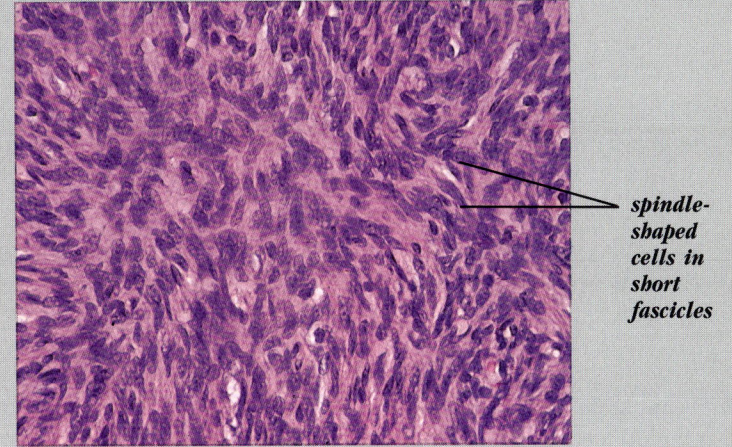

hyperplastic epidermis

normal epidermis

fibrosis

spindle-cell neoplasm in dermis and subcutis

thickened collagen bundles

normal dermis

fibroblasts in haphazard array

interweaving fascicles of spindle cells

coarse collagen fibers

thickened collagen bundles

fibroblasts in haphazard array

spindle-shaped cells in short fascicles

thickened collagen bundle

coarse collagen fibers

ERMATOFIBROMA and dermatofibrosarcoma protuberans are lesions composed of dense infiltrates of spindle-shaped cells that tend to occupy at least much of the thickness of the dermis. Their nuclei are not atypical and mitotic figures are few or absent.

Clinically, dermatofibromas appear as firm, brownish, hairless, nodules on the extremities, especially the lower. They arise secondary to trauma, often in the form of puncture wounds and arthropod (especially mosquito) bites, but sometimes secondary to ruptured follicles or follicular cysts. Therefore, the term dermatofibrosis better describes the lesion, indicating that it is a type of fibrosing dermatitis (a reactive inflammatory process involving fibroblasts), rather than a neoplasm of fibroblasts.

Many synonyms have been given to dermatofibroma, depending upon clinical and histologic nuances. Nodulus cutaneous expresses the clinical nodularity. Fibroma durum describes the hardness of some lesions. During relatively early phases of its development, blood vessels are prominent, thus the appellation sclerosing hemangioma. Later, often secondary to extravasation of erythrocytes, histiocytes arrive in number to ingest hemosiderin and lipid, thus the term histiocytoma. When both histiocytes and fibroblasts are numerous, the lesion is sometimes called a benign fibrous histiocytoma. To very old lesions in which the fibroblasts are decreased in number and the collagen has a homogeneous appearance, the name subepidermal nodular fibrosis (sclerosis) is sometimes applied. Irrespective of histologic variation, these lesions behave in a wholly benign fashion and, in time, slowly regress.

By contrast, dermatofibrosarcoma protuberans begins clinically as a skin-colored to slightly yellowish indurated plaque upon which firm nodules arise in time. The lesion occurs predominantly on the trunk and proximal portions of the extremities. Even though dermatofibrosarcoma protuberans is slow-growing, it may invade deeply into the subcutis and fascia, but rarely metastasizes.

The exact nosologic status of dermatofibrosarcoma protuberans is not yet established with certainty. Some authors hold that it is a fibroblastic neoplasm, whereas others contend that it is a neural one. The presence of melanocytes within some lesions of dermatofibrosarcoma protuberans, the fibrillary collagen, the S-shaped and thin spindle-shaped nuclei, and the often abundant acid mucopolysaccharides indicate that it is probably a neoplasm with neural differentiation.

The limited usefulness of the terms "benign" and "malignant" in the description of cutaneous neoplasms is well illustrated in the case of dermatofibrosarcoma protuberans. Is this neoplasm benign or malignant? If by malignant one means having the potential for metastasis, then dermato-fibrosarcoma protuberans is malignant. But, like basal-cell carcinoma, dermatofibrosarcoma protuberans metastasizes rarely, instead tending to recur locally. In fact, most lesions of dermatofibrosarcoma protuberans, like most basal-cell carcinomas, are not life-threatening to patients.

44. Lichen Amyloidosus

vs. Colloid Milium

Lichen Amyloidosus	Colloid Milium
1. Scalloped surface	1. Domed surface
2. Papillated epidermal hyperplasia with hyperkeratosis overlies amyloid	2. Thinned epidermis with loss of the normal pattern between epidermal rete ridges and dermal papillae
3. Rete ridges form pincers around deposits of amyloid	3. No pincers formed by rete ridges
4. Small deposits within broadened dermal papillae	4. Large deposits within the upper half of the dermis
5. Amyloid in small globules	5. Colloid in large accumulations
6. Amyloid is amphophilic or eosinophilic in sections stained with hematoxylin and eosin	6. Colloid is amphophilic or basophilic in sections stained with hematoxylin and eosin
7. No clefts within the globules of amyloid	7. Clefts within the nodules of colloid
8. Stellate fibroblasts and melanophages intimately associated with globules of amyloid	8. A few thin fibroblasts associated with colloid, but not macrophages
9. Angioplasia associated with amyloid	9. Angioplasia not associated with colloid
10. Solar elastosis not usually seen	10. Solar elastosis always present

Lichen Amyloidosus　　　　Colloid Milium

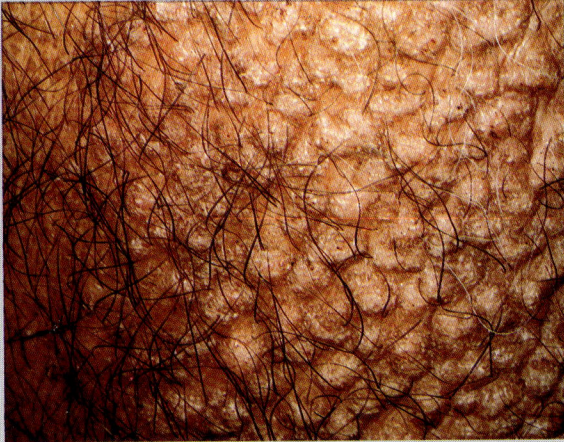 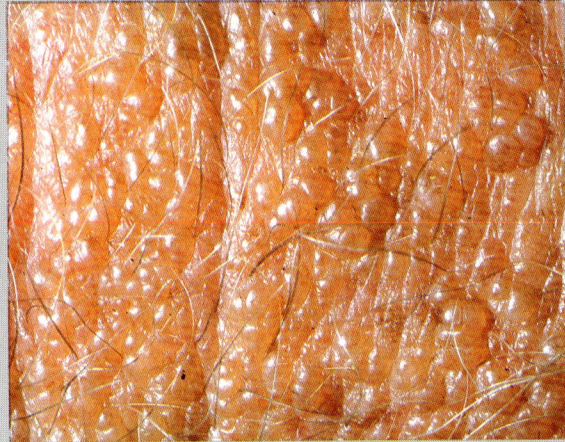

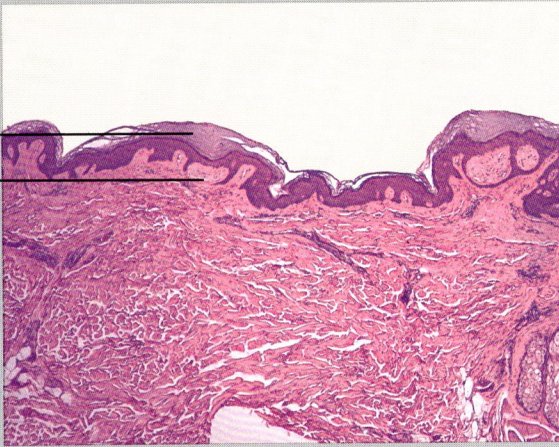

focal hyper-keratosis

globules of amyloid in papillary dermis

normal cornified layer of volar skin

large masses of colloid in reticular dermis

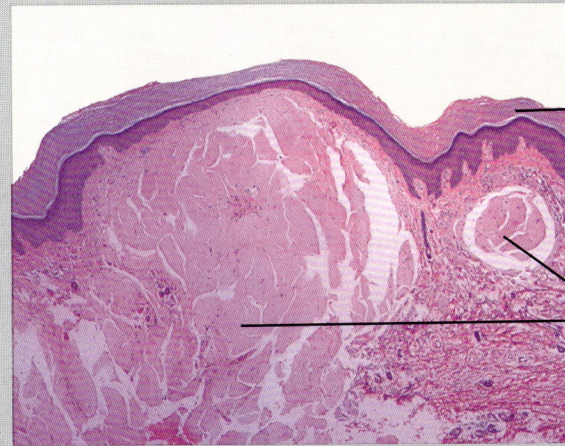

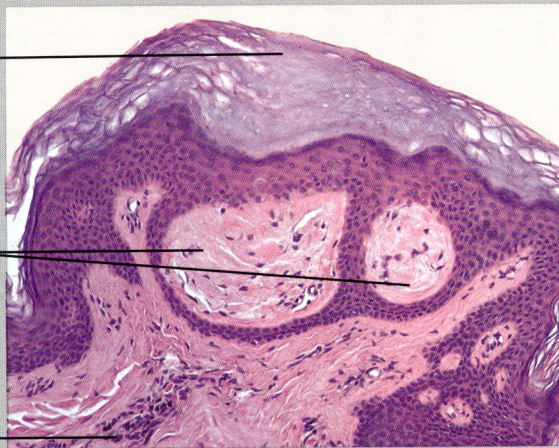

focal compact ortho-keratosis

globules of amyloid surrounded by collarettes of epidermis

lymphocytes and melanophages

mass of colloid

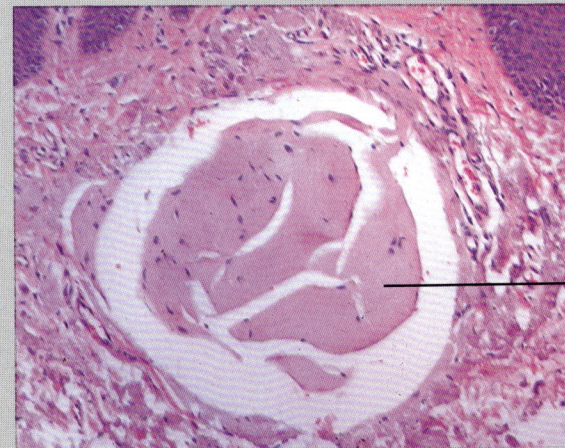

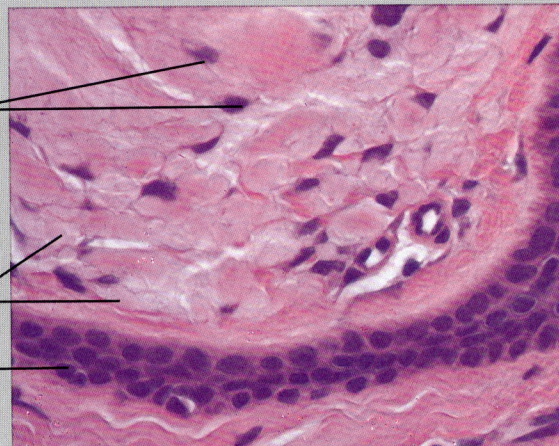

plump fibroblasts

globules of amyloid

epidermal collarette

thin fibroblast

clefts

colloid

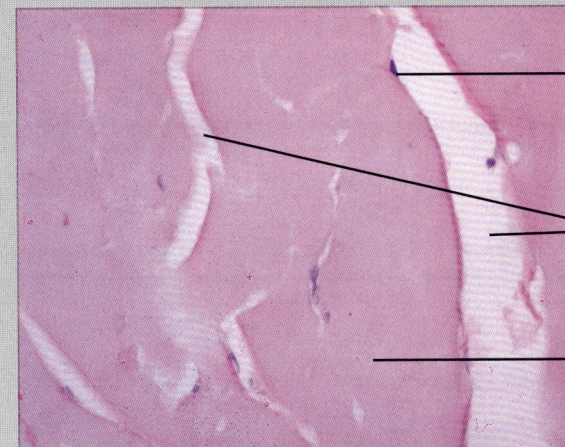

LICHEN amyloidosus and colloid milium are both caused by deposits of homogeneous material of different chemical natures in the upper part of the dermis. Both have fibroblasts within the masses of homogeneous material. It is likely that fibroblasts contribute to the formation of both amyloid in lichen amyloidosus and colloid in colloid milium.

Because of the above listed highly characteristic histologic features, special stains need not be performed routinely to differentiate amyloid from colloid. When necessary for academic completion, Congo red is the most reliable differentiating stain because it is positive for amyloid by dichroism and negative for colloid. Crystal violet stain for amyloid is prettier, but less reliable.

The clinical lesion of lichen amyloidosus consists of closely agminated, discrete, slightly raised, brownish-red translucent papules that are often hyperkeratotic. The condition is intensely pruritic and occurs most commonly on the anterior aspects of the legs, but may be widespread. Macular amyloidosus, as the title implies, begins as flat lesions. In contrast to lichen amyloidosus, macular amyloidosis has a predilection for the interscapular region. The keratotic papules of lichen amyloidosus develop as a result of progressively greater formation of amyloid in the papillary dermis and are the more papular and keratotic from persistent rubbing. In other words, there may be superimposition of lichen simplex chronicus upon lichen amyloidosus. A current hypothesis about the formation of amyloid in the upper portion of the dermis in the lesions of macular and lichenoid amyloidosus holds that the globules of amyloid derive from necrotic keratinocytes in the epidermis and these apoptotic bodies are then acted upon by fibroblasts and macrophages to become amyloid.

Colloid milium consists of discrete, smooth, yellowish, translucent, waxy papules on sun-exposed areas, especially the malar eminences of the face and dorsa of the hands. Sometimes the papules of colloid milium are found only on the left side of the face and on the dorsa of the left hand in persons who spend much of their time driving cars in sunny climates, such as taxi-drivers. At first glance, the smooth translucent papules of colloid milium may be misinterpreted as being tense vesicles or as "juicy" edematous papules of polymorphous light eruption.

Whereas colloid in the skin is found only in colloid milium, amyloid is found in a variety of circumstances other than in the macular and papular (lichenoid) forms of amyloidosus. For example, amyloid is present around blood vessels in the skin and subcutaneous fat of patients with systemic amyloidosis, in large solitary nodules of nodular amyloidosis and, most

commonly, as an incidental finding in a host of inflammatory, hamartomatous, and neoplastic conditions in the skin, especially in seborrheic keratoses
and in basal-cell carcinomas.

45. Pretibial Myxedema
vs. Scleromyxedema

Pretibial Myxedema	Scleromyxedema
1. Epidermis often slightly thickened and hyperkeratotic	1. Epidermis usually normal or only slightly hyperplastic
2. Pathologic changes mostly in the upper half of the dermis in fully developed lesions	2. Pathologic changes often throughout the entire dermis and even into the septa of the subcutaneous fat in fully developed lesions
3. Abundant acid mucopolysaccharides in the upper half of the dermis ("lakes of mucin")	3. Slight and subtle increase in acid mucopolysaccharides throughout the dermis
4. Wide separation of collagen bundles by acid mucopolysaccharides	4. Slight separation of collagen bundles by acid mucopolysaccharides
5. Mast cells markedly increased in mucinous areas	5. Mast cells slightly increased in mucinous areas
6. Fibroblasts slightly increased in number scattered individually within the abundantly mucinous stroma, mostly in the upper part of the dermis	6. Fibroblasts markedly increased in number with long axes parallel to the epidermis and some aggregated into fascicles within the slightly mucinous stroma throughout the entire dermis
7. Fibroblasts both spindle-shaped and stellate	7. Fibroblasts spindle-shaped only
8. No significant increase in amount of collagen	8. Increased amounts of basophilic-staining new collagen
9. Hair follicles spared	9. Hair follicles destroyed
10. No perivascular inflammatory-cell infiltrate	10. Sparse perivascular inflammatory-cell infiltrate around an increased number of dilated blood vessels

Pretibial Myxedema

Scleromyxedema

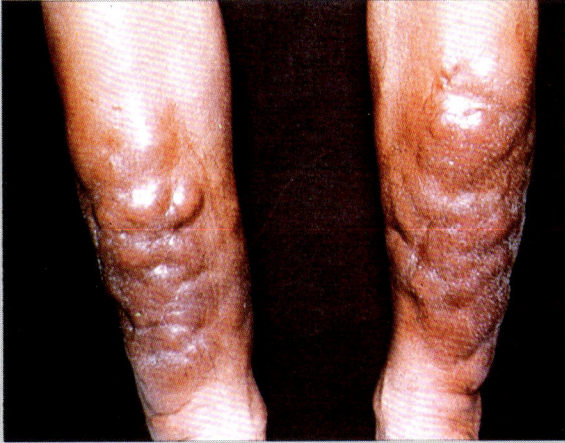
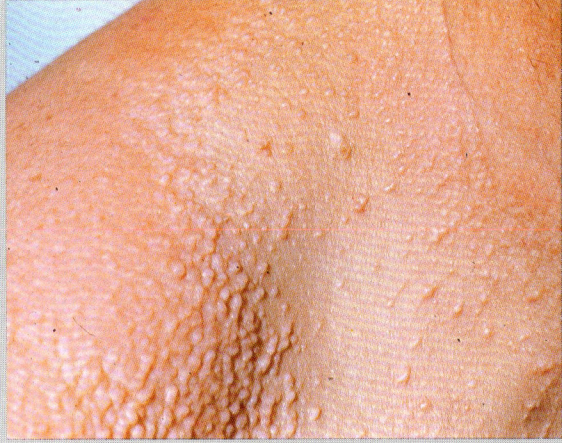

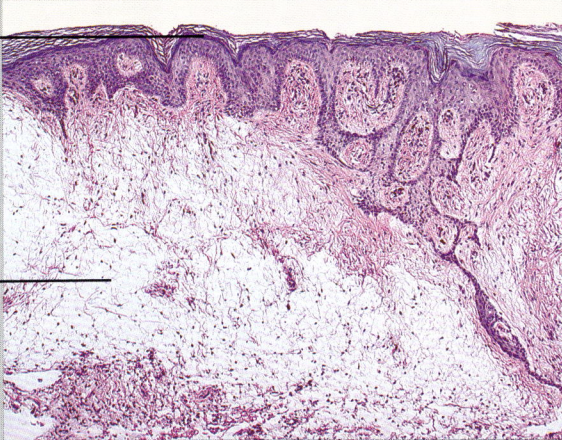

slightly papillated hyperplastic epidermis

abundant mucin throughout reticular dermis

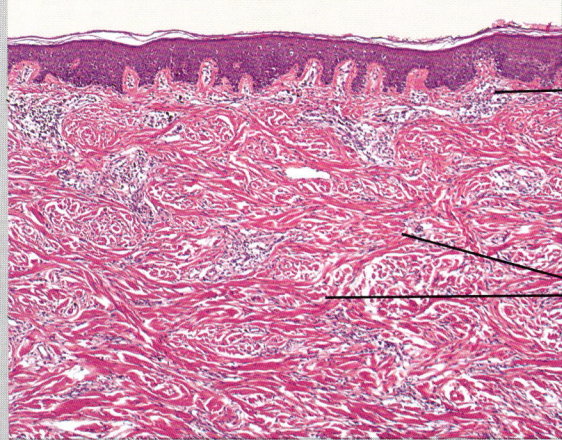

sparse lympho-histiocytic infiltrate

coarse collagen in haphazard array

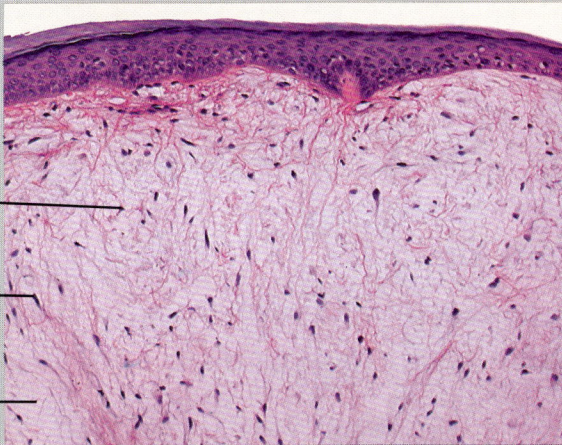

stellate fibroblast

spindle-shaped fibroblast

abundant mucin

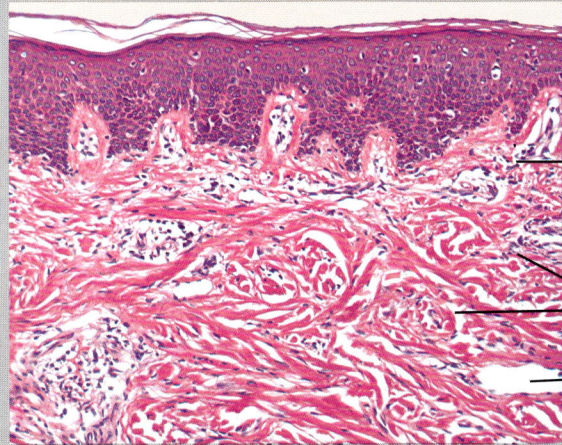

slight perivascular infiltrate

increased numbers of fibroblasts

dilated blood vessel

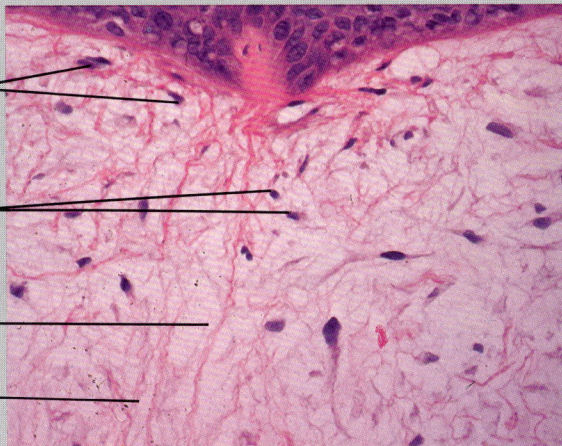

fibroblasts

mast cells

mucin

delicate collagen fibers

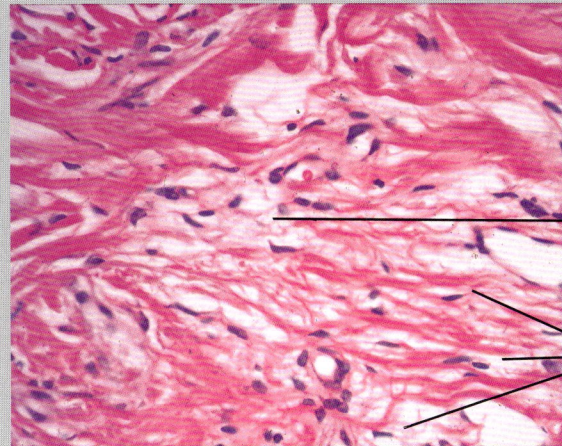

slight mucin

increased numbers of fibroblasts

P RETIBIAL myxedema and scleromyxedema are both cutaneous mucinoses associated with an increased number of fibroblasts and mast cells in the zones of acid mucopolysaccharides (glycoaminoglycans).

Pretibial myxedema may occasionally develop in patients who are euthyroid, but most commonly it is a manifestation of hyperthyroidism. Clinically, the lesions appear on the anterior aspects of the lower extremities and consist of firm, raised, yellow-tan plaques. Other signs of thyrotoxicosis often present concomitantly with pretibial myxedema are exophthalamos and acropathy. The causative factor of this triad is currently thought to be long-acting thyroid stimulator, an immunoglobulin of the IgG class. Pretibial myxedema not uncommonly develops after therapy for thyrotoxicosis.

Scleromyxedema is synonymous with papular mucinosis and lichen myxedematosus. Clinically, severe forms of the disease consist of diffuse erythematous induration and small papules. When the face is markedly involved, as it usually is, the clinical differential diagnosis is scleroderma. Other features of scleromyxedema are light-chain immunoglobulinopathy involving IgG and association with multiple myeloma.

The mucin in both pretibial myxedema and scleromyxedema is hyaluronic acid, because it takes the stains of colloidal iron and alcian blue at pH 2.5 and stains metachromatically with toluidine blue at pH 3.0. Histologically, in sections stained by hematoxylin and eosin, mucin appears as basophilic material that is granular and stringy.

Under scanning power, scleromyxedema appears to be a kind of fibroplasia, whereas pretibial myxedema is clearly a mucinosis.

The histologic differential diagnosis of scleromyxedema includes eruptive xanthoma, because the increased number of fibroblasts interposed between collagen bundles often have pale abundant cytoplasms and therefore resemble foam cells. The histologic differential diagnosis of pretibial myxedema includes generalized myxedema and focal mucinosis, which are different in that the mucin in generalized myxedema is not as massive and in focal mucinosis not as diffuse (i.e., it is circumscribed).

The hardness of the skin in scleromyxedema results from the new collagen formation, whereas the firmness of pretibial myxedema is secondary to abundant deposits of mucin.

Glossary

abscess refers to a collection of neutrophils that may form within the epidermis, hair follicles, dermis, and the subcutaneous fat, or any organ. When the neutrophils undergo degeneration, fat accumulates in their cytoplasms and this fat gives pus its yellow appearance.

acantholytic cell refers to an epithelial cell that has undergone dyshesion, i.e., separation from another epithelial cell, and has consequently become round. Cells in the spinous, granular, and cornified layers may undergo acantholysis.

acantholysis describes the process by which acantholytic cells come into being, namely, by dissolution of intercellular bridges and consequent "rounding up."

acinar means, literally, pertaining to a bunch of grapes; figuratively, in pathology, it refers to spaces lined by epithelium, especially to gland-like or duct-like structures.

acral parts of the skin refers to the distal parts, especially the skin of the fingers and toes, but also nose and ears.

active junctional nevus is a term that should never be used because it has not been defined in a standard way.

amphophilic means having both basophilic and eosinophilic staining qualities.

anagen indicates that part of the hair cycle during which hairs grow and the inferior portion of the hair follicle has a fully developed bulb, a tricholemmal sheath replete with glycogen, and a papilla that contains abundant mucin.

apoptosis refers to a kind of necrosis of keratinocytes in which the necrotic cells are subsequently phagocytized.

arborization describes a tree-like shape as a result of inward turning of epithelial structures of adnexa at the periphery of a common wart or a pyogenic granuloma (around which it is sometimes called an epidermal "collarette"). In truth, the elongated collars of epithelium are eccrine ducts and hair follicles rather than actual epidermal rete ridges.

atopy is applied to a genetic disposition to development of allergic rhinitis, (especially "hay fever"), allergic asthma, atopic dermatitis, and allergic urticaria.

atrophy refers to a decrease in amount of tissue. Clinically, superficial atrophy usually refers to thinning of the skin, shininess, loss of the skin markings, telangiectases, and pigmentary changes that in sum correspond histologically to sclerosis of the papillary dermis with thinning of the epidermis and some loss of the normal pattern between rete ridges and dermal papillae. Deep atrophy may also result from loss of connective tissue, but in the reticular dermis (e.g., anetoderma and stria atrophicans) and from loss of subcutaneous fat (e.g., lipodystrophy).

atypia is applied to nuclei that are large, hyperchromatic, variable in size and shape, and have prominent nucleoli.

ballooning describes intracellular edema, recognizable by swollen, pale cytoplasms of affected cells.

basal-cell hyperplasia refers to an increased number of basal cells as sometimes occurs in focal acantholytic dyskeratosis and in the epidermis above dermatofibromas.

basaloid means resembling the cells of the basal layer of the epidermis such as those that make up seborrheic keratoses and basal-cell carcinomas.

basement membrane denotes an anatomic zone defined as the undulating line between the epidermis and the dermis that takes the PAS stain when viewed by conventional microscopy. It is composed of type IV collagen.

basket-weave pattern of the stratum corneum applies to the normal appearance of the cornified layer (except for that on the palms and soles) in sections of skin viewed by conventional microscopy.

benign is a word that describes the behavior of a neoplasm, namely, one that does not have the potential for metastasis. It should not be used to describe cytologic characteristics.

bulbous designates resembling a bulb in shape, like a light bulb, the bulb of a flower, of an onion, or of the dermal papillae in lichen amyloidosus.

catagen designates the involutional stage of the hair cycle in which the inferior part of the hair follicle is characterized by a thickened, corrugated, glassy membrane.

cholesterol clefts are elongated spaces with pointed ends that presumably represent sites from which crystals of cholesterol have been removed from tissue by the agents used in processing specimens of tissue for histologic examination.

Civatte bodies are necrotic keratinocytes, also termed colloid bodies, hyaline bodies, and apoptotic bodies.

cleft describes a narrow space which is usually an artifact of histologic preparation (e.g., in basal-cell carcinomas, Spitz's nevi, and focal acantholytic dyskeratosis); differentiated from a blister by absence of plasma within the space.

coarse collagen in vertical streaks refers to a diagnostic sign of persistent rubbing of skin in lichen simplex chronicus and its variants prurigo nodularis and picker's nodule, where coarse collagen fibers in a thickened papillary dermis are oriented parallel to one another and to the rete ridges and perpendicular to the skin surface.

collarette of epithelium describes the inward bowing of epithelial structures of adnexa surrounding a pyogenic granuloma, verruca, seborrheic keratosis, etc.

colloid bodies are necrotic keratinocytes, also termed Civatte bodies, hyaline bodies, and apoptotic bodies.

compact orthokeratosis designates the normal configuration of the stratum corneum on palms and soles and in some pathological conditions such as lichen simplex chronicus, wherein the cornified cells are closely packed together.

compendigo refers to a combination of simple lentigo and compound nevus.

compound nevus refers to a lesion composed of nests of melanocytes in the epidermis and nests of nevus cells in the dermis.

connective tissue nevus denotes a congenital malformation of the dermis, either the papillary dermis (where it resembles clinically numerous skin tags) or the reticular dermis (where it involves collagen, elastic tissue, or both), or of the fat (nevus lipomatosus).

cords refers to epithelial cells in rows of two.

cornoid lamellation designates a column of parakeratosis which extends above the epidermis and into it, where vacuolated and dyskeratotic cells are seen; a requisite for the histologic diagnosis of porokeratosis in any of its forms.

crust denotes a collection of plasma containing white blood cells, red blood cells, or both.

cyst signifies an epithelial-lined round or oval space; in skin, almost always lined by epithelium of an adnexal structure and containing its product, e.g., *infundibular cyst* (also termed "epidermoid cyst") lined by epithelium resembling the upper portion of the hair follicle and containing cornified cells in basket-weave or laminated pattern; *isthmus-catagen cyst* lined by epithelium that resembles the isthmic portion of the hair follicle and the epithelium at the base of hair follicles in catagen and that contains cornified cells compactly arranged; *sebaceous duct cyst* (also termed "steatocystoma") lined by epithelium that resembles the duct of the sebaceous gland and that contains sebaceous material; *eccrine duct cyst* (also termed "eccrine hidrocystoma") lined by epithelium that resembles the duct of the eccrine gland and that contains a sweat-like substance; *apocrine gland cyst* (also termed "apocrine hidrocystoma") lined by epithelium that shows "decapitation secretion" and contains apocrine secretion.

degeneration, in classical pathology, refers to certain alterations in the cytoplasms of cells and in intercellular materials, e.g., fatty degeneration and degeneration of collagen.

degeneration of collagen describes loss of the normal structure of collagen as a result of anoxemia or of the action of lysosomal enzymes from leukocytes; seen as granular basophilia in sections stained by hematoxylin and eosin; should not be referred to as necrosis of collagen.

deposit is a substance such as mucin, amyloid, or urate that is not normally present in quantity in the skin.

desmoplasia designates the fibroplasia that develops in response to certain epithelial neoplasms such as malignant melanoma.

differentiation refers to the relative capability of a neoplasm to resemble a normal structure; when successful, neoplasms are designated well-differentiated, and if unsuccessful they are termed poorly differentiated.

digitated refers to one type of papillated epidermal hyperplasia, namely, finger-like projections above the skin surface, as in verruca vulgaris.

DOPA is an acronym for *d*ihydrox*y*p*h*en*y*l*a*lanine which is oxidized by dopa-oxidase in a positive dopa reaction, i.e., one in which melanogenesis occurs.

dyskeratotic cell is one that has cornified prematurely and with a pyknotic nucleus and brightly eosinophilic cytoplasm as in focal acantholytic dyskeratosis or in squamous-cell carcinoma in situ.

ecchymosis is a broad flat purpuric lesion that results from bleeding into the upper part of the dermis.

eddies of squamous cells describes whorls of spinous cells that seem to form around intraepithelial eccrine sweat ducts, especially in seborrheic keratoses and warts that have been irritated; usually signs of biologic benignancy.

elastotic material is synonymous with solar elastosis, i.e., the altered spaghetti-like connective tissue produced by fibroblasts that have been chronically exposed to damaging effects of sunlight.

epidermal hyperplasia refers to increased numbers of spinous cells in the epidermis; we use it as a synonym for acanthosis.

epidermal nevus denotes a congenital malformation characterized by papillated or digitated epidermal hyperplasia with hyperkeratosis.

epidermopoiesis means the making of epidermis; the process of maturation of epidermal basal cells into cornified cells.

endophytic means growing inward from the skin surface.

epithelial structures of adnexa designates derivatives of the embryonal ecto-
derm such as hair follicles, sebaceous glands, apocrine glands and
ducts, and eccrine glands and ducts.

epithelioid tubercle describes a collection of epithelioid histiocytes; when not
surrounded by lymphocytes they are termed "naked tubercles," a characteristic feature of the granulomas of sarcoidosis.

erosion signifies loss of part or all of the epidermis without loss of any
dermal tissue.

exo-endophytic means growing outward and inward from the skin surface.

exophytic means growing outward from the skin surface.

fascicle designates an elongated collection of spindle-shaped cells that tend
to intersect with other bunched cells.

fibrillar denotes arrangement in fibrils, i.e., delicate slender strands of connective tissue.

fibrotic tracts are linear bands of fibrosis that form at sites of permanently
extinct hair follicles.

fibrous tracts are linear bands of fibrous tissue that form normally behind
hair follicles that have retracted in telogen.

focal acantholytic dyskeratosis signifies a focus of suprabasal cleft, above
which there are acantholytic and dyskeratotic cells in the spinous and
granular layers, and above them, columns of parakeratosis.

follicular mucinosis refers to the presence of abnormal collections of acid
mucopolysaccharides within the epithelium of hair follicles, either as a
process sui generis (i.e., alopecia mucinosa) or secondary to other conditions such as mycosis fungoides, other cutaneous lymphomatoses,
and angiolymphoid hyperplasia with eosinophilia.

frond-like means leaf-like.

germinal centers are characteristic structures of lymph nodes which sometimes occur in the skin in pseudolymphomas.

germinative cells designate, among others, the cells in the basal layer of the epidermis, hair matrix, and the matrix of a nail, i.e., those cells that generate "daughter" cells that produce cornified end products, namely, the cornified layer, hair shafts, and nail plates.

glassy membrane is a synonym for the PAS-positive basement membrane that surrounds the inferior part of the hair follicle.

granulation tissue describes highly vascular, edematous connective tissue that contains a mixed cellular infiltrate and forms in response to some traumas to skin such as incisions, puncture wounds, and in ulcerations.

granulomatous dermatitis designates inflammatory infiltrates in which histiocytes predominate. It may be divided into nodular and diffuse types and the nodular type may be subdivided as tuberculoid, sarcoidal, palisaded, suppurative, and foreign body.

guttate means drop-sized and shaped; usually applied to eruptive lesions of psoriasis and to a distinctive type of parapsoriasis.

hematoma is a nodule formed by bleeding into the lower part of the dermis and/or the subcutaneous fat.

horn pseudocysts are whorls of delicate, laminated orthokeratotic cells that form in the absence of well-defined epithelial linings as within some seborrheic keratoses and trichoepitheliomas.

hyaline bodies are necrotic keratinocytes, also termed colloid bodies, Civatte bodies, and apoptotic bodies.

hyperchromasia means "over coloration"; increased intensity of nuclear staining.

hypergranulosis means an increased thickness of the stratum granulosum.

hyperplasia of atypical melanocytes describes increased numbers of melanocytes with atypical nuclei within or above the basal layer of the epidermis and within epithelial structures of adnexa.

ichthyosis is a skin condition characterized by fish-like scales, e.g., ichthyosis vulgaris, X-linked ichthyosis, lamellar ichthyosis, and acquired ichthyosis.

"id" reaction intends to convey papules, papulovesicles, and vesicles that develop at a distant site presumably because of a hypersensitivity reaction of tissue to fungal or other antigens at another site.

"Indian-file" arrangement of neoplastic cells describes atypical epithelial cells arranged as single cells between collagen bundles, especially common in metastatic carcinomas.

"infiltrating" margins is applied to the interposition of neoplastic cells between collagen bundles; a poorly circumscribed neoplasm.

infundibulum of the hair follicle refers to the upper funnel-shaped portion of the hair follicle bounded by the ostium above and the duct of the sebaceous gland below.

intradermal nevus refers to a lesion composed of nests, cords, and strands of nevus cells within the dermis.

invasion is a term that is imprecisely defined in general pathology and, in our opinion, is best reserved for militarists.

"irregularly" psoriasiform denotes elongated rete ridges of uneven lengths, but with preservation of the normal undulating pattern between rete ridges and dermal papillae.

isthmic portion of the hair follicle designates the intermediate portion of the hair follicle that is a bridge between the infundibular portion above and the inferior portion below; bounded by the duct of the sebaceous gland above and the site of attachment of the erector muscle below.

jentigo refers to a combination of simple lentigo and junctional nevus.

junctional activity is a term that should never be used because it has not been defined in a standard way.

junctional nevus refers to a lesion composed of nests of melanocytes confined to the epidermis usually at the dermo-epidermal junction.

lamellar collagen describes collagen fibers in the papillary dermis that are arranged in parallel to themselves, especially beneath melanocytic hyperplasia, such as in simple lentigines; and atypical melanocytic hyperplasias, such as malignant melanomas in situ.

laminated orthokeratosis refers to the configuration of the stratum corneum in some pathological states such as ichthyosis vulgaris and X-linked ichthyosis, wherein the cornified cells are arranged in plate-like fashion.

Langer's lines refer to lines along which surgical incisions gape or fall together depending upon whether made across or parallel to them; charted by Langer, who pierced the skins of cadavers with an awl.

leukocytoclasis refers to the breaking up of leukocytes (karyorrhexis) resulting in nuclear "dust," usually made up of the fragments of the nuclei of polymorphonuclear leukocytes.

lichenification denotes thickening of the skin characterized clinically by induration, hyperpigmentation, and accentuation of the normal skin markings. Histologically, the epidermis is hyperplastic and the papillary dermis is thickened by coarse collagen bundles in vertically arranged streaks.

lichenoid means resembling lichen planus clinically, i.e., flat-topped papules, and histologically, i.e., a band-like infiltrate in the papillary dermis, usually obscuring the dermo-epidermal junction along which there are vacuolar alteration and necrotic keratinocytes.

lobular panniculitis refers to an inflammatory process in the panniculus adiposus, recognizable with scanning magnification, in which the inflammatory-cell infiltrate is situated mostly in the fat lobules.

lymphoid follicles refer to collections of mononuclear cells that resemble germinal centers in lymph nodes.

macule refers to a small flat, nonpalpable spot on the skin, up to 1 cm in size and of different color than that of the surrounding normal skin.

malignant is a word that describes the behavior of a neoplasm, namely, one that has the potential for metastasis. It should not be used to describe cytologic characteristics.

maturation designates (1) the end stage of development of a germinative cell, e.g., cornified cells for basal cells; and (2) the tendency for nuclei of nevus cells to become smaller with progressive descent into the dermis in contrast to melanocytes of malignant melanoma, which usually do not.

melanocytic hyperplasia designates increased numbers of normal-appearing melanocytes in the basal layer of the epidermis and in epithelial structures of adnexa.

melanophage refers to a macrophage that has ingested melanin.

metastasis means "out of place," the spread by blood or lymph vessels of neoplastic cells from a primary neoplasm to distant sites; often the cause of death.

microvesiculation describes small spaces within the epidermis as a result of spongiosis, ballooning, or acantholysis. These spaces are not sufficiently large to be recognized clinically as vesicles or blisters.

mixed inflammatory-cell infiltrate describes an infiltrate composed of different types of cells, i.e., more than simply lymphocytes and histiocytes, but also neutrophils, eosinophils, or plasma cells.

Munro's microabscess signifies a small collection of neutrophils within the epidermis (spinous, granular, and cornified layers) of psoriasis.

necrotic cell is one that has died suddenly with a pyknotic nucleus and brightly eosinophilic cytoplasm as in erythema multiforme or in fixed drug eruptions. Dyskeratotic cells are also dying cells (although more slowly) and a rapidly dying cell cannot be differentiated histologically from a slowly dying cell on the basis of observing merely a single cell. This differentiation requires visualization of the cornified layer to see if it is normal (as is the case when keratinocytes die rapidly) or parakeratotic (when they die slowly).

necrotizing vasculitis is applied to necrosis of endothelial cells and degeneration of collagen in the walls of blood vessels in association with an infiltrate of inflammatory cells within and around the walls of the affected blood vessels. Fibrin is often deposited in the walls of these vessels. Nuclear "dust" may or may not be present.

nests are roundish collections of cells such as melanocytes in melanocytic nevi and atypical lymphocytes in mycosis fungoides.

nevoid means hamartomatous; a malformation. A hamartoma is not always a nevus, but a nevus is always a hamartoma.

nevus is a word that must be modified always, e.g., a hamartoma in the sense of an organoid nevus such as nevus sebaceus of Jadassohn, and a derivative of melanocytes such as a melanocytic nevus.

nevus cell is a cell in the dermis of a compound or intradermal type of melanocytic nevus; fundamentally a melanocyte.

nodule is a dome-shaped solid lesion formed of cells, deposits, or elements of connective tissue.

orthokeratosis designates hyperkeratosis in which nuclei are not retained in the cells of the cornified layer. It may be subclassified as compact, laminated, or basket-weave in appearance.

Paget cell refers to a cell that is specific for mammary and extramammary Paget's disease and is characterized by a large, round, or oval nucleus and abundant pale-staining cytoplasm that contains mucopolysaccharides demonstrable by staining with hematoxylin and eosin and better yet with special stains.

pagetoid cell refers to a cell that resembles the cells of mammary and extramammary Paget's disease by having a large round or oval nucleus and abundant pale-staining cytoplasm, as occurs, for example, in malignant melanoma.

pagetoid pattern describes the scattering, like buck-shot, of Paget or pagetoid cells throughout epithelium as it appears in mammary and extramammary Paget's disease on the one hand, and Bowen's disease and malignant melanoma on the other.

papillated describes nipple-shaped elevations above the skin surface, usually used to designate by microscopy an exophytic type of epidermal hyperplasia.

papillomatosis describes accentuation of the dermal papillae so that they project slightly or markedly above the skin surface as in acanthosis nigricans and some connective tissue nevi. The epidermis overlying the elongated papillae may or may not be hyperplastic.

papillomatous is synonymous with papillated.

papulovesicle describes a combination of a papule (i.e., a small, slightly elevated solid lesion) and a vesicle (i.e., a small, slightly elevated, fluid-containing lesion).

parakeratosis is applied to retention of nuclei in the cells of the cornified layer. This is usually the result of accelerated or faulty epidermopoiesis.

parapsoriasis en plaques is a synonym for the early patch stage of mycosis fungoides.

patch refers to a broad flat lesion.

Pautrier's microabscess denotes a collection of atypical mononuclear cells within the epidermis of lesions of mycosis fungoides; a misnomer because abscess denotes a collection of neutrophils.

pedunculated refers to a polypoid excrescence, i.e., attached to the skin by a stalk.

petechia denotes a pinpoint punctum of extravasated red blood cells in the upper part of the dermis.

plaque refers to an elevated broad lesion, often formed by coalescence of papules.

pleomorphism indicates variation in size and shape of cellular structures, e.g., nuclei in an infiltrate, usually of a neoplastic process.

poikiloderma vasculare atrophicans is a synonym for the late patch stage of mycosis fungoides, i.e., a plaque of mycosis fungoides that has undergone spontaneous regression with residual features of poikiloderma, namely, atrophy, telangiectases, hyperpigmentation, and hypopigmentation.

polymorphic eruption means having more than one type of primary and/or secondary skin lesion, i.e., a combination of macules, papules, vesicles, and so on.

polypoid means like a polyp, i.e., an excrescence above the skin surface having a narrow base and a stalk.

pseudoglandular describes a structure that resembles an authentic gland such as may form in certain squamous-cell carcinomas characterized by suprabasal clefts and acantholytic cells.

psoriasiform means resembling psoriasis clinically, i.e., reddish plaques covered by scales, and histologically, i.e., elongated rete ridges of approximately equal lengths with preservation of the normal undulating pattern between rete ridges and dermal papillae.

purpura refers to the purple color caused by visible hemorrhage in skin.

"pushing" margins is applied to the smooth, rounded borders of a neoplasm that appears to grow centrifugally; a well circumscribed neoplasm.

reticulum-cell sarcoma is an antiquated term for nodular lesions of mycosis fungoides and large cell lymphomas in the skin whose cells resemble histiocytes, but are actually large atypical T-lymphocytes. Newer terms for reticulum-cell sarcoma include histiocytic, centroblastic, lympho-blastic, and immunoblastic lymphomas.

satellitosis signifies a local metastasis and thus may sometimes be apparent in the same tissue specimen as is the primary neoplasm.

scale designates a collection of orthokeratotic cells, parakeratotic cells, or both.

scale-crust describes a combination of a scale (cornified cells) and a crust (serum containing blood cells).

sclerosis refers to a type of fibrosis characterized by homogenization of collagen with decreased numbers of fibroblasts.

sebaceous follicle describes a vellus-hair follicle on the face characterized by a prominent infundibulum, a puny inferior portion, and a large sebaceous gland.

septal panniculitis refers to an inflammatory process in the panniculus adiposus in which the inflammatory-cell infiltrate is situated mostly in the septa rather than mostly in the lobules as viewed with scanning magnification.

sessile means a seated, i.e., broad based, excrescence above the skin surface.

siderophage refers to a macrophage that has ingested iron.

solar elastosis is synonymous with elastotic material, i.e., the altered spaghetti-like connective tissue produced by fibroblasts that have been chronically affected by sunlight.

spongiform pustule describes a collection of neutrophils in the spinous and granular zones of the epidermis. Remnants of cell membranes give the pustule a sponge-like appearance.

spongiosis refers to intercellular edema recognizable by widening of the intercellular spaces and stretching of the intercellular bridges.

spongiotic psoriasiform dermatitis signifies a combination of intercellular edema and a hyperplastic epidermis in which some of the pattern of epidermal rete ridges and dermal papillae is preserved, especially seen in subacute contact and nummular dermatitis.

squamoid means resembling the cells of the spinous zone of the epidermis, like those that make up a verruca or a squamous-cell carcinoma.

strands refer to epithelial cells in single file.

subcorneal pustule describes a collection of neutrophils situated immediately beneath the cornified layer of the epidermis.

supra-papillary plate(s) refers to the portion(s) of the epidermis situated immediately above the summit(s) of the dermal papillae.

telangiectasis signifies a dilated end-vessel, usually a dilated capillary and venule.

telogen refers to the resting stage of the hair cycle in which the inferior part of the hair follicle has retracted to the level of the site of attachment of the erector muscle.

trabecula is a synonym for a fibrous septum, as in the subcutaneous fat.

tricholemmal sheath describes the external or outer root sheath of the hair follicle, which in anagen contains abundant glycogen.

trichomalacia means literally "softening of hair," but refers histologically to pleated hair shafts that contain clumps of melanin as a result of twisting the hairs in trichotillomania.

tumor means a swelling; a term that ideally should not be used synonymously with neoplasm nor to modify cells as in "tumor cell(s);" neoplasm and neoplastic cells are preferable terms.

ulcer indicates loss of the entire epidermis and at least some dermal tissue.

vacuolar alteration describes tiny spaces on either side of the basement membrane at the dermo-epidermal junction; *liquefaction degeneration* is synonymous.

vasculitis means an inflammatory process in which the inflammatory-cell infiltrate is partially localized within the walls of blood vessels; may be subdivided into small-vessel (e.g., allergic and septic) and large-vessel types; the commonest vasculitis in skin is "allergic" (leukocytoclastic) vasculitis.

vegetation is descriptive of a heaped-up collection of scale-crusts, sometimes hemorrhagic, often purulent.

vellus is applied to the fine delicate hairs found on much of the body, e.g., the face, arms, and trunk, in contrast to terminal hairs, which are broader and longer and which are found on the scalp, in the axillae, and in the pubic region.

verrucous means like a verruca, i.e., a rough, finger-shaped lesion clinically and characterized histologically by digitated epidermal hyperplasia or neoplasia.

vesiculobullous denotes a condition in which there are small and large blisters, i.e., vesicles and blisters.

vesiculopustule applies to a lesion that has features of a small blister (containing largely plasma) and a pustule (containing neutrophils in quantity).

villous describes papillated projections that resemble intestinal villi such as the appearance of the dermal papillae in pemphigus vulgaris.